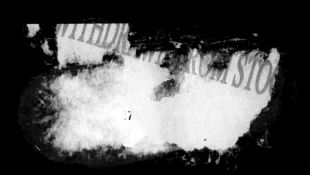
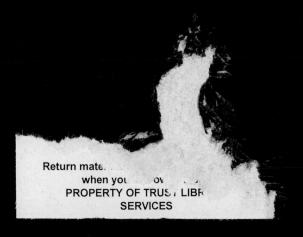

Endoscopy and Gastrointestinal Radiology

Requisites in Gastroenterology
Anil K. Rustgi (ed.)

Books in the series:

Volume 1: Esophagus and Stomach, David A. Katzka, David C. Metz (eds)
Volume 2: Small and Large Intestine, Gary R. Lichtenstein, Gary D. Wu (eds)
Volume 3: Hepatobiliary Tract and Pancreas, K. Rajender Reddy, William B. Long (eds)
Volume 4: Endoscopy and Gastrointestinal Radiology, Gregory G. Ginsberg,
   Michael L. Kochman (eds)

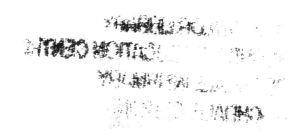

Commissioning Editor: *Rolla Couchman*
Project Development Manager: *Joanne Scott*
Project Manager: *Alan Nicholson*
Designer: *Andy Chapman*

The REQUISITES in

Gastroenterology

Anil K. Rustgi MD (ed.)
Chief, Division of Gastroenterology
University of Pennsylvania School of Medicine
Philadelphia, PA
USA

Volume 4: Endoscopy and Gastrointestinal Radiology

Edited by

Gregory G. Ginsberg, MD
Associate Professor of Medicine
Director, Endoscopic Services
Division of Gastroenterology
University of Pennsylvania School of Medicine
Philadelphia, PA
USA

Michael L. Kochman, MD, FACP
Professor of Medicine
Co-Director, Gastrointestinal Oncology
Endoscopy Training Director
Divison of Gastroenterology
University of Pennsylvania School of Medicine
Philadelphia, PA
USA

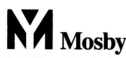
Mosby
An Affiliate of Elsevier, Inc.
Edinburgh • London • New York • Oxford • Philadelphia • St Louis • Sydney • Toronto 2004

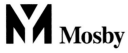

An Affiliate of Elsevier Inc

First published 2004

ISBN 0-3230-1885-8

British Library Cataloguing in Publication Data
A catalogue record for this book is available from the British Library

Library of Congress Cataloging in Publication Data
A catalog record for this book is available from the Library of Congress

Note
Medical knowledge is constantly changing. As new information becomes
available, changes in treatment, procedures, equipment and the use of drugs
become necessary. The editors/contributors and the publishers have taken care to
ensure that the information given in this text is accurate and up to date. However,
readers are strongly advised to confirm that the information, especially with
regard to drug usage, complies with the latest legislation and standards of
practice.

Printed in the USA

The
publisher's
policy is to use
**paper manufactured
from sustainable forests**

Contents

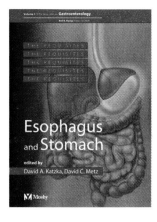
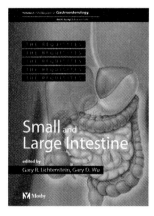
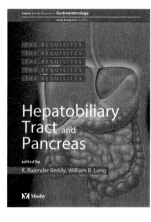
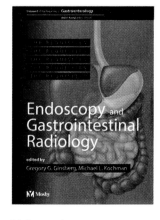
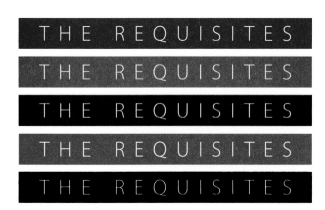

Series Foreword

This exciting and innovative *Requisites in Gastroenterology* series takes a broad-based and fundamental approach to the pathophysiology, diagnosis and management of gastrointestinal, hepatic and pancreatic diseases and disorders. The series is divided into 4 inter-related volumes, each of which in turn is edited by nationally and internationally renowned editors who are supported by excellent contributors. The contributors represent a breadth of disciplines and expertise, and are drawn from a number of different institutions and academic medical centers. At the same time, the University of Pennsylvania provides a 'home' base for the series, and indeed, its gastroenterology, surgery, radiology and pathology departments have been a foundation for clinical care, teaching and investigation for several generations.

Volume 1 deals with diseases and disorders of the esophagus and stomach, edited by Drs David Katzka and David Metz. Volume 2 covers small and large intestinal diseases and disorders, edited by Drs Gary Lichtenstein and Gary Wu. Volume 3 delineates hepatobiliary and pancreatic diseases and disorders, edited by Drs Rajender Reddy and William Long. Finally, Volume 4, edited by Drs Gregory Ginsberg and Michael Kochman, brings together the important diagnostic and therapeutic modalities of endoscopy, interventional endoscopy and radiological imaging that are of direct relevance to topics covered in Volumes 1, 2 and 3. While each volume is self-sufficient, all volumes provide the reader with a focused, cohesive and integrated view of the principles and practice of gastroenterology,

hepatology and pancreatology. Each volume is well illustrated and contains tables and figures that highlight salient features of different topics. Of note, boxes are provided that encapsulate key information covered in each chapter. These collective features are meant to assist the reader. The references are pivotal ones from the literature, and are not meant to be exhaustive.

In the evolution of this series, our collective thinking was to target the audience of medical students, residents, gastrointestinal fellows, allied health professionals (nurses, nurse practitioners, physician assistants), and those physicians (gastroenterologists, hepatologists, oncologists, surgeons, pathologists, radiologists) who require overviews for certifying examinations. The series is unique in the library of books that span the discipline of gastroenterology. The reader will find the volumes 'user-friendly' and will be imparted with expert knowledge and insights, making this an engaging overview and refresher course. We hope and trust that we will succeed in this mission.

The volumes that form the kernel of this series were profoundly influenced on the one hand by students, residents and fellows, and on the other hand, by the pioneering advances of T. Grier Miller, Thomas Machella, Frank Brooks, Sidney Cohen, Richard McDermott, Peter Traber and Ed Raffensperger. It is to these past and future leaders to whom I wish to give my special gratitude.

Anil K. Rustgi, MD
Editor-in-Chief

Preface

Our participation in this new endeavor has been both exciting and challenging. The opportunity of working with the talented contributors in this text has immeasurably increased our appreciation of the complexity of the clinical care that we provide. Hopefully, you will find that this text helps you efficiently to distill the knowledge that these experts have provided.

We have taken some of the major imaging areas within gastroenterology and hepatology and sought out authors who can convey the breadth and depth of their individual expertise, yet place this knowledge in context as one facet of the discipline of gastroenterology. There is no question that the use of imaging, in any of its many forms, is relevant to the modern practice of gastroenterology. Without the ability to diagnose pathology and to treat it definitively (or in some instances with palliation), we would not be able to seek answers or to apply the knowledge that recent advances in basic science have afforded us. The rapid advances in endoscopic and radiologic imaging have created a need for a thorough understanding of the areas in which the various modalities possess unique capabilities and the areas in which their use is complementary – this text clearly provides this understanding. On editing, we were pleased to note that the authors succeeded in transmitting this knowledge and expertise in an orderly and clinically relevant way.

Working on this project has also afforded us the chance to further our skills in time management and cooperation. Without the support of our families, our close collaboration with our colleagues, and Anil Rustgi, who is the editor of this series, this volume could never have come to fruition.

Gregory G. Ginsberg, MD
Michael L. Kochman, MD

Contributors

Poonputt Chotiprasidhi, MD
Clinical Assistant Professor
Division of Gastroenterology
Department of Internal Medicine
University of Michigan Medical Center
Ann Arbor, MI
USA

Douglas O. Faigel, MD
Associate Professor of Medicine
Department of Gastroenterology
Oregon Health and Science University
Portland, OR
USA

Gregory G. Ginsberg, MD
Associate Professor of Medicine
Director, Endoscopic Services
Division of Gastroenterology
University of Pennsylvania School of Medicine
Philadelphia, PA
USA

Michael C. Hill, MB
Professor of Radiology
Director of Body Imaging
Department of Radiology
George Washington University Hospital
Washington, DC
USA

Gordon C. Hunt, MD
Assistant Professor of Medicine
Gastroenterology Division
University of California
San Diego Medical Center
San Diego, CA
USA

Nadia J. Khati, MD
Assistant Professor of Radiology
Department of Radiology
George Washington University Hospital
Washington, DC
USA

Michael L. Kochman, MD, FACP
Professor of Medicine
Co-Director, Gastrointestinal Oncology
Endoscopy Training Director
Division of Gastroenterology
University of Pennsylvania School of Medicine
Philadelphia, PA
USA

Thomas E. Kowalski, MD
Associate Professor of Medicine
Director, Gastrointestinal Endoscopy
Division of Gastroenterology and Hepatology
Thomas Jefferson University
Philadelphia, PA
USA

Jin-Hong Park, MD
Fellow, Division of Gastroenterology and Hepatology
MCP–Hahnemann Hospital
Drexel University School of Medicine
Philadelphia, PA
USA

Stephen E. Rubesin, MD
Professor of Radiology
Department of Radiology
University of Pennsylvania School of Medicine
Philadelphia, PA
USA

Dushyant V. Sahani, MD
Clinical Instructor, Harvard Medical School
Assistant Radiologist,
Division of Abdominal Imaging and Intervention
Department of Radiology
Massachusetts General Hospital
Boston, MA
USA

Sanjay Saini, MD
Professor of Radiology
Harvard Medical School
Director, CT Services
Massachusetts General Hospital
Boston, MA
USA

James M. Scheiman, MD
Associate Professor of Medicine
Division of Gastroenterology
Department of Internal Medicine
University of Michigan Medical Center
Ann Arbor, MI
USA

Ilias A. Scotiniotis, MD
Instructor of Medicine
Harvard Medical School
Division of Gastroenterology
Brigham and Women's Hospital
VA Boston Healthcare System
Boston, MA
USA

Anil Shetty, MBBS
Visiting Research Fellow in Radiology
Division of Abdominal Imaging and Intervention
Department of Radiology
Massachusetts General Hospital
Boston, MA
USA

Michael C. Soulen, MD
Associate Professor of Radiology and Surgery
Division of Interventional Radiology
Department of Radiology
University of Pennsylvania School of Medicine
Philadelphia, PA
USA

David H. Stockwell, MD
Fellow in Gastroenterology
Division of Gastroenterology
Brigham and Women's Hospital
Boston, MA
USA

Robert K. Zeman, MD, FACR
Professor and Chairman of Radiology
Department of Radiology
George Washington University Medical Center
Washington, DC
USA

Dedication

With appreciation to my wife Jane; daughters, Jenny, Kathleen, Elizabeth, and Meg; and my teachers for their patience and guidance.

Gregory G. Ginsberg

To my wife, Mary, and my children, Sidney and Elyse, for their patience and love. To my mentors for their efforts and counsel over the years.

Michael L. Kochman

Chapter 1

Upper Endoscopy

David H. Stockwell and Ilias A. Scotiniotis

Introduction

Rigid endoscopes were first used in the nineteenth century and semiflexible gastroscopes were developed in the 1930s and 1940s. It was not until the 1960s, however, that fiberoptic endoscopes in the west and gastrocameras in Japan went into widespread use. By the early 1970s, endoscopes were long enough to reach the duodenum and had taken their modern form with forward viewing optics and fully maneuverable tips. In the mid-1980s, fiberoptic endoscopes were largely replaced by videoendoscopes which allow the endoscopist to view the image comfortably on a monitor rather than having to look directly into the end of the scope. Today, endoscope design includes the lens system, a light source and video camera, a nozzle for a water jet to wash the lens and for insufflating air, and a channel for suctioning and passing instruments such as biopsy forceps, snares, nets, cautery probes, injection needles, and hemostatic clips. Modern endoscopes are portable, allowing procedures to be performed in either the intensive care unit or emergency room. In addition to standard, single-channel (9 mm diameter) endoscopes, some endoscopes are designed for special purposes. These include the therapeutic, dual channel (11 mm diameter) endoscope, side-viewing duodenoscope, pediatric endoscope, and enteroscope. Specialized endoscopes include the capacity for high resolution, magnification, and detection of fluorescence. In the near future, we may see widespread use of mucosal staining with vital dyes, optical coherence tomography, non-sedated ultrathin endoscopy, and wireless capsule endoscopy.

Box 1.1 Contraindications to endoscopy

Absolute contraindications
    uncooperative patient
    suspected peritonitis or perforation
    cardiopulmonary or hemodynamic instability
    severe injury to the hypopharynx
    any setting in which the apparent risk is greater than the expected benefit
Relative contraindications
    Zenker's diverticulum
    decompensated cardiopulmonary disease
    coagulopathy
    unstable cardiac syndromes and recent myocardial infarction

---

General considerations

Before upper endoscopy is performed, it is critical to take a thorough medical history, including the history of prior procedures, important comorbid conditions, medications, allergies, and bleeding tendencies of the patient. Even when indicated, endoscopy should not be performed in certain settings. Absolute and relative contraindications to endoscopy are presented in Box 1.1. No data support routine pre-procedural laboratory testing prior to elective endoscopy, but testing should be done for patients with known or suspected bleeding disorders. In general, patients should have nothing to drink for at least 4 hours and nothing to eat for at least 6 to 8 hours prior to upper endoscopy.

Informed consent

The purpose and nature of the procedure, its risks and benefits, and alternatives should always be clearly discussed with the patient. When a patient lacks the ability to make decisions, informed consent should be obtained from the patient's proxy.

Prophylaxis for endocarditis

The risk of endocarditis due to endoscopic procedures is generally quite low. Current American Society for Gastrointestinal Endoscopy guidelines recommend antibiotic prophylaxis only for patients with high-risk cardiac conditions who are undergoing procedures that are commonly associated with transient bacteremia (Table 1.1). For procedures in the upper gastrointestinal tract ampicillin, 2 grams

Table 1.1 Antibiotic prophylaxis in endoscopic procedures

Low-risk procedures	Intermediate-risk cardiac conditions
EGD ± biopsy/polypectomy Band ligation of esophageal varices	Other congenital heart disease Rheumatic valvular disease Hypertrophic cardiomyopathy Mitral valve prolapse with mitral regurgitation
High-risk procedures	**High-risk cardiac conditions**
Sclerotherapy of esophageal varices (not band ligation) Esophageal stricture dilation Endoscopic retrograde cholangiopancreatography in the setting of obstruction and/or sphincterotomy Percutaneous endoscopic gastrostomy	Prosthetic heart valves Systemic and pulmonary shunts Complex congenital heart disease History of endocarditis Synthetic vascular grafts less than 1 year old
EGD = esophagogastroduodenoscopy	

Table 1.2 Management of anticoagulants in patients undergoing endoscopic procedures

Low-risk procedures	Low-risk conditions
EGD + biopsy Enteroscopy Endoscopic retrograde cholangiopancreatography without sphincterotomy Endoscopic ultrasound without fine-needle aspiration	Deep venous thrombosis Uncomplicated atrial fibrillation Mechanical aortic valve or bioprosthetic valve
High-risk procedures	**High-risk conditions**
EGD + polypectomy Esophageal dilation Treatment of esophageal varices Percutaneous endoscopic gastrostomy Endoscopic ultrasound with fine-needle aspiration Laser therapy/Argon Plasma Coagulation Endoscopic retrograde cholangiopancreatography with sphincterotomy	Any mechanical valve with a prior thromboembolic event Mechanical mitral valve Atrial fibrillation + dilated cardiomyopathy, valvular disease, or a recent thromboembolic event
EGD = esophagogastroduodenoscopy	

intravenously given 30 minutes prior to the procedure, is adequate. Vancomycin, 1 gram, is substituted in penicillin-allergic patients. In patients with intermediate-risk cardiac conditions, cirrhosis, and ascites, or compromised immune systems, there is insufficient data to make firm recommendations, and a case-by-case approach is recommended. In all other patients, even high-risk procedures do not require prophylaxis. The exception to this rule is placement of a percutaneous endoscopic gastrostomy, in which it has been proven that antibiotics reduce infectious complications and are recommended for all patients. In contrast, antibiotics are not recommended for patients with pacemakers, implantable defibrillators, and prosthetic joints.

Anticoagulation

The upper endoscopic procedures that pose a relatively high risk of bleeding complications are listed in Table 1.2. For high-risk procedures in anticoagulated patients at high risk for thromboembolism, warfarin should be discontinued 3 to 5 days prior to the procedure and consideration should be given to using intravenous or low-molecular weight heparin while the International Normalized Ratio (INR) is below a therapeutic level. For high-risk procedures in those at relatively low risk for thromboembolism, warfarin should be discontinued 3 to 5 days prior to the procedure and reinstituted after the procedure. For low-risk procedures, the American Society for Gastrointestinal Endoscopy recommends no change in anticoagulation therapy. However, elective procedures should be delayed if the INR is above the therapeutic range.

Antiplatelet agents

There is good evidence that it is safe to perform even high-risk procedures in patients taking aspirin or other non-steroidal anti-inflammatory drugs (NSAIDs). However, for elective procedures, standard practice typically includes holding aspirin for 7 to 10 days and holding NSAIDs for 2 to 3 days.

Conscious sedation

Conscious sedation, defined as a decreased level of consciousness attained without the loss of ability to defend the airway, is the standard anesthesia used for endoscopy. Patients who are not alert to begin with or who cannot defend their airway are not candidates for conscious sedation and may need general anesthesia with endotracheal intubation prior to endoscopy. Patients receiving conscious sedation should remain cooperative, oriented, and responsive throughout the procedure.

The goals of conscious sedation are to increase tolerance and acceptance of endoscopy and to minimize anxiety, pain, and agitation during endoscopy. Topical benzocaine or lidocaine (lignocaine) sprays are commonly used to numb the oropharynx. Benzodiazepines are the most widely used intravenous agents because of their sedating and amnesic properties. These include midazolam and diazepam. Fentanyl and meperidine are opiates commonly used in conjunction with benzodiazepines to achieve conscious sedation. Many endoscopists have begun to use propofol because of its ability to induce deep sedation and because of its rapid onset and recovery times. Propofol can, however, induce profound respiratory depression and should only be administered by a specially trained anesthesiologist. Because sedation accounts for much of the cost and most of the complications related to upper endoscopy, there has been recent interest in new, ultrathin endoscopes and in unsedated endoscopy, as is commonly performed in Japan.

Monitoring

Endoscopy is typically performed as an outpatient procedure in specialized centers staffed by a well-trained team of nurses, doctors, and assistants. All patients undergoing upper endoscopy with conscious sedation require intravenous access. The patient's level of consciousness, heart rate, blood pressure, arterial oxygen saturation, and, if indicated, cardiac rhythm, should be monitored before, during, and after endoscopy. Oxygen saturation is a useful monitor for hypoxemia but is not a reliable surrogate of ventilatory status or hypercarbia. Typically, the endoscopy nurse's main responsibilities are to monitor the patient and to administer sedation. After the procedure, patients are monitored in the endoscopy suite until the effects of sedation have worn off. Patients who receive conscious sedation must be accompanied home.

Risks and complications

Upper endoscopy is a remarkably safe procedure with a low complication rate. The overall rate of complications associated with diagnostic endoscopy in the upper gastrointestinal tract is approximately one in 1000 procedures, and the mortality rate ranges from 0.5 to 3 per 10 000 procedures. Most complications of endoscopy are cardiopulmonary and are related to conscious sedation. Common cardiopulmonary complications include hypoxemia, hypotension, hypertension, arrhythmias, and aspiration. Arterial oxygen desaturation is most common, occurring in up to one third of patients, though desaturation to less than 90% occurs in less than 10% of patients. The incidence of oxygen desaturation is significantly reduced by the delivery of oxygen via a nasal cannula during the procedure. Older patients and those with important cardiac and/or pulmonary comorbidities should be evaluated before sedation is given. Some of these patients will tolerate endoscopy without sedation. Others are most safely sedated by an anesthesiologist. In all patients it is reasonable to use supplemental oxygen, light sedation, and intermittent oral suctioning.

Serious complications relating directly to the procedure itself include perforation, bleeding, and infection. With modern flexible endoscopes, the rate of perforation is less than 0.01% and almost always occurs in the hypopharynx or high in the esophagus in the setting of anatomical abnormalities, blind passage of the endoscope, or difficult esophageal intubation. Specific high-risk anatomical abnormalities include Zenker's diverticulum or other esophageal diverticula, esophageal strictures, cervical spurs, and malignancy. While minor bleeding is common, significant hemorrhage in diagnostic endoscopy is rare in the patient without coagulopathy or significant thrombocytopenia. Transient asymptomatic bacteremia with normal oropharyngeal or skin flora may occur in up to 25% of diagnostic endoscopy procedures, but symptomatic infection is rare. Appropriate disinfection of endoscopes eliminates all bacteria and spores from equipment. While transmission of infections from contaminated and poorly cleaned endoscopes is increasingly rare, infection with *Mycobacterium*, *Pseudomonas*, and *Salmonella* species, *Helicobacter pylori*, and hepatitis B and C viruses have been documented, and are attributed to lapses in disinfection protcol. Transmission of the human immunodeficiency virus has not been reported.

Rare complications of upper endoscopy include phlebitis at the intravenous catheter site, local and systemic reactions to drugs, methemoglobinemia due to topical benzocaine or lidocaine (lignocaine) sprays, dislocation of the temporomandibular joint, parotid or submandibular gland enlargement, and incidental tooth extraction.

The complication rate is increased for specific therapeutic procedures such as esophageal dilation, percutaneous endoscopic gastrostomy, treatment of bleeding lesions, and sclerotherapy. In esophageal dilation, perforation occurs in 3.7% to 6% of cases. Perforation is most likely in the setting of radiation-induced or malignant strictures and in the setting of pneumatic dilation for achalasia. The rate of bacteremia with esophageal dilation is reported to be as high as 50%.

The high morbidity initially reported with percutaneous endoscopic gastrostomy (10% to 40%) was mostly accounted for by peristomal wound infection. Periprocedural antibiotics have reduced the rate of this complication to between 4% and 14%. A single dose of an agent effective against gram-positive bacteria given 1 hour before the procedure is adequate. Aspiration is the second most common complication of percutaneous endoscopic gastrostomy. Significant bleeding or bowel perforation occurs in less than 1% of cases. Rare complications include ileus and seeding the stomal tract with cancer in patients with head and neck malignancies. Gastrocolonic fistula is a late complication that typically manifests as diarrhea weeks to months after the procedure.

Sclerotherapy of esophageal varices has a much higher rate of complications than band ligation and is no longer recommended as first-line therapy for either acute variceal bleeding or secondary prophylaxis. Overall complications of sclerotherapy range from 20% to 40%, with strictures forming in 15% to 20%, and bleeding from ulceration in 10% to 15% of cases. Peritonitis is seen in 1% to 3% of cases, and pulmonary complications such as the development of a pleural effusion may also occur. The mortality rate is estimated at 1% to 2%. Other common complications of sclerotherapy include fever, chest pain, bacteremia, and dysphagia.

Normal findings

Each endoscopic examination is performed in a standardized way and follows a routine systematic survey. Under the supervision of the physician and endoscopy nurse, the patient is placed in the left lateral decubitus position and sedated. A mouthpiece or bite-guard is inserted to protect the patient's teeth and the endoscope. With the neck flexed forward, the endoscope is inserted under direct vision with identification of the epiglottis, vocal cords, and piriform sinuses. Gentle pressure allows the scope to pass the upper esophageal sphincter (cricopharyngeus), which is often the most difficult part of the examination for the patient.

Esophagus

The esophagus can be inspected in detail on either the insertion or removal of the endoscope. The upper esophageal sphincter is a high-pressure zone 2 to 3 centimeters in length formed by the cricopharyngeus muscle. The upper esophageal sphincter prevents esophageal contents from refluxing into the airway and prevents air from entering the esophagus on inspiration. The striated, skeletal muscle of the proximal esophagus transitions gradually to the smooth muscle of the distal esophagus. The lower esophageal sphincter is tonically contracted to prevent reflux of gastric contents and relaxes with swallowing. While co-ordinated peristaltic contractions are easily appreciated, endoscopy is no substitute for manometry if a motility disorder is suspected. The squamocolumnar junction (Z-line or ora serrata) is defined as the junction of the white, stratified squamous epithelium of the esophagus and the salmon-colored, columnar epithelium of the gastric cardia (Figure 1.1). The squamocolumnar junction is normally located within the zone of the lower esophageal sphincter. The gastroesophageal junction

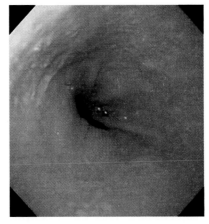

Figure 1.1 Normal esophagogastric junction. The transition between the pearly white stratified squamous mucosa of the esophagus and the pink columnar mucosa of the stomach is seen. The narrowing of the lumen at that level is caused by the lower esophageal sphincter, which relaxes with swallowing to allow the passage of the food bolus.

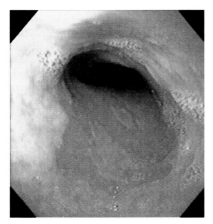

Figure 1.2 Barrett's esophagus. The normal pearly white squamous mucosa is interspersed with "tongues" of salmon-pink colored columnar mucosa. When biopsied, the pink mucosa revealed intestinal metaplasia, confirming the diagnosis of Barrett's esophagus.

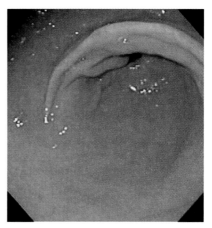

Figure 1.3 Normal antrum and pylorus. The smooth surface of the gastric antrum lacks folds. The pyloric orifice is seen.

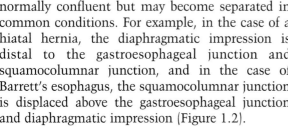

Figure 1.4 Normal second portion of duodenum. The smooth, concentric contour of the duodenal folds is seen. The ampulla of Vater can be seen as a bulge in the wall in the upper left corner. For better visualization of the ampulla, one can employ a side-viewing duodenoscope of the type used for endoscopic retrograde cholangiopancreatography.

is defined as the proximal end of the gastric folds. The third landmark of the distal esophagus is the diaphragmatic impression. These landmarks are normally confluent but may become separated in common conditions. For example, in the case of a hiatal hernia, the diaphragmatic impression is distal to the gastroesophageal junction and squamocolumnar junction, and in the case of Barrett's esophagus, the squamocolumnar junction is displaced above the gastroesophageal junction and diaphragmatic impression (Figure 1.2).

Stomach

Upon entering the stomach, retained gastric contents should be removed immediately to decrease the risk of aspiration. The pylorus, antrum, and incisura angularis (which marks the entrance to the antrum) are inspected with particular care (Figure 1.3). Normal peristalsis begins in the fundus and progresses to the antrum at a frequency of approximately three contractions per minute. Retroflexion is routinely performed in the stomach to allow inspection of the lesser curvature, cardia, and fundus and is the best position for detecting hiatal and paraesophageal hernias.

Duodenum

Once the pylorus is passed, the duodenal bulb is inspected in detail on entry. Passing the superior duodenal angle sometimes requires a blind maneuver, and lesions in this area can be difficult to appreciate. The second (or descending) part of the duodenum is typically the extent of the examination, allowing at least partial visualization of the ampulla of Vater (Figure 1.4).

Indications for upper endoscopy

There is little general consensus on the appropriate uses of endoscopy, with primary care physicians in various trials reporting both overuse and underuse of endoscopic procedures. In addition, there is still debate about the relative merits of upper gastro-intestinal barium studies versus endoscopy. In general, endoscopy is superior for identifying mucosal lesions in the upper gastrointestinal tract, while radiologic studies may be preferable for evaluating anatomic relationships and motility. One of the great advantages of endoscopy is that it allows visualization, biopsy, and therapy in a single session.

Dysphagia

Dysphagia, the sensation of food or liquid "sticking" in the esophagus, may result from a variety of structural, mucosal, or neuromuscular abnormalities of the esophagus and/or oropharynx. Each patient's history should guide initial diagnostic testing. For example, a patient with a history of a recent stroke and the symptom of nasopharyngeal regurgitation suggesting oropharyngeal dysphagia, should have a formal swallowing evaluation and a video swallowing study. On the other hand, a patient with a history of food impaction and dysphagia felt at the level of the xiphoid, suggesting a structural lesion near the gastroesophageal junction, should undergo endoscopy and/or a barium study. Finally, a patient with regurgitation and dysphagia primarily to liquids may require manometric evaluation for a motility disorder.

Patients who present with dysphagia to solid food often have a structural lesion. While most patients with dysphagia to solids have benign lesions, esophageal or gastroesophageal junction cancers are always of the greatest concern and must be excluded (Figure 1.5). Multiple endoscopic biopsies and brush cytology are more than 90% sensitive for diagnosing esophageal cancer, which is typically advanced by the time patients present with symptoms. In about 20% of esophageal cancers, the

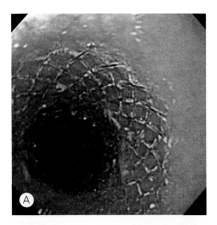

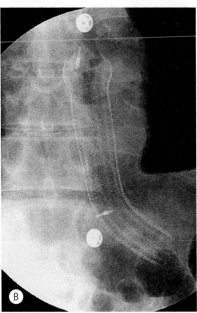

Figure 1.6 Esophageal metal stent for malignant stricture. A) Endoscopic view of the upper end of the metal stent in the esophagus. B) Fluoroscopic image of the stent. Its lower end crosses the esophagogastric junction into the stomach (reproduced with permission from Dr Elon Gale).

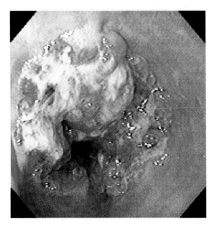

Figure 1.5 Esophageal cancer. A fungating, malignant mass is seen in the distal esophagus. Biopsies revealed squamous cell carcinoma.

stenosis at the time of diagnosis is so tight that it cannot be traversed with the endoscope. If the cancer is deemed unresectable, or if the patient is a poor candidate for surgery, expandable metal stents can be placed endoscopically and are approximately 85% effective in palliating dysphagia (Figure 1.6).

Common benign structural lesions of the esophagus include rings, webs, strictures, and diverticula. The most common benign cause of dysphagia is a mucosal ring in the distal esophagus, termed a Schatzki ring. Peptic strictures (Figure 1.7A) are a common cause of dysphagia in older patients with longstanding symptoms of gastroesophageal reflux disease. The cornerstone of treatment for these benign conditions is endoscopic dilation with tapered bougies, dilators, or balloons (Figure 1.7B and C) followed by acid suppression with proton pump inhibitors. Radiation-induced strictures are often particularly difficult to treat. Rarely, dysphagia is caused by extrinsic compression of the esophagus, for example, by a tortuous aorta. Finally, some patients with mucosal rather than structural lesions of the esophagus from acid reflux, infection, or toxic injury will present primarily with dysphagia.

Patients with motility disorders often present with dysphagia to liquids and solids, as well as regurgitation, chest pain, cough, and aspiration. Two paradigms of esophageal motility disorders are achalasia, with very high lower esophageal sphincter tone, and scleroderma, with very low lower esophageal sphincter tone. In both achalasia and scleroderma, the esophagus is likely to be dilated and non-peristaltic. In achalasia, the esophagus is often filled with food and secretions despite fasting, while in scleroderma, severe esophagitis, *Candida* species, and peptic strictures are common. However, endoscopy is not reliable for distinguishing these conditions, and manometry should always be performed when a motility disorder is suspected. When the diagnosis of achalasia is made, especially in patients older than 50 years, who have weight loss, and have had symptoms for less than 1 year, it is essential to exclude secondary achalasia due to a malignancy at the gastroesophageal junction (pseudoachalasia). Endoscopic treatment options for achalasia include pneumatic dilation and botulinum toxin injection.

Odynophagia

Odynophagia is a common symptom of esophageal ulceration of any etiology. These include infection, medication-induced esophageal injury, radiation-induced esophageal injury, idiopathic esophageal ulceration, bullous disease involving the esophagus, and trauma, including esophageal rupture. An infectious cause should be suspected in patients with odynophagia in the setting of the acquired immunodeficiency syndrome (AIDS) or immuno-

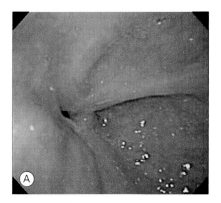

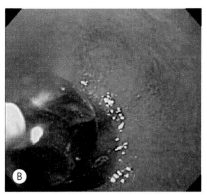

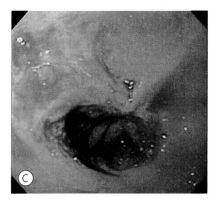

Figure 1.7 Peptic stricture in the distal esophagus. A) A tight, smooth fibrotic stricture is seen in the distal esophagus, B) A dilating balloon has been inflated across the stricture, C) The post-dilation appearance of the area shows disappearance of the stenosis. A mucosal tear has been caused by the balloon at the 9 o'clock position. The normal folds of the gastric cardia can be seen below the esophagogastric junction.

suppression from cancer chemotherapy or organ transplantation. In patients with AIDS, thrush, and odynophagia, candida esophagitis is so common that it should be treated empirically with fluconazole before the endoscopic examination. In patients who fail to respond, endoscopic examination with biopsy and brushing can most often distinguish the white plaques typical of *Candida* species from the large ulcers typical of herpes simplex virus, cytomegalovirus, and aphthous ulceration. While common in the setting of AIDS, it is important to realize that candida esophagitis may also occur in patients with diabetes, those taking steroids or antibiotics, and in those who are not clearly immunosuppressed.

Patients who are elderly, dehydrated, and who take pills without water before bedtime are at particular risk for medication-induced esophageal injury. Such patients typically present with rapid-onset and severe pain, and endoscopy reveals a discrete ulcer with a relatively normal surrounding mucosa. Pill-induced ulcers typically occur at sites of esophageal narrowing such as the aortic arch or gastroesophageal junction and presumably result from prolonged direct contact with caustic substances. Tetracyclines, bisphosphonate, aspirin, iron compounds, potassium chloride, and quinidine are most commonly associated with medication-induced esophageal injury.

Spontaneous esophageal rupture (Boerhaave's syndrome) is a rare cause of odynophagia but should be suspected when patients with a history of severe vomiting present with chest or upper abdominal pain, tachypnea, and dyspnea. Unless the correct diagnosis is made, patients with Boerhaave's syndrome invariably progress to fever, shock, and death. Unfortunately, these patients often have a history of alcoholism or peptic ulcer disease and are typically misdiagnosed. The chest radiograph may reveal mediastinal air or a pleural effusion. The diagnostic test of choice is an esophagram with a water-soluble contrast agent (Gastrograffin®). Endoscopy with insufflation of air can extend the perforation and is contraindicated.

Dyspepsia

Dyspepsia is broadly defined as being discomfort centered in the epigastrium lasting for at least 12 weeks in a 1-year period. It is the most common gastrointestinal complaint of patients presenting to primary care providers and it accounts for enormous health care costs. While many attempts have been made to categorize dyspeptic symptoms in order to determine the etiology, it is probably not useful to classify dyspepsia beyond

- reflux type (in which heartburn and regurgitation predominate)
- ulcer-type (in which epigastric pain predominates)
- motility-type (in which postprandial nausea and vomiting predominate).

The majority of patients have "functional" dyspepsia, meaning that they have no important findings on endoscopy. However, 20% of patients presenting with dyspepsia have peptic ulcer disease, and a small minority have any of a number of other significant pathologic lesions including cancers and premalignant lesions. Most physicians agree that patients with dyspepsia and "red flags" such as age greater than 45 years, dysphagia, odynophagia, recurrent vomiting, weight loss, iron deficiency anemia, early satiety, or guaiac positive stool should undergo endoscopy. There is disagreement, however, on how best to approach young patients with dyspepsia and no alarm signs. In these low-risk patients, the challenge is how best to identify patients with significant underlying pathology while avoiding huge numbers of unnecessary endoscopies.

One strategy that has been endorsed by the American Gastroenterological Association is the "test-and-treat" approach, in which non-invasive testing for *Helicobacter pylori* rather than endoscopy guides treatment. The strength of a "test-and-treat" strategy is that patients with *H. pylori*-associated peptic ulcer disease are treated appropriately while the many patients with "functional" dyspepsia avoid unnecessary endoscopy. On the other hand, current evidence suggests that eradication of *H. pylori* in patients without a discrete ulcer is no better than placebo in eliminating dyspepsia. Because of that, if endoscopy is undertaken, *H. pylori* should not be tested for unless a discrete ulcer is seen. Opponents of the "test-and-treat" approach counter that early endoscopy in patients with dyspepsia serves to reassure those with functional dyspepsia and thus minimizes the subsequent utilization of health care resources.

Gastroesophageal reflux disease

Gastroesophageal reflux disease is a clinical diagnosis based on typical symptoms of heartburn (a burning sensation starting in the upper abdomen

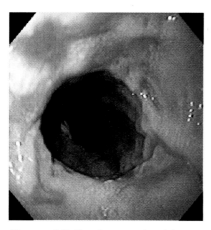

Figure 1.8 Erosive esophagitis caused by gastroesophageal reflux. Patchy erythema and linear erosions are seen in the distal esophagus.

and rising into the chest) and regurgitation of gastric fluid. The best test for documenting abnormal acid exposure in the esophagus, especially as it relates to symptoms, is 24-hour ambulatory pH testing. However, most patients with typical symptoms are appropriately diagnosed by using symptoms and a response to therapy. Endoscopy is sometimes helpful in making the diagnosis of gastroesophageal reflux disease by documenting the diffuse inflammation and ulceration of the distal esophagus typical of erosive esophagitis (Figure 1.8), and endoscopy is often essential in evaluating complications of gastroesophageal reflux disease such as peptic strictures, Barrett's esophagus, and adenocarcinoma.

As in patients presenting with dyspepsia, endoscopy is clearly indicated in patients with gastroesophageal reflux disease and "red flag" symptoms such as age greater than 45 years, dysphagia, odynophagia, recurrent vomiting, weight loss, iron-deficiency anemia, guaiac positive stool, or early satiety. Endoscopy is also indicated in patients who do not respond to medical therapy, and it may be indicated in patients with long-standing or intermittent symptoms or extra-esophageal symptoms such as asthma, chronic cough, hoarseness, or aspiration. In patients with gastroesophageal reflux disease and a poor response to proton pump inhibitors, consideration should be given to predisposing diagnoses such as esophageal motility disorders and Zollinger–Ellison syndrome.

Vomiting

The causes of vomiting are extensive, ranging from gastric-outlet or small-bowel obstruction to motility disorders, acute infection, side-effects of medications, metabolic derangements, pregnancy, eating disorders, and lesions of the central nervous system. Patients with severe or prolonged vomiting of unclear etiology should be evaluated with radiologic studies. These may include abdominal radiographs, upper gastro-intestinal series with small-bowel follow-through, computed tomography (CT), and gastric emptying scintigraphy. Upper endoscopy is typically reserved to rule out mucosal disease or to evaluate lesions identified in the radiologic work-up.

Ingestion of foreign bodies

At least 80% of ingested foreign bodies pass through the gastrointestinal tract spontaneously and require no intervention. For those that do not, the esophagus is the most common site of impaction. In general, mortality from foreign-body ingestion is extremely rare, but certain situations deserve particular attention. Long, pointed foreign bodies, for example toothpicks and fish and chicken bones, are associated with the highest rates of perforation. Other foreign bodies that are particularly dangerous include button batteries, which can rapidly cause corrosive perforation of the esophagus, and narcotic or cocaine packages, which can cause severe toxicity and death if they break. Button batteries should be removed immediately, but drug packets should never be removed endoscopically because of the risk of rupture. Impaction at the level of the upper esophageal sphincter may cause tracheal compression and respiratory compromise. In all ingestions, attention to the airway is the first priority, and impactions high in the esophagus should be treated as a true emergency.

While postero-anterior and lateral radiographs of the neck, chest, and abdomen should always be obtained, normal radiographs do not exclude the presence of an impacted foreign body. Contrast agents such as barium obscure endoscopic visualiz-ation and should be avoided. Water-soluble contrast agents such as Gastrograffin®, should be avoided in the setting of suspected obstruction in the upper gastrointestinal tract because these agents cause a severe chemical pneumonitis when aspirated. In adults, foreign bodies that should generally be removed from the stomach and duodenum include sharp objects, objects longer than 10 centimeters, and objects that have remained in the stomach for more than 1 week. Endoscopy employing combinations of snares, forceps, nets, and overtubes is the method of choice for removing almost all foreign bodies.

Food impaction

The most commonly cause of acute esophageal obstruction in adults is food impaction, typically with meat. Most patients with the so-called "steakhouse syndrome" present to the emergency room with pain and the inability to swallow liquids or solids. For patients with food-bolus impaction who are comfortable and can handle their own secretions, endoscopy need not be emergent. However, no foreign body should be allowed to remain in the esophagus for more than 24 hours because the risk of complications such as transmucosal erosion increases and also meat becomes more difficult to remove as time passes. Approximately 75% of patients with meat impaction have underlying esophageal pathology, usually a Schatzki ring or peptic stricture, and so should be investigated endoscopically even if the obstruction passes spontaneously. Only 1% to 2% are found to have an underlying esophageal malignancy. Most impacted food boluses can be advanced into the stomach by gentle pressure from the endoscope. In a minority of cases, the bolus cannot be coaxed into the stomach and has to be extracted with endoscopic devices.

Caustic ingestions

Caustic ingestions are far less common in adults than in children. In adults, however, ingestions tend to be intentional, of a larger volume, and more severe. Ingestion of alkaline substances such as lye and batteries is both more common and more toxic than ingestion of acid. Emetics and charcoal should not be given. Indications for endoscopy include symptoms such as vomiting, stridor, drooling, odynophagia, ingestion of large quantities of very alkaline (pH above 12.5) or very acidic (pH below 2) substances, and intentional ingestion. The purpose of endoscopy in this setting is to evaluate the severity and extent of mucosal damage, and the initial endoscopic evaluation is best done 24 to 36 hours after the ingestion. Severe burns of the larynx or hypopharynx and respiratory compromise are contraindications to endoscopy. The presence of grade III burns with deep circumferential ulceration and necrosis represents a high risk of perforation and the potential need for surgery. Patients who have had a significant caustic ingestion require ongoing surveillance for the development of long-term complications such as strictures, dysmotility, and carcinoma.

Acute gastrointestinal bleeding

Acute upper gastrointestinal bleeding is a common and potentially life-threatening problem. Endoscopy provides information about the nature of the bleeding lesion, its location, and its activity. Endoscopy allows physicians to make rational decisions about triage and to plan therapy. Two patients with identical presentations of coffee-ground emesis and melena may have very different risks and require very different care. For example, the first patient with a clean-based gastric ulcer on endoscopy may be sent home from the emergency room, whereas the second with a duodenal ulcer containing a visible vessel at its base or with adherent clot requires endoscopic therapy and may be admitted to the intensive care unit.

In all patients who present with acute gastrointestinal bleeding, the first priorities are to establish adequate intravenous access and to resuscitate the patient. The history should focus on understanding the duration and speed of bleeding and on risk factors such as comorbid disease, the use of NSAIDs, and a history of liver disease, heavy alcohol use, or prior gastrointestinal bleeding. In addition to older age and more comorbid disease, markers of increased mortality include bleeding from varices or malignancy, onset of bleeding in the hospital, and recurrent bleeding.

Endoscopy may identify a variety of lesions, but ulcers are the most common, accounting in most series for at least half of all cases of gastrointestinal bleeding. Other common bleeding lesions include erosive esophagitis, esophageal or gastric varices, Mallory–Weiss tears, vascular malformations, and malignancies (Figures 1.8, 1.9). Less common sources of acute upper gastrointestinal bleeding include Dieulafoy's lesions (small arteries that protrude from the mucosal surface), portal hypertensive gastropathy, aortoenteric fistulas, hemobilia (hemorrhage into the bile ducts), and hemosuccus pancreaticus (hemorrhage into the pancreatic duct).

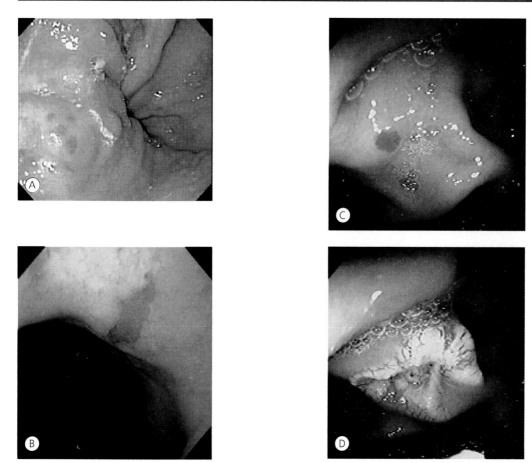

Figure 1.9 Common causes of upper gastrointestinal bleeding. A) Esophageal varix. A bulging variceal column is seen at the lower left corner of the distal esophagus. The red spots on the varix represent a sign of recent or impending bleeding. Normal gastric folds are seen in the upper right corner of the picture. B) Mallory–Weiss tear. A discrete mucosal tear is seen at the esophagogastric junction. The patient presented with dry heaves followed by the onset of hematemesis. C) Vascular malformation of the gastric fundus. D) Endoscopic treatment of vascular malformation. The lesion has been successfully treated with the application of bipolar electrocautery.

Most peptic ulcer disease results from either infection with *Helicobacter pylori* or the use of NSAIDs. However, in the industrialized world the incidence of peptic ulcers that are not related to either of these causes appears to be increasing rapidly. Regardless of their etiology, peptic ulcers can be separated into those with a low risk and those with a high risk of rebleeding based on their appearance (Table 1.3). Clean-based ulcers are not likely to rebleed. Other low-risk stigmata include flat pigmented spots within the ulcer bed, and the risk of rebleeding without endoscopic therapy for low-risk stigmata ranges from 3% to 10% (Figure 1.10A). High-risk stigmata include active arterial bleeding, a non-bleeding visible vessel, and adherent clot. The risk of rebleeding without endoscopic therapy ranges from 25% to 90% for these lesions (Figure 1.10B). Endoscopic treatment of ulcers with high-risk stigmata using an injection of epinephrine (adrenaline) and/or application of bipolar cautery or heater probe has been shown to reduce the rate of rebleeding in high-risk ulcers to about 10%. Recent advances in the treatment of bleeding from peptic ulcers include new endoscopic instruments such as mechanical hemoclips and the adjunctive use of high-dose intravenous proton pump inhibitors (Figure 1.10C). With rare exceptions, the rapid evolution of endoscopic therapy has meant that even severe bleeding from peptic ulcers is now a medical rather than a surgical disease.

Table 1.3 Peptic ulcer rebleeding rates by endoscopic stigmata

	Prevalence (%)	Rebleeding without endoscopic therapy (%)
High risk		
Active arterial bleeding	10	90
Non-bleeding visible vessel	25	50
Adherent clot	10	25–30
Low risk		
Flat spots	10	7–10
Clean-based ulcer	35	3–5

Source: Katschinski B, Logan R, Davis J, *et al*. Prognostic factors in upper gastrointestinal bleeding. *Dig Dis Sci* 1994; 39(4): 706–712

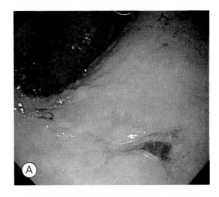

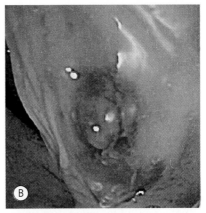

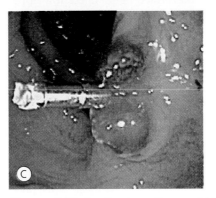

Figure 1.10 Peptic ulcer disease. A) This ulcer in the incisura of the stomach has a flat, clean base and is associated with a risk of rebleeding that is less than 10%. Endoscopic therapy is not warranted. B) This duodenal ulcer shows an adherent clot that is oozing blood. C) This high-risk ulcer has been treated with the deployment of a clip across its base. This immediately stopped the blood oozing with no recurrence of bleeding.

Patients with portal hypertension who present with an initial episode of bleeding from esophageal varices have a mortality rate of 30% to 50% within the following year. Initial bleeding can usually be controlled with sclerotherapy, in which a sclerosing agent is injected into varices, or with endoscopic band ligation, in which elastic bands are deployed onto varices (Figure 1.11). Because of higher complication and rebleeding rates and the need for more endoscopic sessions to eradicate varices, sclerotherapy has largely been abandoned in favor of band ligation. The use of synthetic somatostatin analogs to vasoconstrict the splanchnic circulation and prophylactic antibiotics have been shown to improve short-term outcomes in the setting of acute bleeding. Nonselective beta-blockers have been shown to reduce rebleeding, but not mortality, after an initial bleed. Some patients with refractory bleeding may be managed with transjugular intrahepatic portosystemic shunt, portosystemic shunt surgery, or liver transplantation. Still, despite recent advances in medical, endoscopic, radiologic, and surgical therapy of acute variceal bleeding, mortality from complications such as infection, pneumonia, and renal failure remains high.

Screening for esophageal varices

On average, 40% of patients with compensated cirrhosis have moderate or large esophageal varices. Their risk of a first variceal bleed within 2 years is 20% to 35% but is decreased with appropriate medical therapy. Therefore, the American College of Gastroenterology recommends universal screening endoscopy for all patients with compensated cirrhosis, followed by non-selective beta-blocker therapy for those with varices.

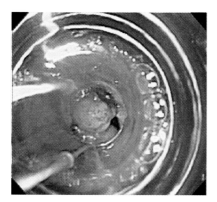

Figure 1.11 Variceal banding. A black rubber band has been deployed around the base of a varix. Three remaining bands can be seen around the transparent cap of the banding device at the end of the endoscope.

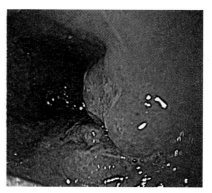

Figure 1.12 Barrett's adenocarcinoma. An ulcerated mass in the distal esophagus is seen to arise within salmon-colored mucosa that represents underlying Barrett's esophagus.

Chronic gastrointestinal bleeding

In patients with chronic gastrointestinal bleeding, the majority of significant lesions are located in the lower gastrointestinal tract. The need for upper endoscopy is dictated by the presence of upper gastrointestinal symptoms such as heartburn, epigastric pain, nausea, and vomiting. If iron deficiency anemia is present and colonoscopy is unrevealing, upper endoscopy should be performed. Upper endoscopy allows diagnosis not only of chronically bleeding mucosal lesions but also of conditions causing iron malabsorption such as celiac sprue. In the absence of iron deficiency or upper gastrointestinal symptoms, the use of upper endoscopy in the evaluation of chronic, occult bleeding is controversial. In at least one large series, endoscopy for occult bleeding identified many lesions in the upper gastrointestinal tract, but very few of these were of clinical importance.

Obscure bleeding is defined as persistent frank or occult bleeding despite unrevealing evaluation with upper and lower endoscopy. Some of these patients have such persistent and severe bleeding that they require intermittent transfusion despite oral iron supplementation. In obscure bleeding, careful repeat upper and lower endoscopy often reveals pathology that was not appreciated on the first examination. In this setting, common lesions in the upper gastrointestinal tract include Cameron's erosions (mechanical erosions inside a hiatal hernia), gastric antral vascular ectasia, portal hypertensive gastropathy, and vascular malformations. Proximal small-bowel enteroscopy should be performed using a dedicated push enteroscope. Capsule endoscopy may also be indicated.

Cancer diagnosis, screening, and surveillance

Endoscopic biopsies typically provide the definitive diagnosis of malignancy in the gastrointestinal tract. Therefore, when a malignancy is suspected on the basis of a patient's history, symptoms, or physical examination, the threshold for upper endoscopy should be low and endoscopy should not be delayed by performing unecessary radiographic procedures.

Commonly discovered mucosal lesions may or may not require endoscopic biopsies. A minority of gastric ulcers are malignant, so all gastric ulcers require follow-up after 8 to 12 weeks of medical therapy to assure healing, and non-healing gastric ulcers should always be biopsied. By contrast, isolated duodenal ulcers are not thought to have malignant potential and do not require biopsies or follow-up. Gastric polyps are frequent incidental findings and are rarely symptomatic. Most are hyperplastic or fundic gland polyps with no malignant potential. However, a minority are adenomas. Therefore, polyps should be sampled and all large gastric polyps should be biopsied and/or excised.

Endoscopy also plays an important role in the surveillance and treatment of premalignant lesions of the upper gastrointestinal tract. The most common of these conditions is Barrett's esophagus, in which the normal squamous epithelium of the distal esophagus is replaced by intestinalized columnar epithelium. By definition, this diagnosis requires histology for confirmation. Barrett's esophagus is associated with gastroesophageal reflux disease and is a risk factor for esophageal adenocarcinoma, which develops in approximately 0.5% of patients with Barrett's esophagus per year (Figure 1.12). The rising incidence of this cancer in the last 50 years is associated with Barrett's esophagus. In patients with Barrett's esophagus, periodic endoscopic surveillance is recommended. After the initial endoscopic diagnosis in patients without dysplasia, four-quadrant biopsies at 2 centimeter intervals should be performed every 2 to 3 years, and in patients with low-grade dysplasia, biopsies should be performed annually. Given their high risk of cancer, patients with Barrett's esophagus and high-grade dysplasia should be considered for esophagectomy, endoscopic therapy, or more intensive endoscopic surveillance.

In the future, biomarkers of malignant potential other than histology are likely to guide recommendations for the treatment of Barrett's esophagus. Another area of ongoing research involves endoscopic methods for the ablation of dysplastic Barrett's epithelium. These are based on the principle that destruction of metaplastic cells can lead to restitution of the normal squamous mucosa as long as acid reflux is well controlled with medication. Techniques that induce such tissue injury include electrocoagulation, laser therapy, argon plasma coagulation, and photodynamic therapy. If a small focus of dysplasia or early carcinoma is identified, it can be resected endoscopically using the technique of endoscopic mucosal resection, in which the tissue is lifted toward the endoscope and then snared at its base. These endoscopic treatments have shown varying degrees of promise, are still under investigation, and should not be used outside large clinical trials.

Endoscopic surveillance for cancer also plays a major role in the rare syndrome of familial adenomatous polyposis. Next to colorectal cancer, these patients die most frequently from adenocarcinoma that develops in upper gastrointestinal tract adenomas. Duodenal adenomas occur most frequently in the region of the ampulla of Vater (Figure 1.13). Surveillance upper endoscopy should be initiated by the third decade of life. Endoscopy should be performed with both forward- and side-viewing instruments to allow for biopsy of the ampulla, even if this has a grossly normal appear-

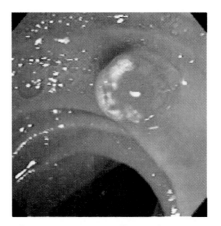

Figure 1.13 Ampullary adenoma. Visualization of the ampulla of Vater with a side-viewing endoscope reveals a friable mass. Biopsies revealed adenoma with high-grade dysplasia.

Box 1.2 Inappropriate or unproven indications for endoscopy

Evaluation of chronic anemia without gastrointestinal symptoms, fecal occult blood positive stool, or iron deficiency
Follow-up of benign lesions such as duodenal ulcers
Evaluation of metastatic carcinoma of unknown primary source
Evaluation of hiatal hernia
Cancer surveillance in the setting of
   achalasia
   atrophic gastritis
   pernicious anemia
   prior gastric surgery

---

ance. Patients with familial adenomatous polyposis should have ongoing surveillance at 1- to 5-year intervals depending on endoscopic findings.

Patients with a history of caustic ingestion are at high risk for developing esophageal carcinoma and should begin endoscopic surveillance 15 to 20 years after the initial injury, surveillance should continue at 1- to 3-year intervals. Several other conditions may be associated with an increased risk of cancer in the upper gastrointestinal tract. However, there are insufficient data to support routine endoscopic surveillance. These include achalasia, a history of gastric surgery, atrophic gastritis, and pernicious anemia. Other inappropriate or unproven indications for endoscopy are presented in Box 1.2.

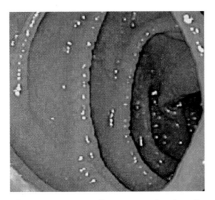

Figure 1.14 Celiac sprue in the duodenum. Endoscopy reveals "scalloping" of the duodenal folds. The diagnosis of celiac sprue is confirmed by showing blunting of the villi on biopsy.

Evaluation of malabsorption

While non-invasive testing of blood and stool is often adequate, some malabsorptive diseases are best diagnosed by small-bowel biopsy. Endoscopy is a useful tool in diagnosing inflammatory, infiltrative, or infectious disorders of the gut. Celiac sprue is increasingly recognized as a common cause of malabsorption, and serologic testing for this disease has become highly sensitive and specific. However, small-bowel biopsy remains the gold standard of diagnosis, revealing blunting and/or flattening of the villi and increased cellularity of the lamina propria. Endoscopically, celiac sprue is suggested by "scalloping" of the duodenal folds (Figure 1.14).

Conclusion

The twentieth century witnessed the birth and rapid evolution of gastrointestinal endoscopy. Endoscopy is now the standard tool for the diagnosis and treatment of most diseases affecting the mucosa of the upper gastrointestinal tract. There is no doubt that endoscopy will continue to evolve, becoming safer and less invasive and allowing physicians access beyond the lumen and to the molecular level.

Further reading

American College of Gastroenterology www.acg.gi.org

American Gastroenterological Association Medical Position Statement: Evaluation of dyspepsia. *Gastroenterology* 1998; 114: 579–581.

American Gastroenterological Association Medical Position Statement: Nausea and vomiting. *Gastroenterology* 2001; 120: 261–262.

American Gastroenterological Association www.gastro.org

American Society for Gastrointestinal Endoscopy www.asge.org

American Society for Gastrointestinal Endoscopy. An annotated algorithmic approach to upper gastrointestinal bleeding. *Gastrointest Endosc* 2001; 53: 853–858.

American Society for Gastrointestinal Endoscopy. Guidelines on the management of anticoagulation and antiplatelet therapy for endoscopic procedures. *Gastrointest Endosc* 2002; 55(7): 775–779.

American Society for Gastrointestinal Endoscopy. The role of endoscopy in the surveillance of premalignant conditions of the upper gastrointestinal tract. *Gastrointest Endosc* 1998; 48: 663–668.

American Society for Gastrointestinal Endoscopy. The role of endoscopic therapy in the management of variceal hemorrhage. *Gastrointest Endosc* 1998; 48: 697–698.

DeVault KR, Castell DO. ACG treatment guideline: updated guidelines for the diagnosis and treatment of gastroesophageal reflux disease. *Am J Gastroenterol* 1999; 94: 1434–1442.

Grace ND. ACG treatment guideline: diagnosis and treatment of gastrointestinal bleeding secondary to portal hypertension. *Am J Gastroenterol* 1997; 92: 1081–1091.

Sampliner RE. ACG treatment guideline: practice guidelines on the diagnosis, surveillance, and therapy of Barrett's esophagus. *Am J Gastroenterol* 1998; 93: 1028–1032.

Chapter 2

Colonoscopy

Gordon C. Hunt and Douglas O. Faigel

History

In 1895 Howard Kelly, a professor of gynecology and obstetrics at Johns Hopkins University, published the descriptions and drawings of the first rigid rectosimoidoscope in the US. These instruments were subsequently referred to as "Kelly tubes". The advent of fiberoptic endoscopes, developed in 1957 by Basil Hirschowitz, allowed for serious consideration of fiberoptic sigmoidoscopy and colonoscopy. Machida and Olympus Corporations introduced market versions of these devices in 1965. In 1970 at the University of Michigan, a longer colonoscope was introduced by Bergein Overholt, which possessed the feature of a four-way tip deflection. This allowed for the appropriate negotiation of the colonic flexures. By the late 1970s almost all endoscopists had accepted that fiberoptic sigmoidoscopes or colonoscopes were clinically superior to any other types in almost all circumstances.

These discoveries are especially important, as colorectal cancer remains the third most commonly diagnosed cancer and the second leading cause of cancer deaths in the US. Each year, more than 130 000 individuals are diagnosed with this condition, and over 50 000 will die from it.

Indications for colonoscopy

A premiere goal of colonoscopy is to decrease the incidence of colorectal cancer by detecting and removing precancerous lesions, or polyps. In the

---

Box 2.1 American Society for Gastrointestinal Endoscopy indications and contraindications for colonoscopy

Diagnostic colonoscopy is generally indicated in the following circumstances.

1. Evaluation of an abnormality on barium enema, which is likely to be clinically significant, such as a filling defect or stricture.
2. Evaluation of unexplained gastrointestinal bleeding (hematochezia not thought to be from the rectum or perianal region, melena of unknown origin, presence of fecal occult blood).
3. Unexplained iron deficiency anemia.
4. Surveillance for colonic neoplasia
   a) examination to evaluate the entire colon for synchronous cancer or neoplastic polyps in a patient with a treatable cancer or neoplastic polyp
   b) follow-up at 3- to 6-year intervals following resection of a colorectal cancer or neoplastic polyp
   c) patients with a strongly positive family history of colon cancer
   d) in patients with chronic ulcerative colitis, colonoscopy every 1 to 2 years with multiple biopsies for detection of cancer and dysplasia in patients with
      • pancolitis of greater than 7-years duration
      • left-sided colitis of more than 15-years duration.
5. Chronic inflammatory bowel disease of the colon if more precise diagnosis or determination of the extent of activity of disease influences the immediate management.
6. Clinically significant diarrhea of unexplained origin.
7. Intraoperative identification of the site of a lesion that cannot be detected by palpation or gross inspection at surgery (i.e. polypectomy site, location of a bleeding source).

Diagnostic colonoscopy is generally not indicated in the following circumstances.

1. Chronic, stable, irritable bowel syndrome or chronic abdominal pain; there are unusual exceptions in which colonoscopy may be done once to rule out organic disease, especially if symptoms are unresponsive to therapy.
2. Acute limited diarrhea.
3. Metastatic adenocarcinoma of an unknown primary site in the absence of colonic symptoms when it will not influence the management.
4. Routine follow-up of inflammatory bowel disease (except for cancer surveillance in chronic ulcerative colitis).
5. Routine examination of the colon in patients about to undergo elective abdominal surgery for non-colonic disease.
6. Upper gastrointestinal bleeding, or melena with a demonstrated upper gastrointestinal source.
7. Bright-red rectal bleeding in a patient with a convincing anorectal source on sigmoidoscopy and no other symptoms suggestive of a more proximal source.

Colonoscopy is generally contraindicated in the following circumstances.

1. Fulminant colitis.
2. Possible perforated viscus.
3. Acute severe diverticulitis.

---

early 1970s, the sequence of colorectal cancers arising from adenomatous polyps was initially proposed. Cancer requires the accumulation of multiple genetic mutations, resulting in hyperproliferation, adenoma development, successive stages of dysplasia, and invasive cancer. The evolution of normal tissue to adenoma formation to cancer generally takes 7 to 12 years. Demographic features including age, gender, and family history determine the prevalence of adenomas, and there is convincing evidence that removing adenomatous polyps prevents colorectal cancer. Only 30% of individuals harbor risk factors for colorectal cancer. These risk factors include family history of colorectal cancer in a first-degree relative, a personal history of colon polyps or colon cancer, a personal history of inflammatory bowel disease, and genetic acquisition of a familial polyposis syndrome (including familial adenomatous polyposis and hereditary non-polyposis colon cancer). Current recommendations of the American Society for Gastrointestinal Endoscopy for proceeding with colonoscopy are listed in Box 2.1.

Table 2.1 Recommendations of the Agency for Health Care Policy and Research Consortium for post-polypectomy surveillance colonoscopy

Findings at index examination	Surveillance interval
Single tubular adenoma	5 years
Multiple adenomas or villous histology	3 years
Numerous adenomas	Consider 1 year
Large sessile adenomas	3 to 6 months to examine the site

Other common indications for colonoscopy include surveillance of either colonic neoplasia or chronic inflammatory bowel disease of the colon. Surveillance interval recommendations for colonic neoplasia are given in Table 2.1. Surveillance recommendations for inflammatory bowel disease are discussed in a separate section below.

If a filling defect or stricture is noted on barium enema study, it should be evaluated without hesitation with colonoscopy. Colonoscopy may also be requested intraoperatively if the surgeon requires precise identification of a lesion that cannot be detected by palpation or gross inspection at surgery.

The role that colonoscopy plays in the evaluation of patients with symptoms of irritable bowel syndrome is less clear. Sigmoidoscopy is recommended for most young individuals (younger than 50 years of age) with presumed irritable bowel syndrome. In constipated patients, sigmoidoscopy may effectively rule out a distal obstructive lesion. In diarrhea-predominant patients, it may rule out inflammatory bowel disease that can mimic irritable bowel syndrome symptoms. In these patients, random biopsies are performed to evaluate for microscopic or collagenous colitis, both of which present with mucosa that appears normal. In patients who are over 50 years and who have the symptoms of irritable bowel syndrome, i.e. abdominal pain and diarrhea or constipation, then a complete colonoscopic examination is recommended because of an increased incidence of colonic neoplasia in this age group. To help differentiate which patients with irritable bowel syndrome should have complete colonoscopy, one should consider duration of symptoms and change of symptoms over time, age and gender of the patient, prior diagnostic studies, family history of colorectal cancer, and degree of psychosocial dysfunction.

Diagnostic colonoscopy is generally not recommended for patients with irritable bowel syndrome whose symptoms are stable. It is also not recommended for any patient with acute limited diarrhea, metastatic adenocarcinoma of unknown primary in a patient without colonic symptoms when the diagnosis will not change the management, routine follow-up of inflammatory bowel disease, or for routine examination in patients who are about to undergo surgery for non-colonic disease. Colonoscopy is not recommended for upper gastrointestinal bleeding in patients with a demonstrated upper gastrointestinal source, or in bright-red rectal bleeding in a patient with a convincing anorectal source on sigmoidoscopy, unless other symptoms suggest a possible proximal source. Colonoscopy is generally contraindicated in fulminant colitis, possible perforated viscus, and in acute severe diverticulitis.

Screening and surveillance recommendations

Screening average-risk individuals

Mounting evidence shows that screening average-risk individuals for colorectal cancer has decreased the incidence and reduced mortality from this disease. Prospective randomized trials have demonstrated a 15% to 33% reduction in colorectal cancer-related mortality in patients screened with fecal occult blood testing. Three expert panels that make recommendations on screening (the American Cancer Society, the United States Preventive Service Task Force, and a consortium of the American Society for Gastrointestinal Endoscopy, American Gastroenterology Association, American College of Gastroenterology, American Society of Colon and Rectal Surgeons, and Society of American Gastrointestinal Endoscopy Surgeons), have all advocated yearly fecal occult blood testing as one option for screening average-risk individuals for colon cancer. Patients are instructed to complete three cards on separate days with stool collection for blood. If any of the cards are positive, it is recommended that the patient have either a colonoscopy or a flexible sigmoidoscopy with double contrast barium enema. Colonoscopy is preferred, however, because of its superior diagnostic characteristics and its ability to remove detected lesions at the time of the examination.

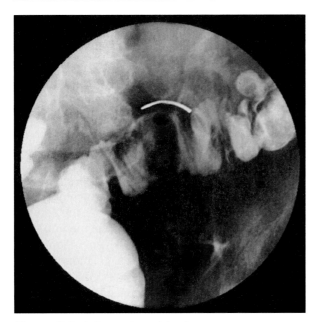

Figure 2.1 A 3-cm sigmoid colon mass as seen on barium enema. The mass was resected and diagnosed as an adenocarcinoma.

In patients aged 50 to 80 years, estimates of the overall reduction in colorectal cancer-related mortality from flexible sigmoidoscopy have been suggested to be 45% in the portion of the colon examined. However, there have been no prospective studies on screening flexible sigmoidoscopy as a test that decreases colorectal cancer-related mortality. Nevertheless, another option for colon screening presented by the three major task forces is flexible sigmoidoscopy every 5 years for patients starting at the age of 50 years. This examination should be combined with either yearly fecal occult blood testing or double contrast barium enema. If any of these examinations are positive, then colonoscopy should be performed. It is not recommended that double contrast barium enema be performed on its own, as it poorly visualizes the rectosigmoid area, it may miss up to 50% of polyps over 1 centimeter in size (data from the National Polyp Study), and double contrast barium enema lacks the sensitivity and therapeutic capabilities of colonoscopy (Figure 2.1). Further, no prospective studies to date have demonstrated that double contrast barium enema significantly reduces colorectal cancer-related mortality. One prospective study found that the sensitivities of barium enema versus colonoscopy for detecting colorectal cancer were 83% and 95%, respectively. Double contrast barium enema is the least expensive screening test that examines the entire colon.

The preferred strategy for colorectal cancer screening is performing colonoscopy every 10 years for patients aged 50 years and older. This test is the "gold standard" for screening as it completely visualizes the entire colon and offers therapeutic potential of polypectomy. A recent prospective study showed that combined screening with flexible sigmoidoscopy and fecal occult blood testing identified 75.8% of subjects with advanced neoplasia of the colon, as determined by colonoscopy. Extrapolating this data, one would hypothesize that screening for colorectal cancer with flexible sigmoidoscopy and fecal occult blood testing would miss one patient in four with advanced neoplasia (defined as an adenoma larger than 10 millimeters, a villous adenoma, an adenoma with high-grade dysplasia, or invasive cancer). A separate prospective study on screening with colonoscopy of a male-dominant population, aged over 50 years, showed 10.5% of asymptomatic patients had advanced neoplasia as defined above. This study also showed that 52% of the 128 patients who had advanced neoplasia proximal to the splenic flexure had no distal adenomas. These studies provide some of the most conclusive and provocative evidence of the feasibility of screening for colorectal cancer with colonoscopy, but the choice of modality for colorectal cancer screening should be discussed between practitioner and patient.

Surveillance intervals

The finding of a neoplastic polyp, defined as a tubular adenoma or villous adenoma, on flexible sigmoidoscopy, is an indication for complete colonoscopy. Approximately 30% to 50% of individuals with a tubular adenoma on sigmoidoscopy will harbor additional polyps, and colonoscopy allows both the detection and removal of synchronous polyps. The incidence of malignancy in a polyp rises as the size and villous component of the polyp increase. Although it is recommended that all neoplastic polyps larger than 1 centimeter should be completely excised, it is controversial whether colonoscopy should be performed to remove neoplastic polyps less than 1 centimeter in size. The occurrence of carcinoma in a polyp smaller than 0.5 centimeters is rare but has been reported. The current recommendations by the American Society for Gastrointestinal Endoscopy and by the Agency for Health Care Policy and Research on the surveillance interval of colonoscopy after polypectomy for a single benign tubular adenoma, is 5 years. Follow-up at 6 years has subsequently been proposed. Table 2.1 shows the current guidelines for surveillance that best reflect the literature, as taken from the Agency for Health Care Policy and Research. Norwegian experts have created substantially different guidelines for post-polypectomy surveillance, they are as follows.

1. After resecting a malignant polyp the recommendations are to examine the resection site at least once within 12 months, and thereafter as for ordinary adenomas.
2. For persons with resected adenomas and with at least one of the following features
   a) high-grade dysplasia or villous components and age less than 75 years, or
   b) size of adenomas 10 millimeters or more, and age less than 75 years,
   the recommendations are for colonoscopy every 10 years.
3. For persons and adenomas with the following features
   a) three or more adenomas of any size and age less than 75 years, or
   b) biopsy-verified adenomas 1 to 4 millimeters left *in situ*, or
   c) features in category (b) plus a history of previous gynecologic cancer,
   the recommendations are for colonoscopy every 5 years.
4. For persons and adenomas with the following features
   a) one or two tubular adenomas less than 10 millimeters in size, or
   b) resected hyperplastic polyps with or without small solitary adenoma, or
   c) age over 75 years at initial polypectomy, or
   d) no remaining adenomas, adenoma remnants, or remaining polyps of unknown histology,
   the recommendations are for no follow-up colonoscopy.

After resection of colon cancer, the incidence of an anastomotic recurrence is between 2% and 3%. Anastomotic recurrences are generally a harbinger of recurrent metastatic disease in the pelvis or abdomen, which is unresectable for cure. Thus, patients with colon cancer should have a clearing colonoscopy preoperatively, or within 2 to 3 months of surgery if obstructed at the time of resection. After the initial postoperative clearing colonoscopy,

this examination should be repeated at 3- to 5-year intervals, or as indicated by associated adenoma findings. The local recurrence rate of rectal cancer is much higher, reportedly between 10% and 35% in most studies. Patients who have had a low anterior resection are sometimes recommended to have surveillance flexible sigmoidoscopies every 6 months for the initial 2 years postoperatively. Anecdotal studies suggest that endoscopic ultrasound may be the best way to detect surgically curable recurrences in a disease where recurrences are usually incurable. The role of endoscopic ultrasound in the detection of local recurrences of rectal cancer has not been evaluated in a randomized clinical trial to date.

Surveillance for cancer in inflammatory bowel disease

The evidence that surveillance with colonoscopy decreases colorectal cancer mortality comes from cohort studies, but there have been no randomized trials to date to evaluate the effectiveness of surveillance colonoscopy in the setting of inflammatory bowel disease. The cost-effectiveness and yield of surveillance of colonoscopy in patients with inflammatory bowel disease is lower than for any other indication for which colonoscopy is performed. The primary difficulty of surveillance in these patients is in detecting dysplasia in flat mucosa. Dysplasia can be a patchy lesion and this creates sampling error. Several studies have shown that for a 90% to 95% confidence level in detecting the highest degree of dysplasia, 33 to 64 biopsies of the colon must be taken. These samples should preferably be from jumbo-forceps biopsies with turn-and-suction technique, taken in four quadrants at every 10 centimeters of the involved colon. Samples should be separated if taken from mass lesions or villiform mucosa. An expert pathologist should confirm high-grade dysplasia discovered in flat mucosa. Patients with chronic colitis and completely resected adenomatous polyps in flat mucosa can be managed conservatively. The presence of a dysplasia-associated lesion or mass that cannot be removed endoscopically or that does not have the typical appearance of an uncomplicated adenoma, is an indication for colectomy. Unifocal low-grade dysplasia in flat mucosa is no longer an indication for colectomy, but should prompt more frequent surveillance and a more intensive biopsy protocol.

Current clinical recommendations are to initiate surveillance after 8 years of pancolitis or after 15 years in left-sided disease. Interval colonoscopy should be performed every 1 to 3 years in patients with colitis of 8- to 20-years duration, annually after 20 years, and potentially even more frequently after 30 years. This is especially true if one has concurrent risk factors such as a family history of colon cancer or sclerosing cholangitis. For Crohn's colitis, the utility of endoscopic surveillance remains to be defined. Most experts recommend surveillance for these patients at similar intervals to those with ulcerative colitis.

Future research should be directed at improving the surveillance yield of colonoscopy in patients with ulcerative colitis and Crohn's colitis. This may involve stool collection for DNA markers, flow cytometry to detect aneuploidy, light-induced autoflorescence, photodynamic detection of aminolevulinic acid uptake in dysplastic tissue, and high-resolution endoscopy.

Procedure for colonoscopy

Preparation

Perhaps the most unpleasant part of colonoscopy for the patient is taking an oral preparation to cleanse the colon. Several preparations involving combinations of diet restriction (i.e. a clear liquid diet the day before) and pill or liquid laxatives, are used clinically. The most popular preparations are polyethylene glycol-based solutions and sodium phosphate oral laxatives. Because of its small volume of oral intake, patients generally prefer sodium phosphate solutions. However, sodium phosphate solutions may induce fluid shifts in patients with renal insufficiency or on renal dialysis, and also is considered unsafe in patients with liver disease and ascites or with congestive heart failure. The ideal preparation from the perspective of both palatability and safety has not yet been developed.

Sedation

Cardiopulmonary events attributed to sedation are the most common complication of colonoscopy, including vasovagal reactions and clinically significant oxygen desaturation. Sedation also accounts for about one half of the costs of colonoscopy, in that it necessitates recovery room costs, additional assessment costs, and costs associated with monitoring and administration of oxygen and other medications. Some studies have shown that most American clinicians would not attempt colonoscopy without sedation, while others show that a small but significant percentage of American clinicians would be willing to attempt unsedated colonoscopy. Predictors of willingness for no sedation include male gender, increasing age, and absence of abdominal pain.

The most common combination of agents used for sedation is a narcotic with a benzodiazepine. Alfentanyl, fentanyl, and meperidine are popular intravenous narcotics, and midazolam is a highly utilized benzodiazepine. Meperidine appears to potentiate the sedative effect of benzodiazepines. Alfentanyl and fentanyl have a quicker onset of action and a shorter duration of effect. Unfortunately, all of these agents may require prolonged monitoring post-procedure, contributing to costs.

Nitrous oxide has been used in a 50:50 mixture with inhaled oxygen for colonoscopy. Its onset of action is short (approximately 1 minute), and recovery is faster than with a benzodiazepine–narcotic combination. However, nitrous oxide is contra-indicated in patients with congestive heart failure, severe cardiopulmonary disease, and increased intracranial pressure. It may additionally impose a long-term health care risk to medical personnel. Nitrous oxide has been shown to be equally effective in sedated colonoscopy when compared to opioids, but not as effective as opioid–benzodiazepine combinations, and has not been endorsed in the USA.

Propofol is a relatively new hypnotic sedative agent that has been shown to be safe and effective when used for sedation for colonoscopy. Its major advantages include rapid onset of action and rapid recovery after discontinuation of the infusion, rapid response to titration of the medication, lack of active metabolites, and cost. A potential danger of this medication is deep sedation, resulting in respiratory arrest. When it was introduced in 1989 it was only used by anesthesiologists and its FDA-approved indications remain for anesthesia and sedation in intubated patients. In some units, endoscopists and endoscopy nurses are using it under strict monitoring conditions. All personnel in the endoscopy room should have advanced cardiac life-support skills if deep sedation is used. Patient-controlled sedation with propofol has also been reported with success in small series, resulting in high patient satisfaction and faster discharge. Future controlled trials involving propofol sedation should determine if it is safe in the conditions stated above and if it is cost-effective.

Instrumentation, accessories, and technique

The standard adult colonoscope is 168 centimeters long and 12.9 millimeters in diameter with a working channel of 3.7 millimeters. Older fiberoptic instruments have been replaced by video-colonoscopes incorporating color charge coupled device (CCD) chips. Total colonoscopy in adults can often be achieved with a pediatric instrument measuring 168 centimeters long, 11.3 millimeters in diameter and with a working channel of 3.2 millimeters. As an alternative to the standard adult colonoscope, a variable-stiffness colonoscope has recently been introduced (Olympus Inc.). This instrument is available in the diameters of both a pediatric colonoscope and a standard adult colono-scope. Some colonoscopists find that the standard smaller diameter "pediatric" colonoscope is too flexible to permit an adequate rate of intubation of the cecum. However, the "softness" of the pediatric colonoscope allows it to be pushed around the colon with a lesser degree of discomfort than the standard adult colonoscope. The ability to stiffen the variable-stiffness pediatric colonoscope allows the physician to traverse more easily the sigmoid bends with a "push" technique, and, once the sigmoid colon has been successfully intubated, the instrument can be straightened and subsequently stiffened to permit further advancement into the proximal colon. Some studies have found that this instrument decreases the overall intubation time, but this difference has not necessarily been found to be statistically significant. The instrument has also been found to decrease the number of times that external abdominal compression needs to be applied. The adult-sized variable-stiffness instrument has an integral water jet to clean debris from the colon.

In addition to technical advances in colonoscopes, monitors are being produced with high photographic definition, and endoscopes are being manufactured with higher resolution capabilities. Colonoscopes with zoom magnification, which is accessible via a rotating dial on the instrument head, have the potential capability of distinguishing adenomas from hyperplastic polyps based on the pit pattern.

Accessories for obtaining biopsies, or for performing polypectomies or other therapies are introduced via the working channel of the colonoscope. Standard items found in every endos-copy unit include biopsy forceps, diathermy snares, and retrieval baskets or graspers. Several novel and recently introduced accessories are of interest to colonoscopists. A "spike-snare" (needle-tip snare) (Olympus, Inc. and Wilson-Cook) has a 1 millimeter-long tip that allows it to anchor the point of the snare to the colon surface. This allows easier and more accurate impaction of the tip into the mucosal surface at the desired location. Other accessories for polyp retrieval include the Roth Basket® and the polyp suction trap. The Roth Basket® is a mesh basket attached to a wire loop of a polypectomy snare, and it is used to capture and retrieve multiple polyp fragments. The polyp suction trap is a trap with four small, fenestrated compartments to allow capture of several polyps from multiple locations, while keeping the fragments from each area separated.

Other newly developed devices include a magnetic imaging apparatus to help determine the real-time location of the colonoscope within the colon. This device produces an image by sensors activated by magnets within the shaft of a colonoscope. This allows depiction of intracolonic looping, paradoxical motion, and proper use of the facility to straighten the instrument.

In addition to colonoscopy, other recent techniques employed to image the colon are CT colonography and chromoendoscopy. These methods are discussed below (see pp. 28–29).

Findings

Colonic neoplasia

Polyps are a frequent and important finding at colonoscopy. Morphologically, polyps may be divided into two main groups – pedunculated (Figure 2.2) or sessile (Figure 2.3). Pedunculated polyps have a classic mushroom appearance with the polypoid lesion extending from a stalk. Competent colonos-copists, using either cutting current or low-powered coagulation current, can remove most pedunculated polyps. Studies have verified that the morbidity, mortality, and cost of colonoscopic polypectomy are significantly less for polypectomy than by laparotomy. The latter is justified only when the experienced endoscopist cannot successfully or

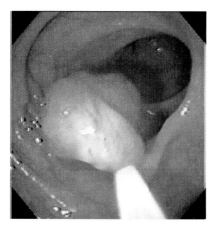

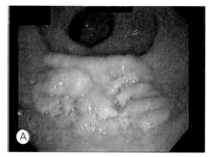

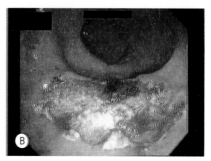

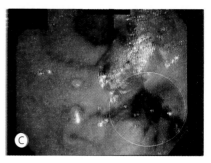

Figure 2.2 Pedunculated polyp. The stalk has been trapped within a polypectomy snare.

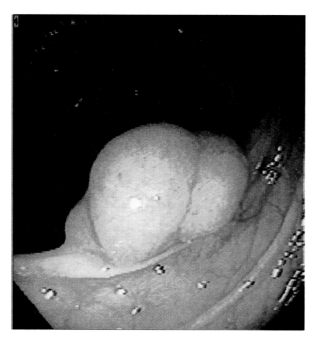

Figure 2.4 A) A large villous adenoma of the rectum. B) After removal by endoscopic mucosal resection and argon plasma coagulation of residual polyp material from the edges. C) A tattoo (circled) has been placed by submucosal injection of India ink to mark the site for future surveillance.

Figure 2.3 A large 2-cm sessile polyp seen in the transverse colon.

safely remove the entire lesion. Cold biopsy forceps may effectively remove very small polyps (1 to 3 millimeters in size), but this technique is not recommended for larger polyps. Other options for removing polyps less than 6 millimeters in size include hot biopsy forceps, monopolar or bipolar electrocautery snares, and cold snare guillotine resection. The use of hot forceps in the right colon as opposed to the left colon is five times more likely to result in complications, notably post-polypectomy hemorrhage or perforation. Snare resection via either hot or cold techniques is the technique least likely to leave residual polyps. Polyps larger than

7 millimeters in size should generally be removed using electrocautery snare resection.

Removal of large sessile polyps is one of the greatest challenges of polypectomy (Figure 2.4). Injection of submucosal saline facilitates the removal of flat adenomas, and theoretically reduces the risk of perforation. This technique of saline injection to aid in strip mucosal resection is termed endoscopic mucosal resection. As a rule, large sessile polyps can be removed via colonoscopy if they do not cross two successive haustral folds, and do not occupy more than one third of the circumference of the colon. In the past Nd:YAG laser was popular for the ablation of sessile polyps larger than 4 centimeters, but its cost and risk of perforation have allowed argon plasma coagulation to supplant

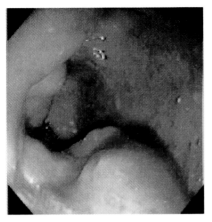

Figure 2.5 Colon cancer. An ulcerated adenocarcinoma of the descending colon.

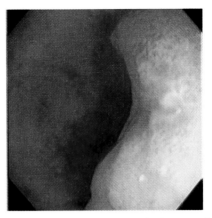

Figure 2.7 Solitary rectal ulcer syndrome presenting as an ulcerated mass.

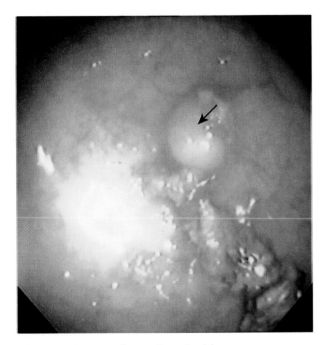

Figure 2.6 A small rectal carcinoid tumor.

its use. Argon plasma coagulation may be used to destroy residual flat polyp material after incomplete electrocautery snare resection in selected patients.

If a polyp is not completely removed, or adenocarcinoma crosses the cautery margin, then injection tattooing may be used to mark the site for subsequent identification at surgery (Figure 2.4C). In western countries, follow-up of adenoma cohorts whose colons have been cleared of polyps by colonoscopy and polypectomy demonstrates dramatic reduction of colorectal cancer incidence and near complete protection from colorectal cancer mortality.

Colorectal carcinomas typically are large sessile masses that may be ulcerated, friable, bleeding, or circumferential (Figure 2.5). Lymphomas rarely occur in the colon but have an appearance similar to carcinomas. Typical submucosal masses include lipomas, gastrointestinal stromal tumors, and carcinoids (Figure 2.6). Lipomas may have a yellowish color and be soft, indenting when probed with biopsy forceps. In women, colonic implants of endometriosis may appear as pigmented submucosal masses. Endoscopic ultrasound is useful in imaging submucosal masses in the distal colorectum.

Non-neoplastic abnormalities

Common abnormalities, which may be recognized on standard digital rectal examination, include internal and external hemorrhoids, rectal prolapse, polyps (especially diminutive hyperplastic polyps), and masses. After digital rectal examination, insertion of the colonoscope generally reveals a richly vascular rectal plexus. On antegrade view of the rectal mucosa, abnormalities that may be visualized include proctitis, prep-induced colitis, and polyps and/or masses. Patients with long-standing constipation, particularly those with prolapse, may have a solitary rectal ulcer, which in some cases can mimic a neoplastic mass (Figure 2.7). At some point during the procedure, routine retroflexion of the colonoscope within the rectum should be performed (Figure 2.8). Retroflexion of the colonoscope should only be avoided when it is technically difficult or impossible because of prior pelvic surgery, or because of exquisite pain experienced by the patient. If retroflexion is avoided or unsuccessful, the reason why it was not

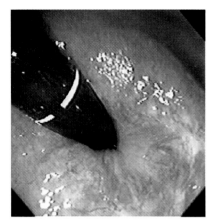

Figure 2.8 Normal retroflexed view in the rectum.

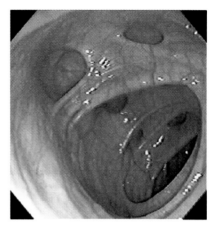

Figure 2.10 Diverticulosis of the sigmoid colon.

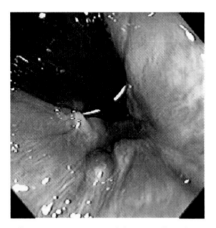

Figure 2.9 Internal hemorrhoids.

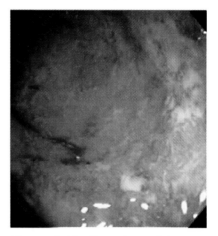

Figure 2.11 Ulcerative colitis.

performed should be clearly documented, as polyps and/or masses may be missed. A common finding on retroflexion is internal hemorrhoids that appear as bluish protuberances at the anorectal junction (Figure 2.9).

As the colonoscope is advanced further into the sigmoid colon, diverticulosis will be a common abnormality visualized within this area (Figure 2.10). In Western cultures, 95% of patients with diverticula have sigmoid diverticula, and diverticula are limited to the sigmoid colon in 65% of cases. Other abnormalities encountered in the sigmoid colon include ischemic, infectious, idiopathic ulcerative, and Crohn's colitis in the distal colorectum. Mucosa afflicted with acute colitis is reddened, edematous, and lacks the normal vascular pattern. Ulceration may be present. In ulcerative colitis the inflammatory changes begin at the rectum and continue proximally for a varying distance that may include the entire colon (pancolitis) (Figure 2.11). Ischemic colitis most commonly involves the vascular watershed of the splenic flexure, descending or sigmoid colon; the rectum is typically spared. Rectal involvement is also spared in Crohn's disease. Crohn's colitis is usually discontinuous with areas of intervening uninvolved colon. Aphthous ulcers of the colon may also be seen (Figure 2.12). Perianal disease (fistulae, abscesses) may also occur in Crohn's disease.

Melanosis coli, a dark-brown, pigmented staining of the colonic epithelium, may develop in patients who chronically take anthraquinone laxatives, it can occur throughout the colon (Figure 2.13). Most frequently, however, melanosis coli is observed in the cecum and rectum.

In patients who have previously had a segmental or partial colectomy for colon carcinoma, one must pay particular attention to the site of surgical

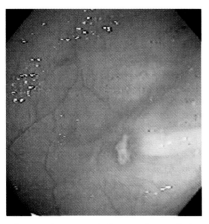

Figure 2.12 Aphthous ulcer of the colon.

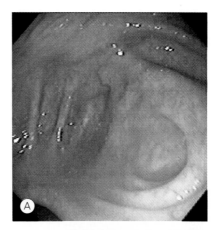

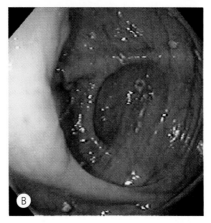

Figure 2.14 Normal cecum. A) Note the normal semilunar appearance of the appendiceal orifice. B) View of the ileocecal valve.

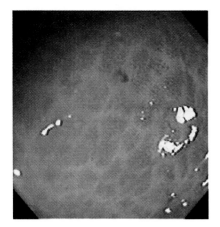

Figure 2.13 Melanosis coli.

anastomosis during initial surveillance colonoscopic examinations. When surgery is performed to resect malignancy, the anastomosis is a potential area for recurrence of cancer, particularly rectal cancer.

There are several anatomic markings of the cecum that define completion of a colonoscopic examination. These findings include direct visualization of the ileocecal valve, the appendiceal orifice, and of the "crow's foot", which is the bridging haustra of the cecum (Figure 2.14). Intubation of the terminal ileum also defines a complete colonoscopic examination, and may be important in patients suspected of having disease in this area (i.e. Crohn's disease, lymphoma).

Arteriovenous malformations, also referred to as angiodysplasias, are most commonly found in the ascending colon and cecum in most series (Figure 2.15). Other findings seen in the cecum and terminal ileum include bacterial infections, such as *Yersinia*

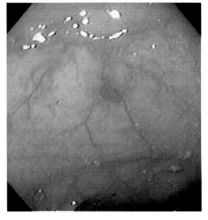

Figure 2.15 An arteriovenous malformation.

spp., *Mycobacterium tuberculosis*, and *Entamoeba histolytica*. Celiac disease may occasionally be diagnosed with random biopsies of the terminal ileum. The appearance of colonic mucosa in microscopic and collagenous colitis is normal. The diagnosis is made in patients with chronic diarrhea, by taking random biopsies from throughout the colon, although the yield may be somewhat higher proximal to the splenic flexure.

Complications

In addition to the previously discussed sedation risks, the major risks during colonoscopy are bleeding and perforation. In the University of Minnesota Colon Cancer Control Study, the risk of serious bleeding and perforation requiring surgery among 12 246 patients undergoing colonoscopy was approximately 0.1%. A study on screening colonoscopy for average-risk individuals reported a rate of serious complications (cerebrovascular accident, bleeding requiring hospitalization, or myocardial infarction) of 0.3% in 3121 patients. The rate of bowel perforation with flexible sigmoidoscopy has been reported to be 0.0014%. Other studies in the 1990s suggested that the perforation rate of diagnostic colonoscopy is 1/3000 to 1/5000. Transmission of infection has been reported to occur in rare cases but was attributed to inadequate processing of the endoscope and its accessories between procedures.

Palliation of colorectal cancer

Colonoscopic palliation may be applied to rectal bleeding and obstructive colorectal cancer. In non-operative patients, non-obstructive tumors which present with rectal bleeding may be treated in several ways. Rectal tumors may be debulked with a polypectomy snare, and the surface may subsequently be coagulated with argon plasma coagulation or laser.

Up to 30% of patients with primary colorectal carcinoma present with large-bowel obstruction. This can be treated by Nd:YAG laser, but this is no longer a frequently used method of therapy, because of its cost and risk of perforation. Photo-dynamic therapy and endoscopic stenting are other methods used for the palliation of malignant colonic obstruction. Placement of a self-expanding colorectal stent may also be utilized for pre-operative decompression (Figure 2.16). For most instances, stenting has become established as the preferred endoscopic treatment for palliation of malignant obstruction. Placing a metal stent in an

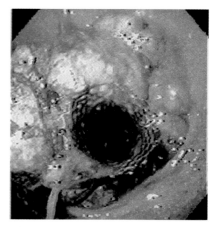

Figure 2.16 A self-expanding metallic stent placed to palliate obstructing rectal cancer.

obstructing lesion allows the acutely ill patient to stabilize clinically with preoperative decompression and subsequent bowel cleansing, enabling a one-step operative procedure. Metal stents may also be placed for palliation in patients with significant comorbidities or widely metastatic disease. Retrospective studies have suggested that placement of metal stents may reduce costs by decreasing the number of intensive care unit and hospital days, and by reducing the number of surgical procedures needed.

Potential complications of expandable colorectal stents include migration, perforation, bleeding, stent malpositioning, and occlusion of the stent by stool. Stents placed low in the rectal vault may cause tenesmus or fecal incontinence. After successful placement of a colorectal stent patients are recommended to consume a low-residue diet, and use stool softeners or laxatives. In the future, expandable metal stents that emit radiation or release chemotherapeutic agents may be used.

Computed tomography colonography

Computed tomographic colonography was initially described in 1994. It has generated much enthusiasm as a new method for screening for colorectal carcinoma, and is typically referred to as "virtual colonoscopy". It utilizes volumetric data acquired by either a single detector or multidetector helical CT scanner. Using specific imaging software, CT colonography creates two-dimensional and three-dimensional images of the colon.

Volumetric data must be obtained twice, once while the patient is prone and once while supine. A purgative colonic preparation is required, as is complete colonic air or carbon dioxide insufflation of the colon. When compared to double contrast barium enema, CT colonography does not require mucosal coating with barium, there are no overlapping segments of the colon and rectum, and it is less time consuming. In limited series, for detecting polyps 1 centimeter or larger in size, CT colonography has a reported sensitivity of 75 to greater than 90%. In comparison to colonoscopy, CT colonography does not require sedation or post-procedural monitoring, and the risk of bleeding, perforation, or death is less. It may detect extra-colonic abnormalities such as renal masses, lung nodules, and abdominal aortic aneurysms. It must be noted that detection of asymptomatic abnor-malities may lead to unnecessary evaluations and patient anxiety.

One of the main drawbacks of CT colonography when compared to colonoscopy is that it does not allow tissue sampling or therapy. Polyps that are detected by this test will require another preparation for colonoscopy and polypectomy. Computed tomography colonography cannot differentiate between polyps and adherent stool. A high positivity rate (30% to 50%) necessitates colonoscopy in almost half of patients undergoing CT colonography, drawing its cost-effectiveness into question. Interpretation of the data may also be time con-suming. Initial reports suggested that the inter-pretation took about 30 minutes, but with further familiarity with the results, radiologists are now reporting interpretation times of 5 to 15 minutes. The radiation dose of abdomino-pelvic CT is not insignificant, with some authors estimating the cancer risk of a single examination to be as high as 1 in 5000. It remains to be elucidated what specific role CT colonography will play as a clinically viable screening test.

Chromoendoscopy

Chromoendoscopy, or spraying of tissue stains during endoscopy, is an investigational technique that may allow better detection and characterization of colonic lesions. When utilized with a colonoscope that magnifies the image (magnification endoscopy), the histology of lesions may be better predicted. The optical system of a magnifying colonoscope differs from the conventional colonoscope, which has a fixed focusing system. Current magnifying colonoscopes have the ability to magnify a colon polyp 10 to 35 times, to an ultrahigh magnification of 170 times.

Chromoendoscopy was initially used in Japanese studies to evaluate early gastric cancer. Indigo carmine (Daiichi Pharmaceutical Corp., Tokyo, Japan) is one stain that is used, it is not absorbed and has no toxicity. It is a blue contrast agent, which accentuates the contours of a lesion, especially flat adenomas. Some studies have shown indigo carmine to be helpful at distinguishing between hyperplastic polyps and adenomatous lesions during colonoscopy.

Crystal violet (gentian violet, Honzo Pharmaceutical Corp., Nagoya, Japan) and methylene blue are vital stains that are preferentially taken up by Lieberkühn's gland openings (crypts) of neoplastic polyps, appearing as dots or pits. A "pit pattern classification" scheme has been described, classifying colonic polyps and flat colonic lesions according to their appearance, structure, and staining pattern. Crystal violet may be most beneficial when combined with magnifying colonoscopy to determine the optimal treatment for early colorectal cancer. It also allows the endoscopist to evaluate a poly-pectomy site for residual polyp tissue. Prior to staining colonic mucosa with any stain, the mucosa should be washed with water, with or without a proteinase.

Chromoendoscopy has mostly been described in the Japanese literature. There is debate as to whether or not Western populations have different pathology (with diminutive polyps) when compared to Japanese populations (where high-grade dysplastic lesions in small and flat polyps appear to be more common). If chromoendoscopy is able to expedite therapy by increasing the ease and efficiency with which diagnoses are made, the cost-effectiveness of colonoscopy may improve.

Training in colonoscopy

Colonoscopists who have not been formally trained in a gastroenterology fellowship program miss more colorectal cancers than do gastroenterologists. Higher complication rates occur in the examiner's first 500 examinations, which is the initial time of training. Studies that use objective criteria for completion and competence have estimated that 100 supervised examinations are required to achieve a 90% success rate. However, a multicenter study involving 14 gastrointestinal fellowship programs and 135 gastrointestinal fellows found that fewer than 3% of fellows were technically competent if they had completed less than 100 supervised examinations. In this study, more than 200 supervised procedures were needed for an individual to be considered technically competent at diagnostic colonoscopy.

Additional data has shown that at least 100 colonoscopies should be completed under supervision prior to assessing one's competency. These guidelines are based on published data as follows. Formally trained and experienced colonoscopists consistently achieve a cecal intubation rate of over 95%, whereas the cecal intubation rate of trainees is only 84%. The learning curves are similar regardless of subspecialty background training. Family physicians with limited training report cecal intubation rates varying from 54% to 83%.

However, the performance of a predetermined number of procedures may not necessarily guarantee competency. Training in colonoscopy includes recognizing and diagnosing lesions and findings, understanding gastrointestinal pathophysiology, and applying appropriate clinical management strategies. The colonoscopist must also competently perform therapeutic procedures such as polypectomy and the treatment of bleeding sites. Proficiency in techniques of conscious sedation is also advocated by the major gastrointestinal organizations. Thus, proficiency should be substantiated by documentation provided by the applicant from Residency Program Directors, Chiefs of Service, or other members of the teaching faculty who have directly observed the applicant performing endoscopy.

Further reading

Baron TH. Expandable metal stents for the treatment of cancerous obstruction of the gastrointestinal tract, *N Engl J Med* 2001; 344: 1681–1686.

Bell GD. Premedication, preparation, and surveillance. *Endoscopy* 2002; 34: 2–12.

Eisen GM, Chutkan R, Goldstein JL, *et al.* Guidelines for colorectal cancer screening and surveillance. American Society of Gastrointestinal Endoscopy. *Gastrointest Endosc* 1999; 50: 921–924.

Fleischer DE. Chromoendoscopy and magnification endoscopy in the colon. *Gastrointest Endosc* 1999; 49: S45–49.

Hoff G, Sauar J, Hofstad B, *et al.* The Norwegian guidelines for surveillance after polypectomy: 10-year intervals. *Scand J Gastroenterol* 1996; 31: 834–836.

Koslin DB. Update on gastrointestinal imaging. *Rev Gastroenterol Disord* 2002; 2: 3–10.

Lambert R, Provenzale D, Ectors N, *et al.* Early diagnosis and prevention of sporadic colorectal cancer. *Endoscopy* 2001; 33: 1042–1064.

Lieberman DA, Weiss DG. One-time screening for colorectal cancer with combined fecal occult-blood testing and examination of the distal colon. *N Engl J Med* 2001; 345: 555–560.

Lieberman DA, Weiss DG, Bond JH, *et al.* Use of colonoscopy to screen asymptomatic adults for colorectal cancer. Veterans Affairs Cooperative Study Group 380. *N Engl J Med* 2000; 343: 162–168.

Rex DK. Colonoscopy. *Gastrointest Endosc Clin N Amer* 2000; 10: 135–160.

Rex DK, Johnson DA, Lieberman DA, *et al.* Colorectal cancer prevention 2000: screening recommendations of the American College of Gastroenterology. *Am J Gastroenterol* 2000; 95: 868–877.

Rex D, Rahmani E, Hasemann J *et al.* Relative sensitivity of colonoscopy and barium enema for detection of colorectal cancer in clinical practice. *Gastroenterology* 1997; 112: 17–23.

Smith RA, Cokkinides V, Levin B, *et al.* American cancer society guidelines for the early detection of cancer. *CA Cancer J Clin* 2002; 52: 8–22.

Wexner SD, Eisen GM, Simmang C. Principles of privileging and credentialing for endoscopy and colonoscopy. *Dis Colon Rectum* 2002; 45: 161–164.

Waye JD, Kahn O, Auerbach ME. Complications of colonoscopy and flexible sigmoidoscopy. *Gastrointest Endosc Clin N Am* 1996; 6: 343–373.

Chapter 3

Small Intestinal Endoscopy

Thomas E. Kowalski and Jin-Hong Park

Introduction

Endoscopy of the small intestine, or enteroscopy, has not shared the success of its siblings, esophagogastroduodenoscopy and colonoscopy, mostly because of the inherent difficulty in examining a freely moving, coiled, twenty-foot conduit, but also because of the notion that pathology of the small intestine is rare. Technological advances however, have closed the gap, making enteroscopy a more accessible diagnostic modality and an effective therapeutic modality for those lesions within the reach of our ever-lengthening push enteroscopes. Although enteroscopy is expected to rapidly evolve and alter our understanding of small-bowel pathophysiology, this chapter will serve as a foundation upon which to relate enteroscopy to the pathology that is common to the small intestine.

Anatomy

Gross features

The small intestine is a structurally and functionally unique segment of gut that courses approximately 600 cm (19.5 ft) between the pyloric sphincter and ileocecal valve. The small intestine is divided into duodenum, jejunum, and ileum. The ligament of Treitz separates the duodenum from the jejunum, but no such demarcation separates the jejunum from the ileum and endoscopically it is impossible to distinguish these segments. By convention, therefore, the jejunum is considered to be the proximal two fifths of small intestine distal to the ligament of Treitz and the remaining three fifths of small bowel is ileum. The ligament of Treitz also defines where the small intestine leaves the confines of the retroperitoneum to become attached solely to the freely mobile mesentery. Unperturbed, the jejunum resides in the left upper quadrant and cephalad periumbilical area while the ileum is located in the right lower quadrant and pelvis. Because of its mobility, this spatial relationship within the abdomen is not maintained during enteroscopy and is often permanently altered by abdominal surgery.

The luminal diameter of the small intestine narrows along its length, measuring 20 to 30 mm in the duodenum, 15 to 20 mm in the jejunum, and 10 to 12 mm in the ileum. Brunner's glands, which secrete mucus and bicarbonate, are often visible in the proximal duodenum, occasionally visible in the distal duodenum, and are rarely noted in the jejunum. The entire small intestine is lined by visible finger-like projections called villi. When compared to the ileum, the duodenum and jejunum have taller villi and larger, more numerous plicae circularis. In contrast, the ileum, particularly the terminal ileum, contains large visible collections of lymphoid follicles (Peyer's patches) that are especially prominent in young patients.

Blood supply, lymphatics, and innervation to the small intestine

The proximal duodenum receives a rich blood supply via the gastroduodenal artery, a branch of the hepatic artery that originates from the celiac trunk. The distal duodenum is supplied by the superior and inferior pancreaticoduodenal arteries, which respectively arise from the gastroduodenal artery and superior mesenteric artery. The superior mesenteric artery supplies the remainder of the small intestine via overlapping mesenteric collaterals denoted as vasa recta in the jejunum and as arcades in the ileum. The venous drainage of the small intestine is via the portal circulation. The superior and inferior pancreaticoduodenal veins drain blood directly from the duodenum into the portal vein, whereas the superior mesenteric vein that collects blood from the jejunum and ileum empties into the splenic vein first prior to joining the portal vein.

Lymphatic drainage occurs via lymph channels and mesenteric lymph nodes adjacent to the superior mesenteric and celiac arteries. Drainage proceeds to the periaortic nodes and into the thoracic duct via the cisterna chyli.

The small intestine is innervated by both sympathetic and parasympathetic nerves.

Sympathetic nerves derive from preganglionic fibers of the T6 to T11 thoracic roots that synapse with postganglionic fibers in the celiac and superior mesenteric ganglion to respectively innervate the duodenum and remaining small intestine. Parasympathetic and sensory innervation is provided primarily by the vagus nerve.

Enteroscopic modalities

Historical perspective

Prior to the mid-1970s examination of the small bowel was limited to barium radiology and surgery. In 1972, Classen introduced "rope-way" enteroscopy. The rope-way method involved the spontaneous passage through the entire gastrointestinal tract of a swallowed guidestring. Once the guidestring extended from mouth to anus, it was exchanged for a slightly larger and stiffer teflon tube, over which an endoscope could be passed. This procedure was onerous for the patient and physician and was quickly abandoned.

Shortly thereafter a very long, thin, flexible endoscope with a distal inflatable balloon was introduced as the Sonde enteroscope. The Sonde enteroscope was passed transorally or transnasally. The inflated balloon allowed the endoscope to advance by peristalsis and the 285 cm length permitted the distal ileum to be reached. Once in the ileum, the enteroscope was slowly pulled back so as to visualize the entire small-intestinal mucosa. The total procedure time averaged from 6 to 14 hours. Unfortunately, despite this long study duration, the distal ileum was infrequently reached and the lengthy procedure was poorly tolerated. Another limitation was the enteroscope's marginal tip deflection that only allowed for an estimated examination of 50% of the luminal surface. In addition, the Sonde enteroscope was relegated strictly to diagnostic applications, as the instrument did not include an instrument channel. For 25 years, Sonde enteroscopy has been performed by a small number of endoscopists mostly at academic centers and, indeed, the tool has taught us much about small-bowel pathology. Fortunately, however, the recent introduction of the capsule enteroscope has made Sonde enteroscopy an obsolete modality of small-bowel interrogation.

Push enteroscopy

The first time an endoscope was pushed past the ligament of Treitz into the jejunum was in 1973, when Ogashi used a specially designed 162 cm endoscope in conjunction with fluoroscopy for this notable accomplishment. Ogashi's paper was soon followed by reports that the pediatric colonoscope could be used safely for this same purpose. This was the advent of push enteroscopy. Unlike other techniques push enteroscopy allowed for visually directed biopsies and immediately replaced suction-tube biopsies, which were cumbersome, time consuming, and risky. Over the years, the push enteroscope has become the workhorse for small-bowel endoscopy. Push enteroscopes have become longer and more sophisticated. The most popular endoscopes used for enteroscopy are the 133-cm pediatric colonoscope, the 218-cm push enteroscope, and the 240-cm push enteroscope. The longer enteroscopes are generously thought to be capable of visualizing up to 50% of the small intestine. A variety of diagnostic and therapeutic tools can be passed through the enteroscope, for example the biopsy forcep, cytology brush, injection needle, snare, thermocoagulation probe, laser fiber, and catheter for argon plasma coagulation. As such, the push enterosocope has become widely used for a variety of purposes.

Perhaps the most frequent indication for push enteroscopy is the diagnosis and treatment of unexplained overt or occult gastrointestinal bleeding. In this setting, push enteroscopy is performed when esophagogastroduodenoscopy, colonoscopy, and barium studies do not reveal a source of blood loss. Push enteroscopy has been able to identify and treat bleeding sites in a significant proportion of these patients. In recent publications, bleeding sites were both identified and treated in 38% and 64% of studied patients. Angiodysplasias have been the most commonly identified pathology and successful endoscopic treatment has led to a significant decrease in blood transfusions as compared to pretreatment periods and as compared to those patients not treated endoscopically.

Push enteroscopy is also used to obtain a tissue diagnosis from lesions discovered by small-bowel barium studies, computed tomography (CT), or capsule enteroscopy, that are considered to be within the reach of the enteroscope. Push enteroscopy has been successfully used for identifying Crohn's disease, malignancies, polyposis syndromes, celiac sprue, lymphedema, and other small-intestinal pathology.

The area that can be examined with the push enteroscope is, of course, limited to the proximal small bowel in general with less than 50% of the small intestines visualized. When passed via the rectum, the push enteroscope can also be used to visualize the most distal 50 to 100 cm of ileum. In most cases however, push enteroscopy will be used in conjunction with capsule enteroscopy or small-bowel barium studies. In one study, when enteroclysis was performed after enteroscopy, an additional 8% of bleeding sources and 50% of mass lesions were diagnosed.

Technical considerations

Push enteroscopy is performed in a similar fashion to esophagogastroduodenoscopy. Fluoroscopy may be helpful but is not necessary. Conscious sedation using a short-acting benzodiazepine in combination with a rapidly acting narcotic analgesic, monitored anesthesia using propofol, or general anesthesia are each appropriate.

The enteroscope may be passed with or without an overtube. The semi-stiff overtube is used to reduce gastric looping that may lead to patient discomfort, vagal bradycardia, and limited jejunal penetration. The resistance of passing the enteroscope through the jejunum invariably surmounts the resistance towards creating a large gastric loop. As a large gastric loop can consume more than 50 cm of endoscope, the distal extent of scope insertion is limited by at least the same amount. Therefore, when the goal of enteroscopy is to gain maximal small-bowel visualization, the use of an overtube is recommended. If used, the overtube is loaded on the enteroscope prior to intubation. Once the scope is passed distal to the third portion of the duodenum, the enteroscope is pulled back to straighten and lift the scope away from the greater curvature of the stomach. At this point, the generously lubricated overtube is advanced over the scope to the pylorus or preferably into the duodenal bulb. Placement can be confirmed fluoroscopically or when bile is seen to reflux from the tube's proximal end.

Unlike esophagogastroduodenoscopy, small-bowel peristalsis aids in the advancement of the enteroscope. Near continuous small movements of the directional knobs, patience at sharp turns, and periodic endoscope straightening facilitate this process. Glucagon should not be used prior to achieving the most distal extension of the enteroscope but should be given prior to initiating withdrawal.

If lesions are known to exist prior to the procedure, preloading of the appropriate instrument (biopsy forcep, APC catheter, thermal probe) through the instrument channel is recommended, as once the target lesion is reached, a tortuous scope conformation may prevent passage of the instrument.

Complications are generally rare and comparable to those of upper endoscopy. Like upper endoscopy, oropharyngeal tears have been reported. Several case reports describe mucosal stripping secondary to the mucosa becoming caught between the enteroscope and the overtube at the time of either overtube insertion or enteroscope withdrawal. The most commonly used enteroscope overtubes have been modified and the literature has since been devoid of such reports.

Intraoperative enteroscopy

Intraoperative enteroscopy is push enteroscopy performed within the opened abdominal cavity so that the surgeon can assist in the visualization of essentially the entire small intestine.

The most common approach to intraoperative enteroscopy is standard laparotomy, although laparoscopic approaches are currently being investigated. A complete diagnostic laparotomy is performed including direct examination of the serosal surface of the bowel as well as its attached mesentery. The room is then semi-darkened and the enteroscope is passed either transorally or via a newly created enterotomy. Overtubes are not used for intraoperative examinations. A non-crushing clamp is placed across the terminal ileum to prevent colonic distention that often makes abdominal closure difficult. Once the enteroscope is well into the jejunum, the surgeon begins to fold contiguous loops of small intestine, in an accordion-like fashion, onto the enteroscope. During this process, the endoscopist examines the mucosal surface while the surgeon examines the transilluminated serosa. Unlike push enteroscopy, careful evaluation must be performed during enteroscope advancement, as mucosal injury that may occur with bowel manipulation may mimic angiodysplasias upon withdrawal. Intraoperative enteroscopy is significantly limited by the presence of adhesions and, surprisingly, is only successful at achieving complete small-bowel intubation in 57% of patients. A prolonged ileus is the most common postoperative complication.

Currently, intraoperative enteroscopy is accepted as the modality of choice for the visualization and treatment of obscure bleeding and lesions distal to the reach of the push enteroscope. Indications for intraoperative enteroscopy are defined by default when less-invasive studies, including esophagogastroduodenoscopy, colonoscopy, small-bowel barium radiology, and push enteroscopy have all failed to identify the source of blood loss.

Obscure overt and occult bleeding that require transfusion are the most common indications for undergoing intraoperative enteroscopy. Published trials find that, after unsuccessful push enteroscopy, intraoperative enteroscopy identified an additional 48% to 74% of the lesions responsible for bleeding. Of these lesions, 40% to 54% were angiodysplasias, with ulcers, polyps, tumors, diverticula, Crohn's disease, and hemangiomas being less common. In one series, 11% of those with obscure bleeding were diagnosed with tumors. Similar results have been reported with intraoperative enteroscopy providing a diagnosis in 77% of studied patients and the associated intervention leading to a long-term success rate of 55%.

Surveillance and removal of polyps in patients with Peutz–Jeghers polyposis syndrome is another indication for intraoperative enteroscopy. Peutz–Jeghers syndrome is a rare autosomal dominant disorder characterized by numerous hamartomatous polyps that are primarily asymptomatic but may present with anemia, overt gastrointestinal bleeding, or small-intestinal obstruction. Furthermore, contrary to previous notions, recent studies demonstrate that some Peutz–Jeghers polyps may have malignant potential, therefore elective polypectomy via esophagogastroduodenoscopy, colonoscopy, push enteroscopy, and intraoperative enteroscopy should be considered. Following elective polypectomy, it has been suggested that surveillance imaging studies be performed every 2 to 3 years. A cohort of Italian patients followed in this manner led to one polyp being removed by retrograde ileoscopy, 12 by push enteroscopy, and 16 by intraoperative enteroscopy. Intraoperative enterotomy followed by enteroscopy has also been performed to allow *en masse* polypectomy in a Peutz–Jeghers patient with numerous small-bowel polyps. Although there are no long-term data, it is assumed that the prophylactic removal of Peutz–Jeghers polyps will reduce future morbidity and mortality.

Although intraoperative enteroscopy has been used in the past for both diagnosis and treatment, new technologies, including capsule enteroscopy and perhaps virtual CT enteroscopy will, in the near future, strictly limit intraoperative enteroscopy to therapeutic indications.

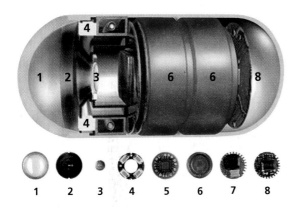

INSIDE THE M2A™ CAPSULE

1. Optical dome
2. Lens holder
3. Lens
4. Illuminating LEDs (Light Emitting Diode)
5. CMOS (Complementary Metal Oxide Semiconductor) imager
6. Battery
7. ASIC (Application Specific Intergrated Circuit) transmitter
8. Antenna

Figure 3.1 M2A capsule enteroscope (Courtesy of Given Imaging).

Capsule enteroscopy

The most recent innovative advance in small-bowel imaging is a disposable, ingestible, wireless, color video camera that transmits over 50 000 images during an 8-hour ambulatory examination. This capsule enteroscope has been developed and marketed by Given Imaging Inc., as the M2A Capsule. The capsule endoscope measures only 11×26 mm and contains a lens, four white-light emitting diodes (LEDs), color-chip camera, radio-frequency transmitter, and two silver oxide batteries (Figure 3.1). The critical development that made the capsule a reality, was the complementary metal oxide silicone chip camera that operates both at low levels of illumination and low power. The capsule moves by peristalsis. The short lens focal length allows circumferential images to be obtained as the optical dome of the capsule sweeps past the gut wall without the need for bowel insufflation. An axicon optical element compensates for the distorted image produced by the conical shape. The optical dome is specially designed to minimize

internal light reflections such that LED flashes do not refract back into the lens of the camera. The shape of the capsule promotes its long axis to be maintained throughout the entire examination with minimal to no tumbling, and similar images are obtained whether the lens of the capsule is oriented forwards or backwards. Images are obtained at a rate of two per second as the capsule traverses the small bowel. The duration of the 8-hour examination is limited only by battery life. Images are transmitted using ultra-high-frequency radio telemetry to an array of antennas worn by the patient. During the capsule examination the patient is alert, awake, and ambulatory and can pursue normal activities. Trigonometric analysis of signal strength allows for the continuous monitoring of capsule position. The image and position data is transferred to a data recorder also worn by the patient. The patient only needs to return to the study center in 8 hours to turn in the data recorder and aerial harness. The capsule itself is disposable and passes in the stool. From the data recorder, the data is downloaded onto a computer workstation loaded with application specific software, to be read by the physician at any time in the future.

Initial studies demonstrate that the mean time the capsule remains in the stomach is 60 minutes (17–280 min) and mean small-bowel transit time is 99 minutes (45–140 min). In nearly all cases, 8 hours was therefore ample time to fully examine the small intestines. Capsule endoscopy has been shown to be statistically superior to barium small-bowel study, push enteroscopy, and Sonde enteroscopy. The first clinical trial compared push enteroscopy to capsule enteroscopy in 21 patients with obscure gastrointestinal bleeding. Push enteroscopy made a diagnosis in 6 of 21 (30%) cases while capsule enteroscopy made a diagnosis in 11 of 21 (55%) cases. In a similar study, Pennazio reported that push enteroscopy identified a bleeding site in 8 of 29 (28%) patients with obscure gastrointestinal bleeding, whereas capsule enteroscopy identified a site in 17 of 29 (59%) patients. Within this group of patients, capsule enteroscopy identified lesions in 12 patients whose push enteroscopy was normal. Similar findings were reported by Delvaux, who demonstrated an additional yield of 45% when capsule enteroscopy was performed in addition to push enteroscopy.

At this point, the capsule is limited to the examination of the small bowel. The capsule is not suitable for the colon because of the colon's greater luminal diameter demanding a brighter light source, the need for stronger batteries with a longer life, and concerns regarding capsule orientation and tumbling. In the near future capsules will have guidance capability and may have mechanisms for obtaining biopsies and performing therapy.

Diseases of the small intestine

Vascular diseases

There are numerous etiologies for diseases of the small-intestinal vasculature. It is therefore unfortunate that no single classification schema has been universally accepted. One schema classifies the disease entity according to the presence or absence of systemic manifestations (Table 3.1) while another distinguishes diseases as either ischemic or hemorrhagic. All etiologies however, may manifest as gastrointestinal bleeding.

Angiodysplasia

By a wide margin the most common vascular abnormality of the small intestine is angiodysplasia which accounts for 40% of all obscure gastrointestinal bleeding. Angiodysplasias are defined as dilated vascular complexes consisting of arterioles, capillaries, and venules found superficially anywhere in the gastrointestinal tract. Endoscopically, angiodysplasias appear as homogeneous, cherry-red spots (Figure 3.2A) or lesions that have a capillary or fern-like pattern (Figure 3.2B).

The pathogenesis of angiodysplasia is not well known. Boley proposed that normal distention of the colon could cause intermittent obstruction of small superficial venous outflow tracts, causing them to dilate. Progression of dilatation would lead to involvement of capillaries creating an arteriovenous malformation. In accordance with Laplace's law, it made sense that this process would occur primarily in the cecum where wall tension is greatest. This theory, however, lacks credence within other areas of the gastrointestinal tract, particularly the small intestine.

Despite being the most common cause of small-intestinal hemorrhage, angiodysplasias are most often discovered incidentally when an endoscopic procedure is being performed for an unrelated reason. Angiodysplasias are most common in patients over 60 years old, and with increasing age their incidence increases in a linear fashion. The incidence of angiodysplasias is increased in patients

Table 3.1

Vascular abnormalities without systemic associations

Angiodysplasia
Venous ectasia
Osler–Weber–Rendu syndrome
Hemangioma
Blue rubber bleb nevus syndrome
Radiation enteritis
Portal hypertensive enteropathy
Dieulafoy's lesion
Hemangiosarcoma
Kaposi's sarcoma

Vascular abnormalities associated with systemic diseases

Diseases involving abnormal vessel structure	*Infiltrative diseases involving vessels*
Osteogenesis imperfecta	Amyloidosis
Ehlers–Danlos syndrome	Sarcoidosis
Marfan syndrome	Tuberculosis
Pseudoxanthoma elasticum	Multiple myeloma
Vitamin C deficiency	
Inflammatory diseases involving blood vessels	*Platelet disorders*
Systemic lupus erythematosus	von Willebrand's disease
Polyarteritis nodosa	Bernard–Soulier syndrome
Henoch–Schonlein purpura	
Churg–Strauss syndrome	
Cryoglobulinemia	*Miscellaneous disorders*
Rheumatoid vasculitis	Klippel–Trenaunay syndrome
Thromoangiitis obliterans	Chronic renal insufficiency
Giant cell arteritis	Turner's syndrome

with chronic renal failure and von Willebrand's disease. Less convincing associations have been described in patients with congestive heart failure, systemic hypertension, blood dyscrasias, and connective tissue disease. Patients with valvular heart disease or valvular prostheses are at no greater risk of developing angiodysplasias than the general population. On the other hand, any disease entity requiring anticoagulation or associated with a coagulopathy, may unmask clinically silent angiodysplasias, increasing the likelihood of symptomatology.

The treatment of angiodysplasias is primarily endoscopic and occasionally angiographic, with surgical intervention, directed by angiography,

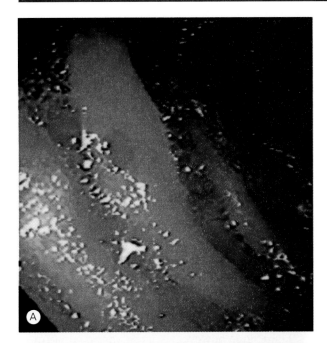

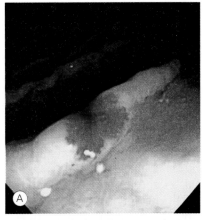

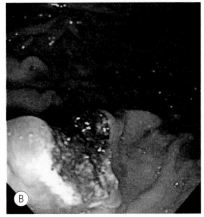

Figure 3.3 View of a small-intestinal angiodysplasia (A) before and (B) after thermal ablation using argon plasma coagulation.

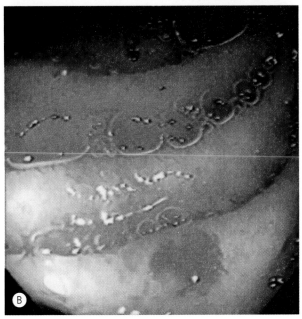

Figure 3.2 Typical small-intestinal angiodysplasias with (A) homogeneous and (B) fern-like appearances.

capsule enteroscopy, or intraoperative enteroscopy, being reserved for complex and potentially life-threatening situations. Angiodysplasias have been successfully treated with all modalities of endoscopic thermal coagulation, including monopolar thermal probe, bipolar thermal probe, Nd:YAG laser, KTP laser, and argon plasma coagulation (APC). Argon plasma coagulation is favored by some as it is a non-contact method that can be applied tangentially

(Figure 3.3) and, when compared to the Nd:YAG laser, has less potential for deep penetration. Endoscopic thermal ablation is generally curative for the lesion that is treated. Bipolar therapy is equally efficacious.

Less common vascular abnormalities

Phlebectasias, or venous ectasias, are dilated submucosal veins that protrude into the gastro-intestinal lumen. Phlebectasias have a bluish-red hue and appear nodular. Most phlebectasias are located in the esophagus and rectum, and are asymptomatic. Bleeding from venous ectasias is distinctly rare.

Telangiectasias, although similar to angio-dysplasias in appearance, are not limited to the gastrointestinal tract and are typified by the Osler–Weber–Rendu syndrome or hereditary hemorrhagic telangiectasia. The Osler–Weber–Rendu syndrome is an autosomal dominant disorder in which the majority of patients present before the age of 30 years with mucocutaneous bleeding. Gastrointestinal bleeding is present in 10% to 40% of these patients usually after the age of 50 years. Argon plasma coagulation or bipolar electrocautery are effective, technically favorable treatment modalities, although new telangiectasias may form only a few weeks following ablation.

Hemangiomas are benign neoplastic proliferations of blood vessels that may occur anywhere in the gastrointestinal tract and are classified as cavernous, capillary, or mixed. Hemangiomas represent 10% of all benign small-intestinal tumors. Bleeding occurs infrequently. Small lesions can be treated endoscopically with little chance of recurrence, while larger lesions require surgical resection.

Hemangiomas may be associated with cutaneous lesions, such as in the blue rubber bleb nevus syndrome. In this syndrome, cutaneous nevi can be found on the face, trunk, and extremities. Within the gastrointestinal tract, the vascular lesions may be located anywhere but are most commonly found within the small intestine. Lesions can be seen endoscopically as blue nodules varying from a few millimeters to many centimeters in size with flat to polypoid morphology. Rupture leads to overt gastrointestinal hemorrhage. Lesions can be treated endoscopically with band ligation, snare polypectomy, injected sclerosant, argon plasma coagulation, Nd:YAG laser, or KTP laser. Surgery is limited to patients refractory to endoscopic therapy. Another rare syndrome with cutaneous features is the Klippel–Trenaunay–Weber syndrome, which is characterized by the triad of cutaneous port-wine stains, varicose veins, and soft-tissue hypertrophy. Varicosities and cavernous hemangiomas associated with this syndrome are typically seen in the colon, but can also involve the small intestines.

Tumors

Overview

Carcinogenesis within the small intestine occurs at a rate that is significantly lower than in other parts of the gastrointestinal tract with primary small-intestinal tumors comprising only 2% of all gastrointestinal tumors despite the small intestine having the largest surface area. Several factors at least partially account for this difference. The small bowel mucosa has less exposure to mechanical, chemical, and biologic irritants, as there is rapid transit of primarily liquid contents containing

Table 3.2 Tumors of the small intestine

Benign	Neuroendocrine	Malignant
Adenoma	Carcinoid	Adenocarcinoma
Leiomyoma	Gastrinoma	Leiomyosarcoma
Lipoma	Somatostatinoma	Other sarcomas
Hemangioma	Vipoma	Lymphoma
Hamartoma	Ganglioneuroma	
Nodular lymphoid hyperplasia		

relatively few bacteria. A higher lymphoid component and expression of secretory immunoglobulin A (IgA) may be protective and small-intestinal enzymes may act to degrade some ingested carcinogens (e.g. benzopyrene).

There are, however, a large variety of tumors arising from the small intestine with an estimated 40 different histologic types of tumors identified (Table 3.2). Almost 75% of small-bowel tumors found at autopsy are benign, whereas tumors resected for symptoms tend to be malignant. Of all benign small-intestinal tumors 25% are leiomyomas. Others such as lipomas, adenomas, hemangiomas, hamartomas, and nodular lymphoid hyperplasia comprise the rest. Approximately 40% of the malignant tumors are adenocarcinomas, 30% are carcinoids, and 15% are lymphomas.

Small-intestinal tumors pose a diagnostic challenge as the initial symptoms include vague intermittent pain and distention that may mimic acid-peptic disease, irritable bowel syndrome, gallstone disease, or genitourinary pathology. Unless anemia, bleeding, or obstructive symptoms are present, these symptoms are often overlooked particularly after a negative esophagogastroduodenoscopy and colonoscopy. Less commonly, tumors present with classic signs and symptoms. In this light, jaundice may suggest ampullary carcinoma, flushing and diarrhea may suggest carcinoid, and nocturnal fever with weight loss may indicate lymphoma.

Gastrointestinal stromal tumors

Leiomyomas, leiomyosarcomas, and leiomyoblastomas have been reclassified under the broader and more embryologically appropriate terminology of gastrointestinal stromal tumor that are characterized by their mesenchymal histologic differentiation. Gastrointestinal stromal tumor with smooth muscle differentiation can be identified based on its histologic findings of smooth muscle components. Gastrointestinal stromal tumor with neural differentiation (previously gastrointestinal autonomic nerve tumors) can be histologically identified by the presence of neurotubules and axon-like cytoplasmic processes as well as a positive immunoreactive staining for S-100 protein and neuron-specific enolase.

Leiomyomas are usually asymptomatic, although some will ulcerate causing occult to massive bleeding, and others will result in obstruction or intussusception. Leiomyomas are most commonly found in the jejunum (Figure 3.4), followed by ileum and duodenum. The malignant potential of a suspected leiomyoma is measured by immuno-reactive staining for c-KIT, CD117, expression of alpha-smooth muscle actin, and the absence of gamma-smooth muscle isoactin, as well as the number of mitotic figures seen per high-power field.

Although larger in size, leiomyosarcomas present in a similar fashion to their benign counterparts. Indeterminant lesions greater than 5 cm should be resected. For known leiomyosarcomas, surgical resection is necessary as endoscopic therapy is not an option. In the past, radiation and chemotherapy have not provided significant benefit and the 5-year survival rate remained at 30%. Recent data with the tyrosine kinase inhibitor, Gleevec®, however, demonstrate promising results.

Adenomas and adenocarcinomas

Adenomas are the most common benign small-intestinal tumor. Adenomas can be located throughout the small intestine but are primarily distributed in the duodenum with a propensity for the periampullary region (Figure 3.5). Histologically, small-bowel adenomas are similar to the tubular, tubulovillous, and villous adenomas found in the

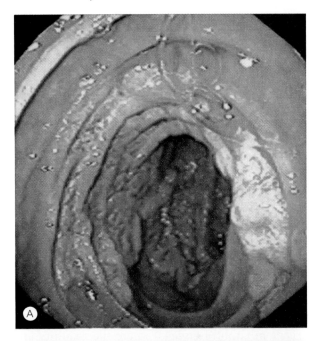

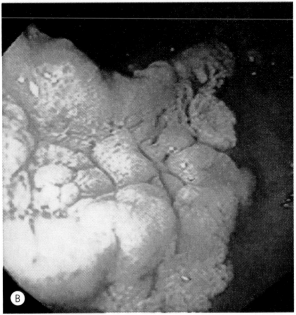

Figure 3.5 Carpet-like duodenal adenoma. (A) Circumferential view demonstrates extent of lesion. (B) Segmental view demonstrates changes in mucosal architecture.

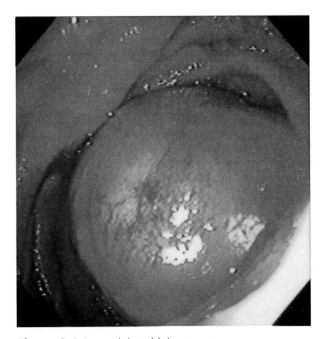

Figure 3.4 Large jejunal leiomyoma.

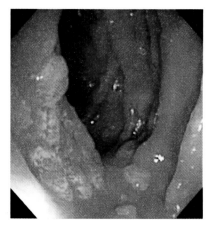

Figure 3.6 Multiple small duodenal adenomas in a patient with familial adenomatous polyposis.

Table 3.3 Relationship between the size of the primary lesion and the metastatic potential of carcinoid tumors

Size of primary lesion	Risk of metastasis
1–5 mm	0%
6–10 mm	15%
11–15 mm	50%
16–20 mm	75%
> 20 mm	95%

colon. Villous adenomas located in the duodenum have a high malignant potential with one large series demonstrating a 42% malignant transformation. For this reason, duodenal villous adenomas require endoscopic removal or ablation. If unsuccessful, surgical resection should be considered.

It follows logically that adenocarcinomas would be the most common small-bowel malignancy and, in fact, they comprise 30% to 50% of all small-intestinal carcinomas. The most common locations for adenocarcinoma is the duodenum and jejunum, except in Crohn's disease, where the majority are found in the ileum. Males are more frequently affected than females, and most adenocarcinomas are seen after the seventh decade of life. Risk factors for adenocarcinomas of the small intestine include familial adenomatous polyposis, Crohn's disease, AIDS, celiac disease, urinary diversion procedures, heavy alcohol use, and neurofibromatosis.

The presence of familial adenomatous polyposis greatly predisposes patients to the development of small-bowel adenomas, and an astounding 80% of this group of patients develop these lesions. Duodenal adenomas, in familial adenomatous polyposis patients, are often numerous (Figure 3.6) and carry a 5% risk of malignant transformation. Untreated, therefore, familial adenomatous polyposis patients have a relatively high risk for developing duodenal adenocarcinoma. To exemplify this fact, familial adenomatous polyposis patients have been shown to have a 100-fold higher risk of developing ampullary adenocarcinoma as compared to the general population. These patients therefore require compulsive endoscopic therapy with subsequent surveillance enteroscopy performed every 3 years. Therapy includes endoscopic mucosal resection,

snare polypectomy, and ablation with thermal modalities. Jejunal and ileal adenomas may be found in 30% of familial adenomatous polyposis patients. Fortunately, the malignant transformation of these lesions is low and screening, treatment, and surveillance, beyond the ligament of Trietz, are not recommended.

Carcinoid tumors

Carcinoid tumors are the second most common malignant tumors in the small intestine with a peak incidence between the sixth and seventh decades. Carcinoid tumors are found primarily in the appendix and the ileum with 40% being within 2 feet of the ileocecal valve. Thirty-five percent of patients have multiple lesions at the time of diagnosis. The risk of metastatic disease is directly related to the size of the primary tumor (Table 3.3). Small-intestinal carcinoids are often asymptomatic but may present as intermittent crampy abdominal pain, partial small-bowel obstruction, gastrointestinal bleeding, segmental ischemia, or intussusception. Only 6% of all intestinal carcinoid tumors and only tumors that are already metastatic to the liver will manifest the carcinoid syndrome characterized by flushing, diarrhea, bronchospasm, and tricuspid valve regurgitation. Endoscopically, carcinoids can appear nodular mimicking Crohn's disease, or polypoid with normal overlying mucosa. Diagnosis is made using histologic findings as well as serum levels of serotonin, 5-hydroxy-indolacetic acid, and serum chromogranin A. Standard imaging studies do not readily identify the locations of the tumors, but somatostatin-receptor nuclotide scintigraphy has shown sensitivities as high as 90%. Surgical excision is the treatment of choice. Lesions less than 1 cm in size can be treated locally while lesions larger than 2 cm must be considered for en-block resections that include locoregional lymph nodes. The 5-year survival for all small-intestinal carcinoids is 65%.

Lymphomas

Lymphomas are the third most common malignant tumors of the small intestine and constitute 15% to 30% of all small-intestinal tumors. Non-Hodgkin's B-cell lymphomas constitute the vast majority of small-intestinal lymphomas. T-cell lymphomas are primarily seen in association with celiac sprue, B-cell mucosal lymphomas (MALT lymphomas) are related to *Helicobacter pylori* infection, and primary small-bowel Hodgkin's lymphomas are extremely rare. Other diseases that have been associated with small-bowel lymphomas include Crohn's disease and Waldenström's macro-globulinemia. Unlike their gastric counterparts, small-intestinal MALT lymphomas are of inter-mediate to high-grade histology and have a 5-year survival as low as 25%. The "western-type" of B-cell MALT lymphoma should be differentiated from its "Mediterranean" variant, designated immunoproliferative small-intestinal disease, an IgA-secreting B-lymphocyte hyperproliferation associated with an alpha-heavy chain paraproteinemia.

The presenting symptoms of small-intestinal lymphoma are vague and include crampy abdominal pain, fatigue, fever, and weight loss. Bleeding, obstruction, and perforation are uncommon. Chronic diarrhea and malabsorption may be presenting symptoms in patients with immuno-proliferative small-intestinal disease. The endoscopic appearance of small-bowel lymphoma runs the entire gamut. Lymphomas may be mucosal or extramucosal, focal or diffuse, nodular, ulcerative, or they may appear as single or multiple mass lesions of varying size and morphology. Staging is performed according to the recently revised European–American lymphoma classification, a modification of the Ann Arbor classification.

Peutz–Jeghers syndrome

Peutz–Jeghers syndrome is an autosomal dominant inherited disorder characterized by mucocutaneous pigmentation in association with hamartomatous polyps. Hamartomatous polyps are disorganized but mature small-intestinal tissues characterized by fibrous smooth muscle bands expanding the muscularis mucosa. The jejunum is the most common small-intestinal site for the polyps,

followed by the ileum, and duodenum. Polyps may also be seen in the stomach and colon. Although Peutz–Jeghers polyps have been thought to have no malignant potential, patients do appear to have an increased risk of small-intestinal adenocarcinoma. It remains unclear as to whether the hamartomas undergo malignant transformation or if there is a coexisting increased risk of developing adenomas *de novo*. Regardless, the relative risk of developing adenocarcinoma of the small intestine is 18 times higher in those with Peutz–Jeghers syndrome as compared to the general population. Peutz–Jeghers syndrome is also associated with an increased risk of other cancers including those of pancreatic, breast, uterine, and ovarian origin.

Patients affected by this syndrome commonly present with symptoms of intussusception, small-intestinal obstruction, and bleeding. Undiagnosed patients are invariably treated with emergency surgery. In the previously diagnosed patient, the need for emergent surgery can probably be reduced by the performance of elective push and/or intra-operative enteroscopy. At this time, push enterscopy should be considered every 2 to 3 years for the surveillance and removal of polyps and elective intraoperative enteroscopy may be considered for those patients with persistent anemia or bleeding. In the near future, capsule enterscopy will certainly have a role toward directing the management of these patients.

Inflammatory diseases

Crohn's disease

Crohn's disease is a systemic disease that can involve any portion of the gastrointestinal tract. Although the disease primarily maintains an ileocolonic distribution, as many as 10% to 30% of patients demonstrate involvement of other small-bowel sites. Other diagnostic modalities including upper endoscopy, colonoscopy, small-intestinal barium radiographs, and CT scans are often adequate to establish the diagnosis and develop a treatment course. Push enteroscopy and capsule enteroscopy (Figure 3.7) may play a role in the estimated 10% to 30% of Crohn's patients with non-classical involvement of the small intestine in early disease, in children, or in patients with non-diagnostic studies. This group includes patients with malabsorption in whom upper endoscopy with duodenal biopsies and small-bowel barium

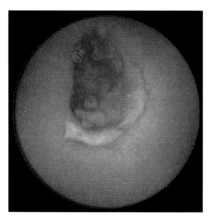

Figure 3.7 Small-bowel Crohn's disease as seen by M2A capsule enteroscopy.

radiographs are normal. Two recent studies revealed that in such patients with unexplained malabsorptive symptoms, enteroscopy may lead to the diagnosis of Crohn's disease in up to 50% of cases. Mucosal biopsies are recommended despite a grossly normal-appearing mucosa. Early Crohn's-related mucosal changes must be differentiated from other etiologies including infection, vasculitis, and non-steroidal anti-inflammatory drug (NSAID) related lesions. Endoscopic therapy has been successfully employed to manage carefully selected strictures in some patients with Crohn's disease. In one series of 55 Crohn's patients with symptomatic strictures, long-term success was achieved in 34 patients with endoscopic treatment.

Non-steroidal anti-inflammatory drug enteropathy

Non-steroidal anti-inflammatory analgesics are highly effective and commonly used agents for the treatment of musculoskeletal disorders. The most common side effects relate to the gastrointestinal tract, with the sequelae of these effects resulting in approximately 20 000 US hospital admissions per year. Gastric and duodenal lesions are the most common and can be easily identified and treated, if necessary, by esophagogastroduodenoscopy. Non-steroidal anti-inflammatory drug-induced pathology in the jejunum and ileum defines NSAID enteropathy. Post-mortem studies have identified such lesions in 8.4% of persons chronically taking NSAIDS. Although potentially symptomatic, NSAID enteropathy remains under-recognized, as securing a definitive diagnosis is difficult. Small-bowel pathology related to NSAIDs has been identified more often in women than in men.

The mechanism of NSAID-induced enteropathy stems from altered or leaky tight junctions that allow bile and bacteria to infiltrate the mucosa, triggering an inflammatory response and eventual ulceration.

Non-steroidal anti-inflammatory drug-induced enteropathy may manifest in several ways, the most common of which is iron-deficiency anemia. In patients on NSAIDS with iron deficiency anemia and positive fecal occult blood testing, Upadhyay found gastric and duodenal lesions in only 35%, suggesting that jejunal and ileal pathology may affect more patients than previously thought. Presentation with overt hemorrhage, perforation, and obstruction are less common.

Push enteroscopy is the preferred evaluation in patients with suspected NSAID enteropathy, because of its therapeutic capabilities. By this method, superficial jejunal erosions, ulcers, and strictures can be identified, biopsied, and treated, precluding the need for further investigation. Diagnosing NSAID enteropathy is important as it affects both clinical management and outcome. In a retrospective analysis, anemic patients identified with NSAID-associated lesions demonstrated a significant improvement in hemoglobin with the administration of misoprostol. In the future, capsule enteroscopy may become the study of choice to evaluate the entire small intestine, determine the need for push enteroscopy, and to formulate a therapeutic plan.

Further reading

Agarwal A: Use of the laparoscope to perform intraoperative enteroscopy. *Surg Endosc* 1999; 13:1143–1144.

Aliperti G, Zuckerman GR, Willis JR, *et al* Endoscopy with enteroclysis. *Gastro Endosc Clin N Am* 1996; 6:803–810.

Askin M, Lewis B: Push enteroscopic cauterization: Long-term follow-up of 83 patients with bleeding small intestinal angiodysplasia. *Gastro Endosc* 1996; 43:580.

Berner J, Mauer K, Lewis B. Push and sonde enteroscopy for the diagnosis of obscure gastrointestinal bleeding. *Am J Gastroenterol* 1994; 89:2139.

Chong J, Tagle M, Bank JS, Reiner DK. Small bowel push-type enteroscopy for patients with occult gastrointestinal bleeding or suspected bowel pathology. *Am J Gastroenterol* 1994; 89:2143.

Chong J, Tagle MK, Barkin J, Reiner D. Small bowel push-type fiberoptic enteroscopy for patients with occult gastrointestinal bleeding or suspected small bowel pathology. *Am J Gastroenterol* 1994; 89:2143.

Chung RS: Laparoscopy assisted jejunal resection for bleeding leiomyoma. *Surg Endosc* 1998; 12:162.

Classen M, Fruhmergen P, Koch H. Peroral enteroscopy of the small and large intestine. *Endoscopy* 1972; 4:157.

Foutch PG, Sawyer R, Sanowski R. Push-enteroscopy for diagnosis of patients with gastrointestinal bleeding of obscure origin. *Gastro Endosc* 1990; 36:337.

Lewis BS, Waye JD. Total small bowel enteroscopy. *Gastro Endosc* 1987 33:435–438.

Ogoshi K, Hara Y, Ashizawa S. New technique for small intestinal fiberoscopy. *Gastro Endosc* 1973; 20:64.

Parker H, Agayoff J. Enteroscopy and small bowel biopsy utilizing a peroral colonoscope. *Gastro Endosc* 1983; 29:139.

Seensalu R: The Sonde Examination. *Gast End Clin N Am* 1999; 9:37–59.

Tada M, Akasaka F, Misaki F, *et al*. Pediatric Enteroscopy with a Sonde-Type Small Intestine Fiberscope. *Endoscopy* 1977; 8:33–38.

Wilmer A, Rutgeerts P: Push enteroscopy. Technique, depth, and yield of insertion. *Gastro Endosc Clin N Am* 1996; 6:759–776.

Chapter 4

Endoscopic Ultrasound

Poonputt Chotiprasidhi and James M. Scheiman

Introduction

Intraluminal endoscopic ultrasound (EUS), also termed endosonography, is a relatively new technology in the US. It can be considered as an adjunctive endoscopic imaging study for patients with previously identified lesions of the gastrointestinal tract and surrounding organs, including the pancreas and biliary tree. Endoscopic ultrasound combines two modalities, endoscopic visualization and high-frequency ultrasound. This permits precise delineation not only of the individual layers of the gastrointestinal tract (Figure 4.1), but high-resolution images of adjacent structures such as the pancreas (Figure 4.2) and mediastinum. This represents a great advantage over other imaging modalities. The technique allows loco-regional staging of gastrointestinal malignancies, determination of the origin of submucosal lesions, and differentiation of other gut-wall abnormalities. The addition of EUS-guided fine-needle aspiration (FNA) has expanded the diagnostic potential for extraluminal lesions,

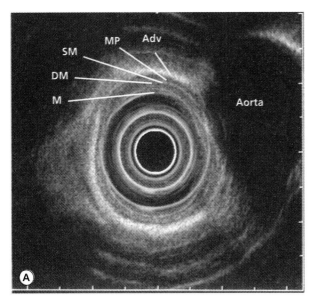
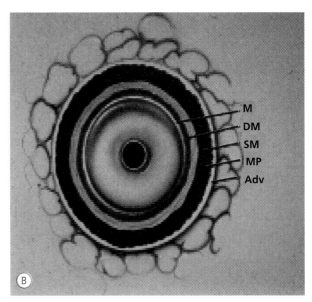

Figure 4.1 (A) Endoscopic ultrasound appearance (Olympus radial image) of the normal esophagus and (B) corresponding drawing of the histology correlation. The wall can be resolved into a five-layer structure. M mucosa; DM deep mucosa; SM submucosa; MP muscularis propria; Adv adventitia (modified from the *ASGE Slide Atlas of Endosonography*).

the pancreas, and lymph nodes, especially in the chest and upper abdomen.

Endoscopic ultrasound makes possible the acquisition of information that was not previously available even with the most sophisticated transabdominal studies such as CT and magnetic resonance imaging (MRI). This unique modality has spawned extensive research and a wide variety of clinical applications have been established. Endoscopic ultrasound, by expanding diagnostic and therapeutic capabilities, provides enhanced patient care, decision making, and treatment.

Endoscopic ultrasound is a technically challenging endoscopic procedure to learn, as ultrasound images are more difficult to interpret than routine endocopic images. Therefore mastering EUS requires extensive training, and the quality of EUS imaging is highly dependent on the skill of the operator. Despite the development of animal and computer models for teaching novice endosonographers, there is no substitute for direct mentored training in an EUS center of excellence.

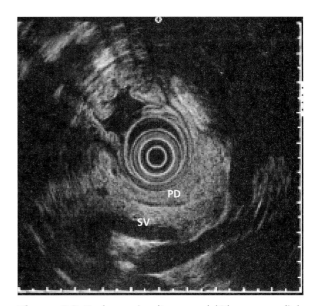

Figure 4.2 Endoscopic ultrasound (Olympus radial image) of the pancreas body imaged from the stomach. Note the high resolution with which the gland is seen, including the 2 mm pancreatic duct (PD).

Instruments

The fiberoptic and videoechoendoscopic devices that are commercially available at present are manufactured by the Olympus Corporation and the Pentax Corporation. The two basic systems are radial array imaging and curved linear array. The Olympus radial scanning system consists of dedicated endoscopes that utilize a mechanical transducer that rotates 360 degrees in a plane perpendicular to the long axis of the endoscope. An ultrasound processor for image capture then reconstructs the ultrasound image. The recently developed and marketed Pentax electronic radial echoendoscope is a forward-viewing endoscope. The instrument uses a curved array scanning transducer with variable frequency (5.0, 7.5, and 10.0 MHz) and has color doppler/B mode capability. Imaging with this intrument provides images similar to the mechanical radial instrument.

The initial curved linear array instruments were developed by Pentax, they utilize an electronic transducer coupled to a 160 cm forward oblique viewing videoendoscope that produces a 100 degree sector scan parallel to the long axis of the endoscope. All Pentax echoendoscopes are utilized in conjunction with a Phillips or Hitachi ultrasound processor. These scanning systems also can perform pulse and color Doppler studies, which enhance the identification of structures such as adjacent blood vessels. This instrument allows the performance of ultrasound-guided FNA, using Doppler to avoid inadvertent vascular injury. Olympus also manufactures curved linear array ultrasound instruments with color doppler imaging capability allowing real-time FNA. Previous models from both companies were fiberoptic endoscope based, they remain in use but have an inferior endoscopic image. Olympus manufactures an ultrasound colonoscope, but most centers use the upper gastrointestinal instrument for rectal cancer imaging. Blind ultrasound probes are also available for the staging of rectal tumors from these and other manufacturers.

Olympus, Fujinon, and other manufacturers have developed ultrasound probe systems that can be placed in the endoscope channel without the need for a dedicated instrument. They provide higher ultrasound frequencies, providing detailed structural analysis of gut-wall lesions, but have a limited depth of penetration. They can be useful for evaluating intraductal (biliary or pancreas) or superficial gut-wall lesions.

Indications for endoscopic ultrasound

The currently accepted indications for EUS are listed in Box 4.1. The absolute contraindications for upper and lower EUS are few, and include

1. lack of patient cooperation
2. known or suspected perforated viscus
3. acute diverticulitis
4. fulminant colitis.

Box 4.1 Current indications for endoscopic ultrasound

Esophagus
  cancer staging
  characterization of submucosal tumors
  biopsy of mediastinal lymph nodes (gastrointestinal tumors)
Stomach
  cancer staging
  characterization of submucosal tumors
  biopsy of paragastric/retroperitoneal lymph nodes (gastrointestinal tumors)
  lymphoma staging
  evaluation of large gastric folds
  post treatment cancer surveillance
Pancreato–biliary
  cancer staging
  suspected chronic pancreatitis
  differential diagnosis of cystic lesions
  localization of neuroendocrine tumors
  suspected choledocholithiasis
  biopsy of retroperitoneal lymph nodes
  pancreatic biopsy for suspected malignancy
Colorectum
  cancer staging
  characterization of submucosal tumors
  lymph node biopsy
  evaluation of pelvic and perianal disease
Non-gastrointestinal disease
  lung cancer staging
  lymphadenopathy of unknown cause
  evaluation of mediastinal masses
Therapeutic endoscopic ultrasound
  celiac plexus neurolysis

Relative contraindications include

1. the lack of availability of an experienced endosonographer
2. high-grade esophageal stricture where risk of dilation is felt to be too great to justify the procedure
3. unstable cardiac or pulmonary disease.

Impact of endoscopic ultrasound on patients with specific diseases

Esophageal carcinoma

Endoscopic ultrasound continues to be the most accurate non-surgical modality for the local staging

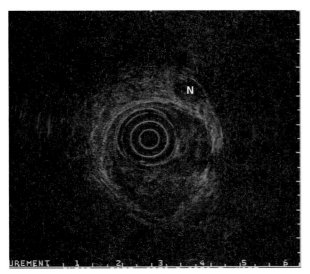

Figure 4.3 Endoscopic ultrasound image of a T3 (penetrating musularis propria) N1 (adjacent node: N) esophageal adenocarcinoma.

of esophageal cancer (Figure 4.3). The EUS accuracy for assessing both the depth of wall invasion by the tumor (T stage) and lymph node involvement (N stage) has consistently been reported to be greater than 80%, significantly superior to staging with CT or MRI. This information greatly impacts surgical decision making, avoiding unnecessary resections in cases of adjacent structure invasion (such as the aorta) and assists in the selection of patients for preoperative radiation therapy. High-grade stenosis may preclude a complete EUS examination with a dedicated echoendoscope in approximately 25% of patients. Dilation of a stricture prior to EUS has been reported to result in a high complication rate in some (20%) studies, but no complications in other studies.

Studies have demonstrated a close correlation between EUS staging and survival rates, thus underscoring the importance of correct preoperative staging when contemplating surgical resection. Traditionally, invasion of an adjacent structure (T4 disease) has generally been considered as not amenable to surgical resection. Although multimodal therapy with chemoradiotherapy has not yet been shown to be clearly superior to conventional surgical resection, many institutions have adopted this promising approach.

The ability of EUS to restage esophageal cancer following neoadjuvant chemoradiotherapy has been investigated. While the accuracy of T staging following such therapy is less accurate than pretherapy, studies have confirmed the ability of EUS to predict survival in this setting.

Malignant involvement of celiac axis lymph nodes is considered as a distant metastasis in patients with esophageal carcinoma. The sensitivity of EUS for the detection of malignant celiac adenopathy is 83% with 98% specificity. Endoscopic ultrasound-guided FNA to confirm the presence of malignant cells may be performed.

Mediastinal masses and lymph nodes

Mediastinal lymph nodes can be detected by EUS in a variety of clinical conditions apart from esophageal and lung cancer. The distinction between benign and malignant lymph nodes is crucial, but not always reliable using imaging criteria and morphological appearance alone. Cytological and/or histological confirmation is often needed.

The sensitivity of EUS and FNA in non-gastrointestinal mediastinal adenopathy is 90% with 100% specificity and 95% accuracy. Endoscopic ultrasound with FNA can diagnose primary and metastatic lesions, in patients both with and without previously diagnosed tumor.

Endoscopic ultrasound and FNA may therefore impact the management in a high proportion of patients with a variety of mediastinal lesions (lymphoma, leiomyosarcoma, paraganglioneuroma, leiomyoma, metastatic cancer, and abscess).

Non-small cell neoplasms of the lung

The staging of non-small cell lung cancer has emerged as a valuable application for EUS and FNA. It is feasible, safe, and accurate when compared to other modalities such as mediastinoscopy and mediastinotomy. It is also cost effective compared to traditional staging with cross-sectional imaging studies and bronchoscopy. Endoscopic ultrasound thus offers a favorable alternative to more invasive approaches. The staging of non-small cell lung cancer using EUS and FNA is superior to EUS without FNA and to CT scan. The results of EUS and FNA have been shown to result in a change of management in 80% of patients.

Gastric adenocarcinoma

For the staging of gastric epithelial cancers, the sensitivity and specificity of EUS for T and N stage are superior to CT scanning (80%–90% and

77%–90% for T and N staging respectively). The accuracy of EUS in staging gastric carcinoma may not approach that of esophageal carcinoma because of the inherent inability of EUS to differentiate between the subserosal and serosal layers, which is problematic in distinguishing T2 (invasion of the muscularis propria) and T3 (invasion of the serosal layer) lesions. Understaging because of microscopic deposits and overstaging because of tumor-associated fibrosis or inflammation can occur. Because many patients undergo palliative resection, in addition to the lack of clear value of adjuvant therapy, EUS has limited impact in clinical decision making for advanced gastric cancers, but it does provide important prognostic information.

Gastric mucosa-associated lymphoid tissue lymphoma

Endoscopic ultrasound is quite useful and superior to other imaging techniques in the detection of destruction of the gastric wall due to lymphoma, linitis plastica, and other infiltrative disorders. However, histopathologic confirmation by various endoscopic biopsy techniques is still required.

Endoscopic ultrasound is also useful both in assessing surgical resectability and monitoring treatment response among patients with gastric lymphoma.

The absence of deep mucosal invasion on pretreatment EUS imaging is the most critical predictor for the success of antibiotic therapy for gastric mucosa-associated lymphoid tissue lymphoma (MALT lymphoma). Other predictors of poor response to *Helicobacter pylori* eradication therapy alone include the presence of high-grade histology and the presence of perigastric lymphadenopathy seen by EUS.

Submucosal tumors of the gastrointestinal tract

Endoscopic ultrasound can resolve the gut wall into a five-layer pattern which corresponds to the histological layers of the gut wall (Figure 4.4). The innermost layer corresponds to the superficial mucosa, the second hypoechoic layer corresponds to the deep mucosa and the muscularis mucosa, the third hyperechoic layer corresponds to the submucosa, the fourth hypoechoic layer is the

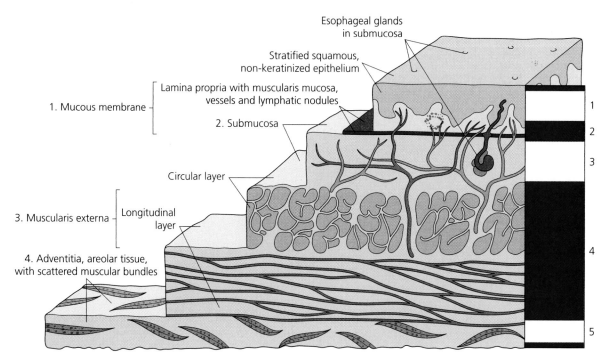

Figure 4.4 Correlation of echolayers, seen by endoscopic ultrasound, and the histology of the gut wall (modified from the *ASGE Slide Atlas of Endosonography*).

muscularis propria, and the fifth hyperechoic layer (which may not be discernible depending on what tissue is adjacent) is the subserosa and serosa.

For benign lesions of the gastrointestinal tract, EUS is particularly good at evaluating subepithelial masses by determining both the layer of origin and the echotexture of the lesion. Examples include esophageal and gastric leiomyomas and lipomas. Endoscopic ultrasound can determine if these endoscopic appearances are due to extrinsic compression, for example splenomegaly bulging into the stomach, or are actually vascular structures, for example gastric varices. Standard endoscopic biopsy specimens of subepithelial lesions are usually inadequate to identify the lesion, as they only sample the overlying normal mucosa. Many benign subepithelial masses have characteristic ultrasonic appearances. An important caveat to remember, however, is that differentiation between benign and malignant processes may require surgical resection, particularly with mesenchymal lesions such as leiomyomas, as 100% certainty cannot be achieved in many cases by forceps biopsy or FNA with cytological confirmation.

Endoscopic ultrasound as an adjunct to endoscopic mucosal resection

In many endoscopic centers endoscopic mucosal resection has become a standard approach for removal of superficial neoplastic lesions of the gut. Endoscopic mucosal resection provides a non-surgical treatment option for local resection of these tumors, including early cancers. With the assistance of high-frequency catheter probe endoscopic ultrasonography, it is now possible to obtain an accurate assessment of the depth of the lesion, and in some cases resect submucosal tumors if the propria layer is uninvolved. Although popular in the Orient, where there is a high incidence of superficial neoplasia, limited data are available on the use of endoscopic mucosal resection in the US.

Rectal carcinoma

Endoscopic ultrasound has become clinically established as the most accurate pretreatment local staging modality for rectal cancer (Figure 4.5). Accurate staging is required to determine which tumors are resectable and which require pre- or

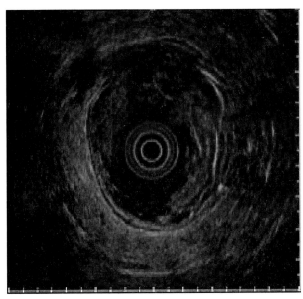

Figure 4.5 Endoscopic ultrasound image of a T3 rectal adenocarcinoma involving muscularis propria.

Table 4.1 Endoscopic ultrasound and rectal cancer management	
$T_1 N_0$	tumor in submucosa or mucosa local excision (endoscopic or transanal) 10% of rectal carcinoma
$T_2 N_0$	surgical resection 10%–20% risk of nodal involvement
$T_2 N_1$ or $T_3 N_0$	surgical resection ± pre-op radiation therapy or chemoradiotherapy
$T_3 N_1$	pre-op radiation therapy or chemoradiotherapy followed by surgical resection
$T_4 N_0$ or $T_4 N_1$	pre-op radiation therapy or chemoradiotherapy followed by surgical resection

postoperative adjuvant chemoradiotherapy. Table 4.1 lists the role of EUS in guiding stage-related patient management strategies. The sensitivity in staging is reported to be in the range of 70% to 90% for T staging with more than 90% specificity, while in N staging it approaches 70% for both sensitivity and specificity. A key limitation is the inability to stage and traverse stenotic tumors and the differentiation of inflammatory from neoplastic adenopathy. Miniprobe ultrasound may be a viable option for preoperative staging of stenotic tumors with accuracy rates equivalent to those of standard echoendoscopes.

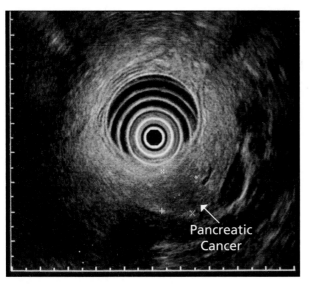

Figure 4.6 Adenocarcinoma of the pancreas.

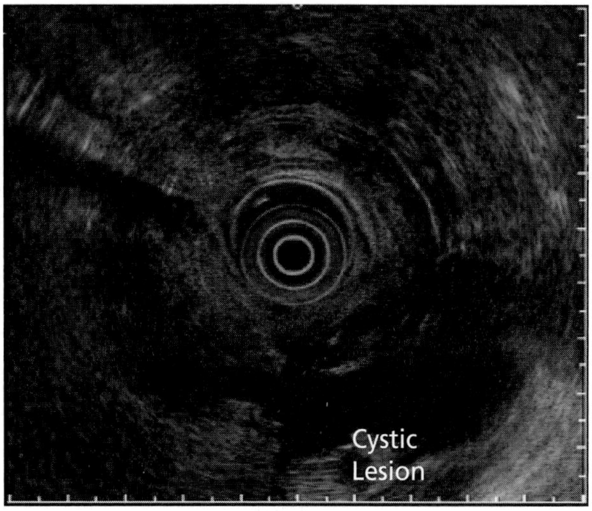

Figure 4.7 Endoscopic ultrasound image of a mucinous cystic pancreatic neoplasm.

Accurate preoperative T staging for colon cancer is less important than for rectal carcinoma because surgical resection is usually indicated regardless of the stage of disease in order to prevent subsequent colonic obstruction. Endoscopic ultrasound may be helpful for prognosis but does not direct the therapeutic approach for colon cancer unlike the situation for patients with rectal cancer.

Pancreatic cancer

Adenocarcinoma of the pancreas is the fourth leading cause of cancer death in the US. On presentation the disease is usually advanced and only 15% of patients have localized tumors amenable to curative resection. The prognosis for the 85% of patients with unresectable disease remains dismal with a median survival of 6 months. The primary therapeutic goal for these patients is palliation. Surgical morbidity and mortality, whether for palliation or curative resection, has been markedly reduced in the last decade. The goal of any imaging modality is to provide greater accuracy in the staging of these cancers in a manner that is both cost effective and as non-invasive as possible. It is hoped that this will lead to a greater degree of curative resections and fewer unecessary laparotomies.

The emergence of endoscopic palliation of biliary obstruction has underscored the importance of preoperative staging and selection of patients for surgery. Candidates for curative surgery should have no evidence of distant metastatic disease and

be free of tumor invasion into the major peripancreatic vascular structures. Computed tomography and, more recently, laparoscopy have become indispensable for detecting intra-abdominal (occult hepatic and peritoneal) metastatic disease. Computed tomography is a reliable method of documenting both distant disease and locally invasive disease as is the case in more than 80% of cases of pancreatic cancer. Because of this and the fact that CT is non-invasive, it has remained the preferred *initial* imaging procedure.

The EUS appearance of most pancreatic tumors (Figure 4.6) is a distinct, typically hypoechoic lesion distinguishable from the hyperechoic homogeneous echo pattern of the normal gland. The presence of hyperechoic areas, including those with shadowing consistent with calcification, seen with lesions associated with chronic pancreatitis may be indistinguishable. This points out the importance of tissue sampling when cancer is suspected. Large lesions may not be completely visualized because of the limited depth of penetration with EUS. Pancreatic cancers typically lead to post-obstructive dilation of the pancreatic and biliary ductal systems. Masses due to other tumors secondarily involving the pancreas, such as lymphoma, do not have characteristic features that reliably distinguish them from primary pancreatic neoplasms, again emphasizing the value of cytological evaluation. Cystic tumors of the pancreas may have a variety of appearances, including a focal collection of multiple small cysts surrounded by a mass, or a single large cyst (Figure 4.7) with an irregularly thickened wall surrounded by a pericystic inhomogenous mass.

Endosonography appears most useful in cases where CT fails to demonstrate a lesion. In the case of tumors measuring 3 cm or less, EUS has been reported to be 100% accurate in tumor detection, far superior to CT (55%) and even endoscopic retrograde cholangiopancreatography (ERCP) (90%). Endoscopic ultrasound is useful in the visualization of the pancreas in the case of a failed ERCP, or in the evaluation of ductal strictures seen at ERCP with a brush cytology sample negative for malignancy. If a mass is found in association with a stricture, EUS can sample the lesion and provide resectability information with a single examination.

Peripancreatic lymph node metastases can be identified by EUS using either the criteria of size (> 5 mm) and/or echo features. Malignant lymph nodes are reported to be hypoechoic, rounded, and well demarcated. The accuracy of EUS in identifying malignant adenopathy is 75% to 80% and is far superior to all other imaging modalities. Aspiration of the node may be performed to confirm malignant nature. This, however, is not always necessary in the case of pancreatic tumors, where vascular invasion and potential resectability is paramount.

The most important criterion for assessment of resectability by all imaging procedures is tumor involvement with the major peripancreatic vessels: the portal venous system (portal vein, confluence with the superior mesenteric vein, and the splenic vein) and the celiac axis with common hepatic and splenic arteries. Traditionally, the detection of tumor invasion of the portal and mesenteric vasculature has relied on mesenteric angiography or CT. However, EUS has emerged as an innovative pancreatic imaging modality with an accuracy greater than 90% in the local staging of pancreatic cancer, and it is superior to angiography and CT for defining vascular invasion. Three reliable criteria for vascular invasion by tumor seen on EUS have been described. These include

1. tumor within the vessel lumen
2. abnormal vessel contour with loss of the vessel–parenchymal hyperechoic interface
3. venous collaterals in the area of a mass that obliterated the normal anatomic location of a major portal confluence vessel.

Endoscopic ultrasound has been reported to be as accurate as 90% in tumor (T) and node (N) staging of pancreatic cancer. In a series of 60 patients with pancreatic and ampullary carcinoma, EUS was 95% accurate in determining portal vascular involvement, whereas angiography and CT were 85% and 75% accurate respectively. Not all studies have confirmed these results and the differentiation of vascular invasion from adherence remains problematic.

Whether the employment of innovative techniques such as helical CT scanning can challenge the results of EUS remains to be definitively determined. At the University of Michigan, we have prospectively compared the ability of helical CT scanning to EUS for the staging of ampullo-pancreatic tumors. In a series of 42 patients, all with the imaging results confirmed at the time of surgery, we found helical CT highly specific but with low sensitivity for detecting vascular invasion by small peripancreatic tumors. Endoscopic ultrasound was more sensitive than helical CT in detecting vascular invasion and was also more accurate in overall T staging. The high specificity of helical CT suggests that further staging procedures with CT evidence of vascular invasion are unnecessary. We recommend that EUS should be employed in patients without CT evidence of an unresectable peripancreatic tumor.

The utilization of endosonography for directed pancreatic tissue sampling using curved linear array ultrasound endoscopes is a safe and effective approach to defining the nature of pancreatic lesions and confirming the diagnosis to facilitate preoperative treatment planning. A 23 gauge 10 cm needle (GIP/Medi-Globe Villmann type EUS needle, Medi-Globe Corp., Tempe, AZ) is employed through the biopsy channel of the Pentax instrument. The Olympus curved linear array scope uses a needle developed by the manufacturer, and Wilson-Cook manufactures a needle that can be used in either instrument. The presence of a cytopathologist to examine the aspirate during the procedure has been shown to improve accuracy. The accuracy of EUS-guided real-time FNA biopsy has been reported to be in the range of 75% to 95%. The complication rate associated with the procedure is less than 1%.

Pancreatic neuroendocrine tumors

Functioning pancreatic neuroendocrine tumors are diagnosed by clinical symptoms related to pathological hormone secretion. Non-functional tumors usually present with advanced disease and may be confused with adenocarcinonas. The functioning tumors vary in their malignant potential. Based upon long-term follow-up, 5% to 10% of insulinomas and 50% to 90% of the other tumors are reported to be malignant. Gastrinomas are diagnosed by elevation in plasma gastrin levels and a positive secretin stimulation test. A serum calcium should be measured to exclude multiple endocrine neoplasia type 1 syndrome. Sixty per cent of gastrinomas are malignant, and metastatic disease is present in 50% of patients. Gastrinomas are typically (80%–90%) located in the "gastrinoma triangle", the area bounded by the confluence of the cystic and common bile ducts, the junction of the head and body of the pancreas, and the distal end of the second portion of the duodenum. Surgical cure is possible in up to 60% of patients, and preoperative localization is therefore *essential*.

Insulinomas are diagnosed by elevation of plasma insulin and C-peptide levels in the face of recurrent hypoglycemia. Ten per cent of insulinomas are part of the multiple endocrine neoplasia type 1 syndrome. Ninety per cent of insulinomas are under 2 cm in size, 86% are single and benign, and up to 40% are less than 1 cm in size, making preoperative localization challenging. Nearly all insulinomas occur within, or are attached to, the pancreas.

Imaging studies are important to localize the primary tumor and exclude metastatic disease precluding surgical cure. Localization of the tumor with traditional imaging studies such as US, CT, MRI, and angiography fail in 40% to 60% of cases. Magnetic resonance imaging may prove more sensitive than CT for localization of liver metastases.

Endoscopic ultrasound, because of its ability to provide high-resolution images of the pancreas and surrounding structures, has proven ideal for the localization of these small tumors. The EUS appearance of these tumors is typically a hypoechoic to isoechoic homogenous well-demarcated mass within the gland (Figure 4.8). Cystic lesions may also be seen. Precise localization within the gland may be achieved by examining relationships with the large vessels and duct.

At our center, EUS rapidly replaced selective venous sampling as the initial imaging modality for pancreatic neuroendocrine tumors. This approach has proven highly cost effective. At our most recent review, 44 individuals underwent surgical exploration, EUS had an overall sensitivity of 83% and accuracy of 89% in pancreatic neuroendocrine tumor localization. Endoscopic ultrasound was more sensitive for pancreatic gastrinoma versus insulinoma. In our experience, a negative pancreatic EUS in the gastrinoma patient guided surgical exploration and was predictive of extrapancreatic tumor location.

Acute and chronic pancreatitis

The role of EUS in acute pancreatitis is to determine whether the patient has concomitant choledocholithiasis without the risk of ERCP-related pancreatitis. The sensitivity and specificity of EUS in this setting exceed those of magnetic resonance cholangiopancreatography (MRCP). In the evaluation of the inflamed pancreatic parenchynma, EUS is unable to differentiate inflammation from neoplasia.

Pancreatic histology remains the gold standard for the diagnosis of chronic pancreatitis. The absence of tissue examination in most comparative studies makes it difficult to compare various diagnostic modalities, and confirmation of the diagnosis can be elusive. Subtle morphologic changes in early disease can make the diagnosis of chronic pancreatitis problematic. Alternatively, advanced chronic pancreatitis, particularly when focal in nature, may be impossible to differentiate from adenocarcinoma.

The EUS features of chronic pancreatitis vary with the severity of the disease. Parenchymal changes such as heterogeneity of the gland with a speckled or mottled pattern may be seen. Calcifications within the gland may be seen as echogenic foci with secondary shadowing. Other EUS features in chronic pancreatitis include dilation or irregularity of the main pancreatic duct or its side branches, calculi, and hypodense cystic areas. Cysts with debris or irregular walls raise

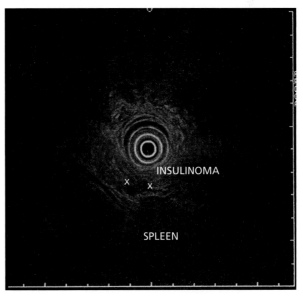

Figure 4.8 Typical endoscopic ultrasound appearance of an insulinoma in the tail of the pancreas.

concern for cystic tumors and should undergo aspiration for cytology and tumor marker levels. Early chronic pancreatitis may only have parenchymal changes without any ductal changes, and hence, ERCP may be normal.

In patients with chronic pancreatitis, EUS is most helpful in defining the presence of disease in the face of a normal ERCP, delineating strictures identified by ERCP, or when ERCP fails. Prospective comparisons of EUS with ERCP in patients with suspected chronic pancreatitis have concluded that EUS can be positive in cases with normal ERCP, EUS can readily identify stones as the cause of ductal obstruction, but differentiating focal pancreatitis from malignancy remains a challenge. While EUS-guided FNA is helpful, the negative predictive value remains a source of concern, and surgical exploration may be required in equivocal cases.

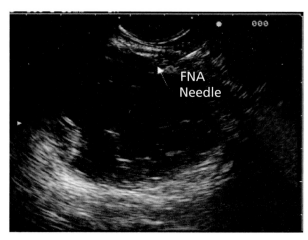

Figure 4.9 Fine-needle aspiration (FNA) of a pancreatic cystic neoplam (same lesion as Figure 4.7). Note the different orientation of the curved linear array instrument (Pentax).

Pancreatic pseudocysts and cystic neoplasms of the pancreas

Endoscopic ultrasound is commonly employed prior to, and to perform, endoscopic drainage of pseudocysts. Prior to performance of endoscopic cystogastrostomy or duodenostomy, EUS is employed to evaluate the distance between the cyst and gut wall, and to verify the absence of intervening large vessels. The use of EUS in this situation has proven useful in changing the endoscopic management approach.

Cystic neoplasms of the pancreas represent a rare but diverse collection of tumors with varied malignant potential and clinical presentation. With the increasing early use of abdominal CT in patients with abdominal symptoms, these lesions seem to be detected with increasing frequency. Differentiating these lesions from the much more common ductal adenocarcinoma or benign pancreatic pseudocysts can be challenging and it is estimated that CT provides correct characterization of cystic pancreatic lesions in only 60% of cases. In one large series, incorrect diagnosis of cystic neoplasms delayed appropriate surgical treatment or led to an inappropriate intervention in up to 37% of cases. Furthermore, these tumors vary greatly from one another and from the more typical adenocarcinoma of the pancreas in their pathologic behavior, clinical course, and prognosis making a precise diagnosis critical in directing treatment.

The approach to the patient with a pancreatic cystic lesion begins with a detailed history. A history to suggest prior pancreatitis or trauma is important. A careful review for symptoms of a hormone excess state should be sought, such as difficult to manage peptic ulcer, diarrhea, hypoglycemia, rash, or flushing. In the absence of a history of pancreatitis, pseudocyst is quite unlikely and the concern of a cystic neoplasm is paramount. In general, all symptomatic lesions should proceed to appropriate surgical resection. If preoperative characterization of the lesion is desired, EUS ± FNA for cytology and fluid analysis can provide information of diagnostic and prognostic value. For those patients with lesions that appear benign, such as classic appearance of a serous cystadenoma, a decision regarding the patient's willingness to observe the lesion should be developed in collaboration with a pancreatic surgeon. Though controversial, EUS ± FNA (Figure 4.9) with cytology and fluid studies (cytology, CEA levels) can provide evidence to support the approach of watchful waiting and carefully monitor the patient with serial examinations to exclude change in size. Endosonographers will continue to play an important role in the differential diagnosis and management of these lesions that seem to be detected increasingly often in clinical practice.

Gallstones and related diseases

Transabdominal ultrasound is highly sensitive and specific for detecting cholelithiasis, since the calcium present within the gallstones is a strong reflector of ultrasound waves. In contrast, for choledocholithiasis or common bile duct stones, transabdominal ultrasound is not sensitive but may be specific.

Endoscopic ultrasound can be an alternative to ERCP in the preoperative evaluation of patients with gallstone disease prior to laparoscopic cholecystectomy. The sensitivity of EUS is as good or better than ERCP (in prospective studies more than 95% sensitivity), and can be used when the likelihood of common bile duct stones is not high, avoiding the risk of pancreatitis. Endoscopic ultrasound is superior to conventional ultrasound and has also been shown to be a cost-effective initial screening study, in place of ERCP for patients with a low or intermediate risk of bile duct stones, although EUS does not have the therapeutic capacity.

Magnetic resonance cholangiopancreatography is a promising non-invasive alternative to EUS for imaging the bile duct, although it may not be as accurate. In our study of a patient population with a low disease prevalence, EUS was superior to MRCP for choledocholithiasis. Endoscopic ultrasound was most useful for confirming a normal biliary tree, and we belive it can be considered to be a low-risk alternative to ERCP. Although MRCP had the lowest procedural reimbursement, the initial EUS strategy in our study had the greatest cost effectiveness by avoiding unnecessary ERCP examinations.

Portal hypertension

In patients with cirrhosis and portal hypertension, EUS can demonstrate a dilated azygos vein and a dilated thoracic duct. Large peri-esophageal veins may predict the development or recurrence of esophageal varices. However, the clinical applications of these EUS findings are unclear.

Endoscopic ultrasound is more sensitive than diagnostic endoscopy in the diagnosis of gastric varices, and it may be a consideration for patients with portal hypertension who have upper gastrointestinal bleeding in the absence of esophageal varices.

Intraductal ultrasound of the biliary tree and pancreas

While CT, MRI, and transabdominal ultrasound can detect biliary dialtation, they are less specific for the location and cause of the obstruction. Endoscopic retrograde cholangiopancreatography with or without cytology and/or biopsy is usually required to establish the diagnosis. Unfortunately, the diagnosis remains unclear in approximately one third of patients.

Intraductal ultrasound is a new development in EUS technology. It can usually be performed easily and safely at the time of ERCP. It provides high-resolution detailed images of ductal and periductal tisssues. The information obtained may assist in the selection of appropriate candidates for surgery. Intraductal ultrasound is more sensitive than ERCP for the diagnosis of choledocholithiasis, and may help differentiate benign from malignant strictures. The role of intraductal ultrasound in pancreatic duct stricture, intraductal papillary mucinous tumors, pancreatic carcinoma, neuroendocrine tumors, and SOD is still under investigation.

Fine-needle aspiration and endoscopic ultrasound-guided therapy

In addition to its role as a standard diagnostic approach to pancreatic cancer and metastatic adenopathy, EUS–FNA techniques can also be used to deliver medications. Celiac plexus block is typically performed by an anesthesiologist using fluoroscopic landmarks for injecting the neural plexus to control severe pain arising from the upper abdomen. Endoscopic ultrasound can easily demonstrate celiac axis in the majority of patients, and EUS-directed celiac neurolysis can be an effective method to decrease pain among patients with advanced pancreatic carcinoma. The long-term efficacy of this technique is yet to be proven in patients with chronic pancreatitis.

The future for EUS–FNA is bright, with active investigation on the horizon evaluating directed therapy into pancreas with immune agents, chemotherapy, and possibly radiofrequency ablation to treat either patients with small pancreatic tumors or those patients who are non-operative candidates.

Conclusions

Local staging of gastrointestinal malignancies (esophageal, stomach, pancreatic, colorectal) is the best established indication for EUS. Endoscopic ultrasound provides the most accurate information regarding the depth of tumor penetration (T stage). Assessment of lymph node involvement (N stage) can also be assessed. It is accurate and cost effective in determining the resectability of pancreatic adenocarcinoma. Endoscopic ultrasound allows differentiation of submucosal masses, thickened folds, and extrinsic compression. However, when the ultrasonic features do not clearly distinguish between a malignant and benign entity (e.g. chronic pancreatitis versus cancer), a definite diagnosis can be obtained only by EUS–FNA. Endoscopic ultrasound is the best preoperative test to localize pancreatic endocrine tumors. Endoscopic ultrasound as the sole preoperative examination is highly cost effective and accurate.

In summary, EUS has established itself as an important diagnostic modality, mainly for the detection and staging of gastrointestinal tumors. However, it is not simply a diagnostic modality, it is now becoming a therapeutic modality for many gastrointestinal conditions.

Further reading

Anderson, MA, Carpenter S, *et al*. Endoscopic ultrasound is highly accurate and directs management in patients with neuroendocrine tumors of the pancreas. *Am J Gastroenterol* 2000; 95(9):2271–2277.

Brugge, WR. The role of EUS in the diagnosis of cystic lesions of the pancreas. *Gastrointest Endosc* 2000; 52(6 suppl.):S18–S22.

Byrne MF, Jowell PS. Gastrointestinal imaging: endoscopic ultrasound. *Gastroenterology* 2002: 122:1631–1648.

Scheiman JM, Carlos RC, *et al*. Can endoscopic ultrasound or magnetic resonance cholangiopancreatography replace ERCP in patients with suspected biliary disease? A prospective trial and cost analysis. *Am J Gastroenterol* 2001; 96(10):2900–4.

Tierney WM, Francis IR, *et al*. The accuracy of EUS and helical CT in the assessment of vascular invasion by peripapillary malignancy. *Gastrointest Endosc* 2001; 53(2):182–188.

Wallace, MB, Hawes RH. Emerging indications for EUS. *Gastrointest Endosc* 2001; 52(6 suppl.):S55–S60.

Endoscopic Retrograde Cholangiopancreatography

Ilias A. Scotiniotis and Gregory G. Ginsberg

Introduction

Endoscopic retrograde cholangiopancreatography (ERCP) remains the "gold standard" for imaging the pancreaticobiliary tree. An array of tissue sampling techniques and the application of endoscopic therapies offer advantages over purely diagnostic imaging studies. This chapter will review the role of ERCP in the evaluation and management of pancreaticobiliary diseases, emphasizing therapeutic applications.

Technique of endoscopic retrograde cholangiopancreatography

Endoscopic retrograde cholangiopancreatography is a technically demanding procedure. In experienced hands, it is a safe and well-tolerated procedure that can usually be performed on an out-patient basis. The procedure is performed with the patient in a modified prone position to enhance visualization of the pancreaticobiliary systems, and imaging is obtained with a fluoroscopic unit. Conscious sedation is administered, typically with intravenous midazolam and meperidine or fentanyl. Propofol administration by an anesthesiologist is used increasingly for patients who are difficult to sedate. Duodenoscopes used for ERCP are specially designed with side-viewing orientation to offer an "en face" view of the major papilla. The outer diameter of a duodenoscope is 10.5 to 12.5 millimeters. It should be noted that the side-viewing orientation of the endoscopes used for

ERCP allow only a cursory examination of the esophagus, stomach, and duodenal bulb. A duodenoscopic examination is therefore not a substitute for examination with a forward-viewing upper endoscope.

Once the endoscope is positioned in the second portion of the duodenum, the major papilla is inspected for gross abnormalities (Figure 5.1). A cannulation catheter is then passed through the working channel of the endoscope. By maneuvering the tip of the endoscope and angling the tip of the catheter with an "elevator" lever, selective cannulation of the bile duct or pancreatic duct is performed. Radiopaque dye is then injected under fluoroscopic inspection. Selective cannulation requires considerable endoscopic skill and experience. Successful cannulation should be achieved in more than 90% of cases. A variety of catheter designs and guidewires are available to assist in cannulation. Reaching the papilla can be a challenge if the patient has had a prior gastrectomy with Billroth II anastomosis, since the endoscope must ascend the length of the afferent limb in a retrograde direction. Pyloric or duodenal stenosis or a Roux-en-Y gastrojejunostomy may make it impossible to reach the papilla.

Endoscopic sphincterotomy

Endoscopic sphincterotomy utilizes an electrocautery wire to transect the sphincter muscle surrounding the distal bile duct or pancreatic duct (Figure 5.2). It is performed as primary therapy for sphincter of Oddi dysfunction or to facilitate access to the bile

duct or pancreatic duct for therapeutic interventions such as stone extraction.

Indications

Indications for ERCP are listed in Box 5.1. It is indicated for the evaluation of disorders related to the pancreaticobiliary systems. Purely diagnostic

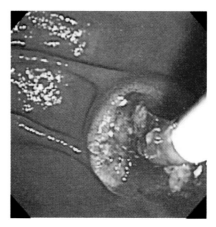

Figure 5.2 Endoscopic sphincterotomy. The bowed wire of the sphincterotome is used to cut the sphincter along the direction of the bile duct toward 11 o'clock.

Box 5.1 Indications for endoscopic retrograde cholangiopancreatography

Biliary tract diseases
1. obstructive jaundice
2. extrahepatic cholestasis
3. cholangitis
4. postoperative and traumatic biliary complications, e.g. bile leaks, fistulas, strictures
5. evaluation of sphincter of Oddi dysfunction by manometry
6. obtaining bile for diagnosis of microlithiasis
7. sphincterotomy for complications of gallstone disease when the gallbladder will be left *in situ*

Pancreatic diseases
1. acute biliary pancreatitis, if severe or with persistent biliary obstruction
2. suspected pancreatic cancer
3. suspected chronic pancreatitis
4. endoscopic therapy of known chronic pancreatitis
5. evaluation of pancreatic trauma
6. pancreatic duct 'road map' prior to surgery

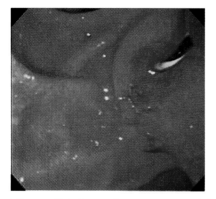

Figure 5.1 Normal appearance of the normal major papilla. A transverse duodenal fold is seen draping over the upper margin of the papillary mound. The bile duct has been cannulated and a guidewire has been left in place after removal of the catheter.

ERCP may be indicated for the evaluation of abnormal liver-associated enzymes and unexplained pancreatitis, however, most ERCP is performed with some therapeutic intent or for tissue sampling. These therapeutic maneuvers include sphincterotomy, stone extraction, stent placement, and/or dilation. Tissue-sampling techniques include brush cytology, forceps biopsy, fluid collection, and fine-needle aspiration.

A major indication for ERCP is the evaluation of suspected biliary obstruction. In jaundiced patients, it should only be undertaken when there is a high index of suspicion for obstruction. The distinction between obstructive and non-obstructive jaundice can usually be made on the basis of the pattern of liver-enzyme elevation in combination with bile-duct diameter on transabdominal ultrasound. A normal common bile duct should be less than 8 millimeters in diameter when the gallbladder is in place. Transabdominal ultrasound is therefore a useful initial test in the evaluation of a patient with jaundice or cholestasis. Two instances in which biliary obstruction may not be accompanied by ductal dilatation on ultrasound are (a) obstruction of recent onset, in which the duct has not had time to accommodate, and (b) primary sclerosing cholangitis, in which diffuse scarring of the ducts prevents dilation. The broader indications for ERCP include pancreatic disorders as well as the application of endoscopic therapy within the biliary or pancreatic ducts.

Table 5.1 Complications of endoscopic sphincterotomy.[1]

Type of complication	Percentage with complication	Percentage with severe complication
Pancreatitis	5.4	0.4
Hemorrhage	2.0	0.5
Perforation	0.3	0.2
Cholangitis	1.0	0.1
Cholecystitis	0.5	0.1
Miscellaneous[2]	1.1	0.3
Any complication	9.8	1.6

[1] Modified from Freeman ML, Nelson DB, Sherman S, et al. Complications of endoscopic biliary sphincterotomy. *N Engl J Med* 1996; 335: 909-918.
[2] Includes cardiopulmonary complications, ductal perforations by guidewire, stent malfunction, antibiotic-induced diarrhea, indeterminate fluid collection, and infection of pancreatic pseudocyst.

Complications

Complications associated with ERCP are listed in Table 5.1. The complication rate for ERCP is about 5% overall, but increases to 9% to 10% if therapeutic maneuvers such as endoscopic sphincterotomy are performed (Table 5.1). Complications related to ERCP can be divided into those that are inherent to any prolonged endoscopic procedure and those that are specific to ERCP and sphinctorotomy. The former include aspiration pneumonia, adverse cardiovascular or neurologic events related to sedation, drug reactions, and perforation. The most common ERCP-specific complication is pancreatitis, occurring in 5% of patients undergoing sphincterotomy, and accounting for more that half of the total complications. The presence of pancreatitis-like pain is important in defining this complication, since 50% to 75% of all patients will have an elevation in amylase or lipase levels after ERCP. Bleeding from the sphincterotomy site, which occurs in 2% of cases, can usually be managed endoscopically using injection, electrocautery, or mechanical hemostasis and only rarely requires angiographic or surgical therapy. The mortality rate related to endoscopic sphincterotomy is 0.4%.

Sphincterotomy has been shown to permanently abolish sphincter pressure. This may lead to bacterial colonization of the bile duct through reflux of duodenal contents, but long-term studies extending beyond 15 years have demonstrated that this does not lead to an increased risk of bile-duct stones or cancer in these patients. Sphincterotomy is therefore considered to be safe in the long term even in young patients.

The normal cholangiogram

Once bile-duct cannulation has been accomplished, care is taken to define all aspects of the biliary tree, including intra- and extrahepatic ducts, as well as the cystic duct and gallbladder (Figure 5.3). The origin and course of the cystic duct can be highly variable. If its take off is very low, the catheter may inadvertently enter the cystic duct instead of the common bile duct. The common hepatic duct extends from above the take off of the cystic duct, then bifurcates into the left and right hepatic ducts before entering the liver. The left hepatic duct is slightly longer than the right hepatic duct. With the patient in the usual semi-prone position during

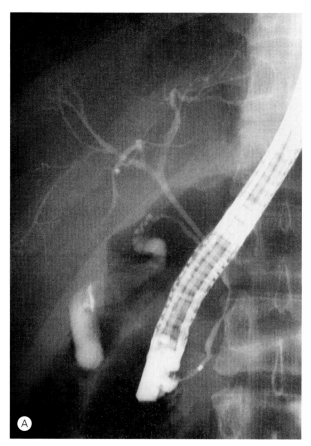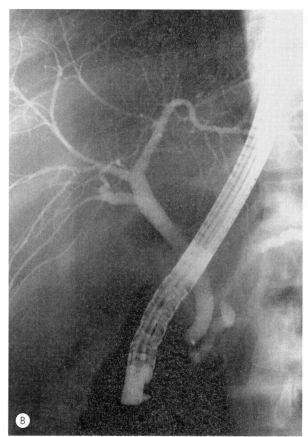

Figure 5.3 Normal cholangiograms. A) A young patient: a catheter has been placed in the distal common bile duct for contrast injection. The cystic duct is seen leading to the gallbladder. The bifurcation of the common hepatic duct into left and right hepatic ducts is demonstrated. B) An elderly patient: advanced age is associated with a "fuller" appearance of the biliary system. The diameter of the bile duct can be compared to the 12 mm outer diameter of the duodenoscope. As seen, the left hepatic duct is often longer than the right. There is opacification of the distal pancreatic duct, seen coursing to the right of the distal common bile duct. The cystic duct and gallbladder have not filled with contrast.

ERCP, the left hepatic duct is in a dependent position compared to the right hepatic duct, and therefore fills preferentially with contrast.

Biliary tract disease

Choledocholithiasis

Bile-duct stones represent the most common malady of the biliary tract and the most common indication for therapeutic ERCP. Endoscopic retrograde cholangiopancreatography is highly sensitive for detecting common-bile-duct stones, although a small stone may be missed because of excessive opacification of the duct. Choledocholithiasis is the most common cause of cholangitis, a condition in which prompt drainage by ERCP has reduced mortality to 10%, compared to a figure of 30% to 50% in the era when an infected biliary system had to be decompressed surgically.

Successful stone extraction from the bile duct usually requires sphincterotomy. Balloon sphincteroplasty, as an alternative to sphincterotomy is reserved for patients with uncorrectable coagulopathies. Stones are extracted by balloon-tipped or basket catheters. A balloon-tipped catheter is advanced past the stone under fluoroscopic guidance. The balloon is then inflated and withdrawn pulling the stone into the duodenum (Figure 5.4). Balloons are available in a variety of sizes, chosen according to the size of the stone and

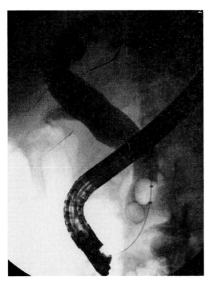

Figure 5.4 Stone extraction using a balloon-tipped catheter. A balloon has been inflated within a dilated bile duct proximal to a stone. The balloon will then be withdrawn across the sphincterotomy to extract the stone. The radiopaque tip of a guidewire is seen within the left intrahepatic ducts.

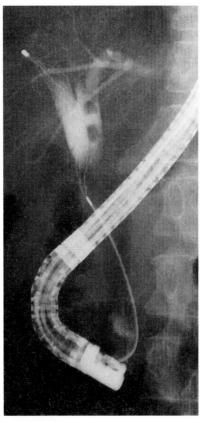

Figure 5.5 Stone extraction using a basket catheter. A basket has been opened adjacent to two stones, seen as filling defects just below the bifurcation of the left and right hepatic ducts. The basket can be manipulated to capture the stones and extract them by withdrawing across the sphincterotomy.

diameter of the bile duct. An alternative technique of stone extraction involves a catheter containing a closed basket. This is advanced into the bile duct under fluoroscopic observation, the basket is opened, and the stone is coaxed into it (Figure 5.5). The basket with the stone in it is then withdrawn from the duct.

Larger stones may prove difficult to extract despite an adequate sphincterotomy. One solution is mechanical lithotripsy, in which a specialized basket is advanced through the endoscope channel, opened to engage the stone, and then cranked closed against an unyielding metal sheath, fragmenting the stone within the bile duct. Mechanical lithotripsy is successful in the majority of cases in which it is employed. However, some stones will prove refractory to endoscopic extraction because of their large size or because of difficult anatomy of the duodenum or bile duct (Table 5.2). In these cases, it is important to obtain biliary decompression by means of a nasobiliary drain or a stent passed proximal to the calculus. Stent placement facilitates subsequent stone extraction by repeat ERCP at a later date. It is thought that contact between the stone and the plastic stent causes a gradual softening and fragmentation of the stone. Complete clearance can be achieved in more than 80% of cases on repeat ERCP 2 to 3 months later. Alternative techniques such as extracorporeal shock wave

Table 5.2 Problem stones encountered at endoscopic retrograde cholangiopancreatography

Large stones (> 25 mm)	Tortuous bile duct
Intrahepatic duct stones	Disproportionate bile duct/stone
Large number of stones	Juxta-ampullary diverticulum
Impacted stones	Previous Billroth II
Dual pathology (stone/ stricture)	Duodenal stricture

lithotripsy or electrohydraulic lithotripsy have also had success in fragmenting refractory stones. Thus, the armamentarium available in specialized centers against "difficult" stones is only rarely exhausted.

Endoscopic retrograde cholangiopancreatography and cholecystectomy

It is generally safe to perform cholecystectomy in the same hospital admission after ERCP and stone extraction. Alternatively, cholecystectomy may be deferred until the inflammation of cholecystitis or pancreatitis has subsided, since sphincterotomy offers significant protection against further episodes of common-bile-duct obstruction. Long-term follow-up of patients whose gallbladder was left in place following sphincterotomy has shown a 10% rate of recurrence of biliary symptoms over an 8- to 10-year period. In elderly patients, it is reasonable to follow a non-operative approach after sphincterotomy, since the risks of cholecystectomy may outweigh the risk of symptom recurrence.

It is also safe to perform ERCP in the immediate post-cholecystectomy period. This may be necessary if pain or enzyme elevation recur following cholecystectomy, suggesting a "retained" stone in the bile duct, or if intraoperative cholangiography demonstrates such a stone. In fact, at a time when cholecystectomy was still performed as an open procedure, the initial indication for ERCP was the demonstration of a retained common-bile-duct stone on intraoperative cholangiogram. Endoscopic stone extraction eliminated the cumbersome process of open bile duct exploration.

After cholecystectomy, common-bile-duct stones may still form *in situ* in the bile duct. These stones are rich in calcium bilirubinate (called "pigment stones"), in contrast to cholesterol-rich stones originating in the gallbladder. Pigment stones may have a softer consistency than cholesterol-rich stones. Juxta-ampullary duodenal diverticula and dilated common bile duct are risk factors for recurrent bile-duct stones.

Cholecystectomy is the most common cause of iatrogenic injury to the bile ducts. The important role of ERCP in the management of these injuries is discussed below.

Benign biliary strictures

Benign biliary strictures are most commonly attributed to primary sclerosing cholangitis, chronic pancreatitis, and postoperative bile-duct injuries. Less common causes include AIDS-associated cholangiopathy and parasitic infections. AIDS cholangiopathy, which can mimic primary sclerosing

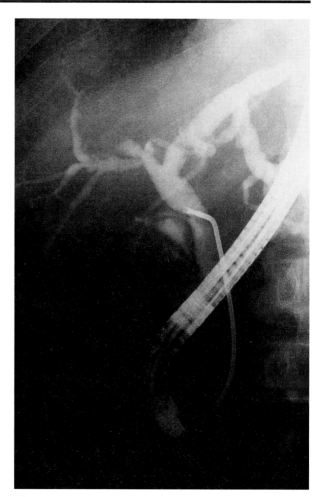

Figure 5.6 AIDS cholangiopathy. The irregular contour and dilation of the bile ducts is seen, giving an appearance that can mimic primary sclerosing cholangitis. A biopsy catheter has been advanced into the bile duct. Biopsies of bile duct epithelium in this patient stained positive for *Cryptosporidium* spp.

cholangitis, has been described associated with cytomegalovirus, *Cryptosporidium*, pneumocystis, and/or microsporidium infections of the bile duct (Figure 5.6). Parasitic infections with *Ascaris lumbricoides* and *Clonorchis sinensis* occur commonly in Asia and Africa but are rarely seen in the US.

Primary sclerosing cholangitis

Primary sclerosing cholangitis is a chronic cholestatic disorder of unknown etiology characterized by fibrosing inflammation of the intrahepatic and extrahepatic biliary tree. The natural history of primary sclerosing cholangitis is variable but may be progressive, leading to cirrhosis, portal hypertension, liver failure, and death within 12 years of diagnosis. The diagnosis of primary sclerosing cholangitis should be suspected in a patient with chronically elevated alkaline phosphatase levels. A high index of suspicion should be present in patients with inflammatory bowel disease, since this underlies 50% to 75% of cases of primary sclerosing cholangitis. Endoscopic retrograde cholangiopancreatography is the gold standard for the diagnosis of primary sclerosing cholangitis, and its availability has led to more patients being diagnosed in the asymptomatic, preicteric phase. Magnetic resonance cholangiography shows promise for the diagnosis of primary sclerosing cholangitis.

The classic picture of primary sclerosing cholangitis is one of diffuse, multifocal strictures of the intrahepatic and extrahepatic bile ducts, with areas of ectasia giving a "beaded" appearance (Figure 5.7). Because of the increased risk of procedure-related cholangitis, ERCP should be performed judiciously in patients with known primary sclerosing cholangitis. One of the most important and difficult differentiations to be made on cholangiography is between benign strictures of primary sclerosing cholangitis and cholangiocarcinoma, which can arise as a complication of primary sclerosing cholangitis in 10% to 15% of cases. Brush cytology of strictures done at the time of ERCP has a sensitivity of 60% for the detection of cholangiocarcinoma. This is an important finding in patients with primary sclerosing cholangitis who are awaiting liver transplantation, since the presence of an occult cholangiocarcinoma is associated with a dismal outcome post-transplantation. Routine surveillance of primary sclerosing cholangitis patients for cholangiocarcinoma using ERCP at regular intervals is not recommended, however, since no effective therapy for this complication is available.

Endoscopic retrograde cholangiopancreatography therapy for primary sclerosing cholangitis is limited to a subgroup of all primary sclerosing cholangitis patients who have a "dominant" stricture, that is, a discrete site of high-grade extrahepatic obstruction with limited involvement elsewhere. Repeated dilation of this type of stricture can improve symptoms of pruritus, jaundice, and fatigue, and may also favorably alter the rate of progression of disease and thus impact on long-term mortality.

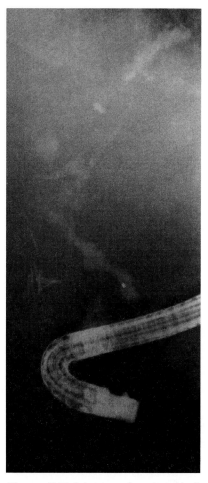

Figure 5.7 Primary sclerosing cholangitis. The classic "beaded" appearance of irregular structuring of the intra- and extrahepatic bile ducts is seen, with areas of dilation. Surgical clips are present from a prior cholecystectomy.

Chronic pancreatitis

Common-bile-duct stenosis due to inflammation and scarring of the pancreatic head is commonly seen in chronic pancreatitis. When there is bilirubin elevation, the risk of secondary biliary cirrhosis exists. The appearance of these strictures on ERCP is often long and tapered. Brushings should always be obtained, since chronic pancreatitis is one of the established risk factors for pancreatic adenocarcinoma. Benign strictures associated with chronic pancreatitis can be temporarily drained by plastic stent placement, but require surgical bypass for long-term therapy.

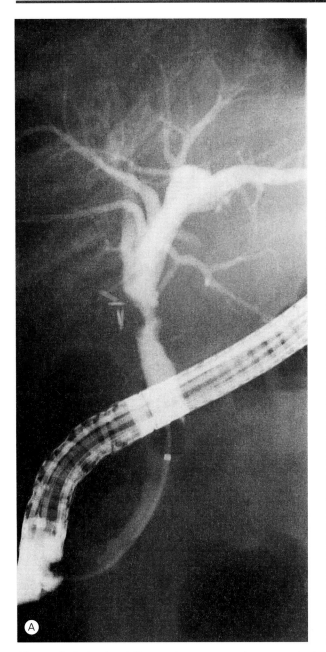

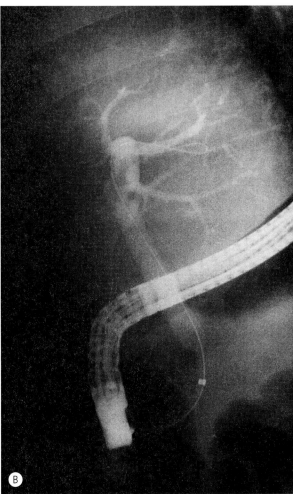

Figure 5.8 Benign biliary stricture occurring post-cholecystectomy. A) The benign stricture is noted as a stenosis of the bile duct adjacent to the surgical clips. B) Balloon dilation of a benign stricture. The smooth, contrast-filled structure in the bile duct is a long balloon used to dilate the stricture (see following page for Fig 5.8, part C).

Postoperative bile-duct injuries

Postoperative bile-duct injuries occur in two forms, bile leaks and biliary strictures, which may coincide. The incidence of these injuries has risen recently because of two factors. The first is the widespread acceptance of laparoscopic cholecystectomy, during which identification of some biliary and vascular structures may be challenging, especially given the high frequency of variant anatomy. The second is the rise in orthotopic liver transplantation which requires a biliary-to-biliary anastomosis.

Bile leaks present in the early postoperative period with abdominal pain, tenderness, and fever. Computed tomography may show evidence of a fluid collection in the right upper quadrant, and nuclear scintigraphy may demonstrate leakage of

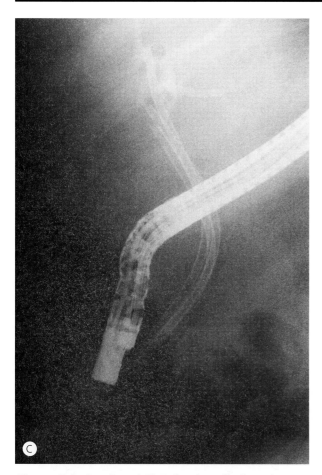

Figure 5.8 *Continued* C) Following dilation, three plastic stents have been placed in parallel across the stricture to prevent restenosis. Repeated dilations and stent exchanges every 3 months for a year have resulted in good long-term patency rates in post-operative biliary strictures.

bile, but ERCP is crucial in defining the exact site of the leak and in treating it. Bile leaks complicate laparoscopic cholecystectomy in 0.5% to 5% of cases. Most are from the cystic duct stump, although leakage can occur anywhere in the extrahepatic biliary tract including small ducts draining directly into the gallbladder (ducts of Luschka) that are not recognized at the time of surgery. Bile leak following liver transplantation usually occurs at the site of the bile-to-bile duct anastomosis or at the site of a T-tube that is placed in the bile duct for a short period after surgery. Treatment of all these types of bile leak involves reduction of intraductal pressure by placement of a biliary stent at the time of ERCP. The stent is then removed 3 to 6 weeks later, allowing adequate time for the site of the bile leak to heal.

Postoperative biliary strictures can be significantly more difficult to treat, since they denote injury to the duct itself or to its vascular supply (Figure 5.8). Until recently, most postoperative bile-duct strictures required surgical revision. However, dilation followed by placement of multiple stents which are upgraded every 3 months has achieved long-term success in 80% of patients. These results are comparable to surgery.

Malignant biliary obstruction

In patients who present with painless jaundice due to malignancy, 85% of tumors are pancreatic carcinomas, 6% are cholangiocarcinomas, and 4.5% each are duodenal and ampullary carcinomas. Given the overall poor prognosis of patients with malignant biliary obstruction, palliation is the goal in most patients. Endoscopic biliary stent insertion is now a widely available means of achieving palliation of biliary obstruction (Figure 5.9). Successful biliary drainage by this method can be achieved in 80% to 90% of cases with low procedure-related morbidity and mortality. An endoscopically placed stent is more likely to achieve long-term biliary drainage than a percutaneously placed stent, and is associated with lower morbidity and short-term mortality than surgical biliary bypass via choledochoduodenostomy or choledochojejunostomy.

The average patency of the commonly used 10 French (3.3 millimeter) diameter plastic stent is 6 months. For about four fifths of patients with malignant biliary obstruction, this surpasses life expectancy. For those patients with a predicted survival longer than 6 months, who may be expected to require stent changes, expandable metal stents are a good alternative (Figure 5.10). While the diameter of plastic stents that can be placed through a duodenoscope is limited by the size of the channel of the scope, metal stents overcome this limitation by being compressed onto a thin delivery device and expanding to a diameter of 10 millimeters upon deployment. By virtue of their larger diameters, metal stents offer a longer mean patency of 9 to 12 months. This can justify the five-fold increase in the cost of a metal stent by avoiding repeated stent exchanges or hospitalizations.

The drawback of metal stents is that they generally cannot be removed once deployed and become embedded into the bile-duct wall. Thus,

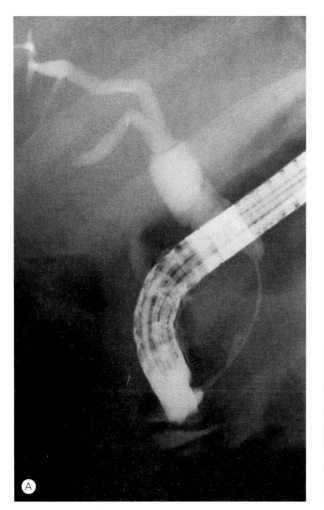
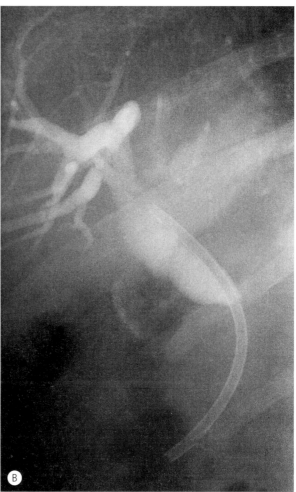

Figure 5.9 Malignant biliary stricture. A) Tight stricture caused by adenocarcinoma of the pancreatic head: a catheter has been placed across the stricture and contrast has been injected into a dilated proximal biliary system. B) An angled plastic stent has been placed across the stricture.

the management of an occluded metal stent can be quite challenging. Occlusion can be due to the accumulation of biliary sludge, dietary fiber, tumor in-growth, epithelial hyperplasia, or a combination of these elements. For this reason, metal biliary stents are not indicated for the management of benign biliary strictures, where long-term patency becomes an issue.

Pancreatic disease

Pancreatic cancer

More than 80% of pancreatic carcinomas originate from the pancreatic-duct epithelium. Endoscopic retrograde pancreatography (ERP), which enables examination of the main pancreatic duct, as well as the secondary and tertiary side branches, is a sensitive and specific means for evaluating pancreatic carcinoma. The normal pancreatic duct measures 2 to 4 millimeters in the head and body

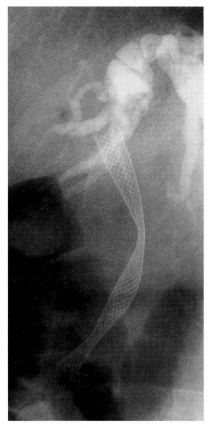

Figure 5.10 Metal stent for palliation of malignant biliary obstruction. The distal tip of the metal stent extends into the duodenal lumen, which is seen as the air-filled structure at the lower left side of the image.

of the pancreas tapering to 1 to 2 millimeters in the tail. The majority of pancreatic cancers involve the head (75%), causing an abrupt cut-off of the duct, or stenosis with proximal dilation. Body and tail lesions make up 20% and 5% of cases respectively. As discussed earlier in this chapter, carcinoma of the pancreatic head may cause stricturing of the common bile duct by direct invasion or by extrinsic compression. Concomitant stenosis or obstruction of the bile duct and the pancreatic duct, the radiological "double-duct sign", is seen in approximately 80% of cases. The double-duct sign was initially proposed as a specific indicator of pancreatic cancer, but may be seen in benign disease such as chronic pancreatitis. Differentiating benign from malignant strictures can be particularly challenging in chronic pancreatitis, which is a risk factor for pancreatic cancer. Ductal brushings and biopsies obtained at ERCP have a sensitivity of only around 60% for malignancy, and further tissue sampling of the pancreas can be performed under endoscopic ultrasound (EUS) guidance if necessary.

Unfortunately, the majority of pancreatic cancers are unresectable at the time that they become clinically apparent. Small tumors of the ampulla are an exception because they can present with obstructive features at an early stage. In general, ERP offers no staging information as it is an inaccurate means of assessing tumor size or extent, nor does it provide information regarding resectability,

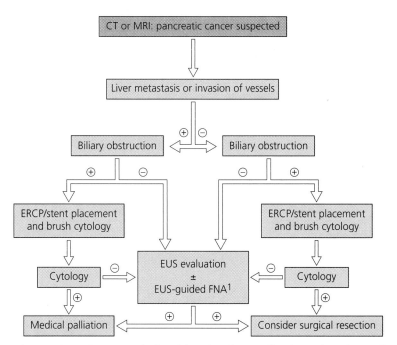

[1]Endoscopic ultrasound-guided fine needle aspiration (EUS-guided FNA) is indicated if (a) a mass is suspected on CT/MRI but biliary obstruction is not present, (b) a mass is seen on ERCP, but attempts at brush cytology are non-diagnostic

Figure 5.11 Suggested algorithm for the application of endoscopic retrograde choliopancreatography (ERCP) and endoscopic ultrasound (EUS) in the evaluation of patients with suspected pancreatic cancer.

nodal involvement, or distant metastases. The emergence of EUS and EUS-guided fine needle aspiration has improved the accuracy of cytologic diagnosis and staging in pancreatic cancer and has diminished the role of ERCP as a purely diagnostic tool. Therefore, ERCP is reserved for cases where placement of a stent for biliary obstruction is anticipated. A suggested algorithm for the application of ERCP and EUS in the evaluation of patients with suspected pancreatic cancer is presented in Figure 5.11.

Acute pancreatitis

Initial studies supported emergent ERCP early in the course of acute pancreatitis attributed to gallstones. More recent studies suggest that improved outcome from ERCP and endoscopic sphincterotomy resulted from a reduction in the incidence of biliary sepsis rather than a direct impact on the course of pancreatitis (Table 5.3). ERCP in the setting of acute pancreatitis should therefore be limited to those patients in whom radiographic or laboratory data suggest the presence of ongoing biliary obstruction and/or cholangitis.

Idiopathic recurrent pancreatitis

Endoscopic retrograde cholangiopancreatography plays a role in the diagnosis of patients in whom no apparent etiology for recurrent episodes of pancreatitis is identified. Diagnostic ERCP with the addition of sphincter of Oddi manometry and biliary crystal analysis can provide information about the cause of pancreatitis in the majority of these patients.

Table 5.3 Randomized trials of early endoscopic retrograde cholangiopancreatography (ERCP) in acute biliary pancreatitis

Study	n	Significant reduction Morbidity	Significant reduction Mortality	Comments
Neoptol 1988	121	+	–	Patients with severe pancreatitis only
Fan 1992	195	+	–	Reduction in biliary sepsis
Nowak 1995	205	+	+	ERCP within 24 hours
Folsch 1997	238	–	–	Excluded if bilirubin > 5

Abnormalities revealed by these studies include small pancreatic tumors, pancreatic-ductal lesions, biliary microlithiasis (biliary sludge), pancreas divisum, choledochocele, and hypertensive sphincter of Oddi. In one study, detection of biliary sludge (a suspension of cholesterol monohydrate crystals or calcium bilirubinate granules typically found in the gallbladder) in bile aspirated from the bile duct on ERCP was predictive of patients that benefited from cholecystectomy or endoscopic sphincterotomy. Patients treated in this way had fewer recurrences of acute pancreatitis during follow-up (up to 7 years) than untreated patients. This supports the notion that biliary sludge is an underestimated cause of acute recurrent idiopathic pancreatitis.

Pancreas divisum is an anatomic variant in which the main pancreatic drainage is provided through the minor papilla rather than the major papilla. This occurs in 5% to 7% of the general population but is found in 7% to 50% of patients with acute recurrent idiopathic pancreatitis. Uncontrolled studies have suggested that minor duct sphincterotomy reduces recurrent episodes of acute pancreatitis.

Endoscopic treatment for pain in chronic pancreatitis

Diagnostic ERCP is indicated when patients with chronic pancreatitis have pain that does not respond to initial standard therapies. Prior to undergoing a surgical drainage procedure for pain control, such as Puestow lateral pancreaticojejunostomy, pancreatography is useful in defining variants in which there is no ductal dilatation or the disease is localized to the head, body, or tail; these patients are not suitable for drainage procedures and resection is the only surgical option.

Potential findings on pancreatography in chronic pancreatitis include tumor, strictures, and stones. Endoscopic management of pancreatic-duct strictures and stones involves modifications of biliary techniques, but results have not been as encouraging. Pancreatic sphincterotomy, for example, carries a higher risk of hemorrhage and perforation than its biliary counterpart, and long-term results of dilation and stent placement for pancreatic strictures have been poor. These approaches may be attempted, however, in patients who are not operative candidates and those preferring an alternative to surgical therapy.

Pancreatic fistulas

A pancreatic fistula is a disruption of the wall of the pancreatic duct, leading to extravasation of pancreatic secretions. The majority of these occur as a complication of acute pancreatitis, with the remainder caused by chronic pancreatitis, trauma, or operative injury to the pancreas. Endoscopic retrograde cholangiopancreatography is the gold standard for the diagnosis of a pancreatic fistula. Many patients with a pancreatic fistula respond to conservative medical therapy (limiting of oral intake, administration of somatostatin analogs, pancreatic enzyme replacement) or placement of internal or external drains. Recent series have suggested that endoscopic placement of a trans-papillary stent in the pancreatic duct can lead to resolution of duct disruption in about 60% of cases. A stent bridging the duct disruption, such that the proximal end of the stent is upstream from the disruption, can lead to a successful outcome in 90% of patients. This is a technically demanding procedure, however, that can only be accomplished in specialized endoscopic centers.

Ampullary tumors

Adenomas and adenocarcinomas arising from the major papilla constitute a distinct pathologic entity. They may be sporadic or associated with familial adenomatous polyposis syndromes. Biliary obstruction is the most common presentation. Patients may also present with pancreatitis and/or anemia. The location of these tumors at the narrowest point of the extrahepatic biliary system leads to obstruction at an early stage, and consequently rates of surgical cure for these lesions are significantly higher than for pancreatic carcinomas or cholangiocarcinomas.

The diagnosis is usually made endoscopically with a side-viewing duodenoscope (Figure 5.12). Forceps biopsies of the suspicious looking papilla often yield the diagnosis, but biopsies obtained deep in the papilla after sphincterotomy can increase the yield. Papillary inflammation attributed to pancreatitis or the passage of gallstones (ampullary pseudotumor) can be distinguished from neoplasia by histology. In non-operative candidates endoscopic stenting is an effective palliative therapy, either alone or with adjunctive endoscopic tumor ablation therapy. When carcinoma is confirmed, treatment depends on the stage. Endoscopic ultrasound is the most accurate modality for staging ampullary tumors. The standard therapy for an invasive papillary tumor is surgical pancreaticoduodenectomy (Whipple procedure). Ampullary adenomas confined to the mucosa may be resected by endoscopic snare papillectomy or "ampullectomy". In snare papillectomy, temporary stenting of the pancreatic and bile duct is performed post-resection to reduce the risk of pancreatitis and cholangitis. This procedure should be reserved for those with experience and proficiency in pancreatic-duct stenting.

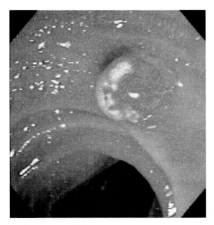

Figure 5.12 Ampullary adenoma in a patient who presented with early biliary obstruction. This friable lesion, visualized through a side-viewing duodenoscope, yielded high-grade dysplasia on biopsy.

Further reading

Barkun AN, Rezieg M, Mehta SN, *et al.* Postcholecystectomy biliary leaks in the laparoscopic era: risk factors, presentation, and management. *Gastrointest Endosc* 1997; 45:277–282.

Brugge WR, Van Dam J. Pancreatic and biliary endoscopy. *N Engl J Med* 1999; 341:1808–1815.

Carr-Locke DL. Endoscopic therapy of chronic pancreatitis. *Gastrointest Endosc* 1999; 49:S77–80.

Desilets DJ, Dy RM, Ku PM, *et al.* Endoscopic management of tumors of the major duodenal papilla: refined techniques to improve outcome and avoid complications. *Gastrointest Endosc* 2001; 54:202–208.

Foelsch UR, Nitsche R, Luedtke R, *et al.* Early ERCP and papillotomy compared with conservative treatment for acute biliary pancreatitis. *N Engl J Med* 1997; 336:237–242.

Freeman ML, Nelson DB, Sherman S, *et al.* Complications of endoscopic biliary sphincterotomy. *N Engl J Med* 1996; 335:909–918.

Chapter 6

Contrast Radiology

Stephen E. Rubesin

Introduction

With the advent of ultrasound, CT, MRI, endoscopy, and EUS, studies of the gastrointestinal tract using barium or water-soluble contrast agents have been relegated to a clinical backwater. Rather than understanding the complementary nature of barium studies and endoscopy, clinicians view barium radiology and endoscopy as competing examinations. Clinicians, and even radiologists, need to be reminded of the importance and cost effectiveness of contrast studies, and the times when barium studies are the best examination for a specific clinical concern. This chapter will first present general principles of contrast studies, then describe the indications, preparation, and technique of specific studies.

General principles

Barium studies are superior to endoscopy in some respects and inferior in others. Barium studies are safer than endoscopy, with lower risk of perforation or bleeding. There are no anesthetic risks with barium studies, as there are with endoscopy. Contrast studies provide the "big picture", showing the size, shape, and position of organs (Figures 6.1 and 6.2). For example, it is of little help to the radiation therapist when the endoscopist says that there is a cancer 27 cm from the incisors. In comparison, the radiologist can say that there is a 2.0 cm sessile lesion of the upper thoracic esophagus centered at the level of the clavicle (Figure 6.3). Barium studies are superior to endoscopy in evaluating the location of a lesion (Figure 6.4), the distribution of disease, bowel motility, and the presence of obstruction or perforation in all areas of the gastrointestinal tract. Contrast studies are complementary to endoscopy in the assessment of extramucosal lesions and the presence of fissures and fistulas.

Endoscopy can assess color and superficial vascular changes in the mucosa that barium studies cannot. However, endoscopy is not always superior to barium studies in the evaluation of even the superficial portions of mucosa. In some cases, barium studies are superior in the evaluation of subtle elevations or depressions not seen on

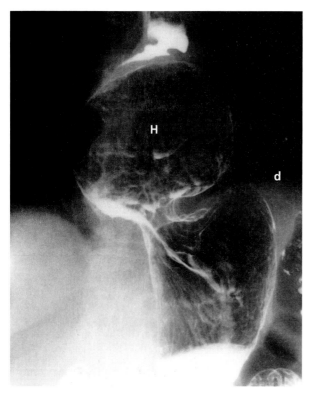

Figure 6.1 The "big picture". An upright radiograph demonstrates a large hiatal hernia (H) above the level of the left hemidiaphragm (d). The hernia does not reduce, even while the patient is standing (reproduced with permission from Rubesin SE. *Principles of Performing a Double Contrast Upper Gastrointestinal Series*. Westbury, NY, E-Z-EM, 2000; 1–29: Fig. 22).

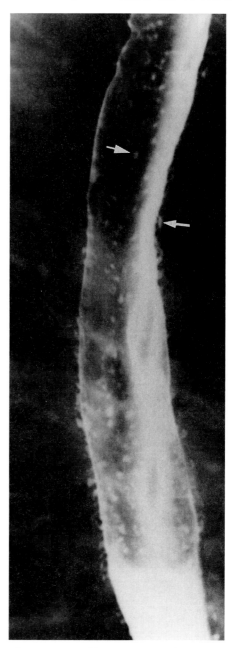

Figure 6.2 Diffuse intramural pseudodiverticulosis. Spot radiograph of the upper and mid-esophagus shows numerous 1 to 2-mm flask-shaped outpouchings (thick arrow) from the lumen of the esophagus. En face, a pseudodiverticulum (thin arrow) mimics an ulcer.

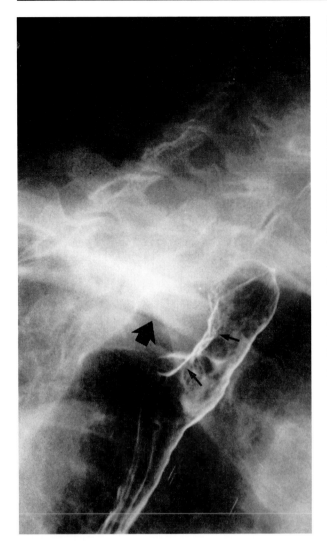

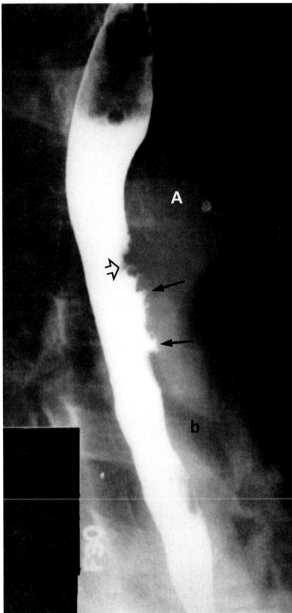

Figure 6.3 Squamous cell carcinoma at the junction of the cervical and thoracic esophagus. There is a 2.0 cm polypoid mass "etched in white" (thin arrows) on the anterior wall of the cervicothoracic esophagus. The radiation therapist is interested in the relationship of the tumor to the surrounding structures. The radiograph shows that the polypoid mass is at the level of the clavicle (thick arrow).

Figure 6.4 Squamous cell carcinoma in mid-esophagus. Spot radiograph shows a tumor 3.0 cm in length extending from the level of the aortic arch (A) to the level of the left mainstem bronchus (b). The tumor is manifest in the column of high-density barium as areas of focal ulceration (arrows) and mucosal nodularity (open arrow).

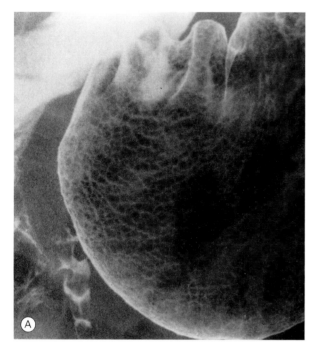

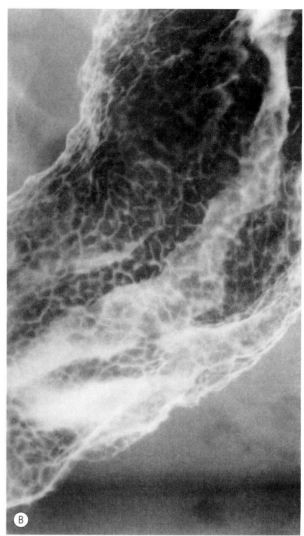

Figure 6.5 Areae gastricae. (A) The mucosa of the stomach is divided into polygonal tufts by a barium-filled groove pattern. The tufts are the areae gastricae. (B) In this patient, the areae gastricae pattern is prominent because of *Helicobacter pylori* gastritis. Five years later this patient developed a MALToma.

endoscopy. By washing the mucus off the mucosa, a barium study may depict mucosal detail not seen by the endoscopist, such the areae gastricae of the stomach (Figure 6.5) or the surface pattern of a tumor (Figure 6.6).

The great advantage of endoscopy is its ability to obtain material for pathologic diagnosis by biopsy. Biopsy is not infallible, however (Figure 6.7). Small biopsy fragments are not always diagnostic for mucosal diseases that have a patchy distribution. Biopsies are unable to assess the depth of a mucosal tumor. Biopsies do not evaluate extramucosal processes very well.

Contrast agents

Water-soluble contrast agents are used to detect perforations in the gastrointestinal tract (Figure 6.8). Non-ionic contrast agents (such as iohexol – Omnipaque, Nycomed Inc., Princeton, NJ) do not draw fluid into the lumen of the gastro-intestinal tract. These agents are designed primarily for vascular or cerebrospinal fluid injection. When there is moderate to severe risk of aspiration, however, non-ionic contrast agents may be used in the upper gastrointestinal tract. Most gastrointestinal studies that require the use of a water-soluble

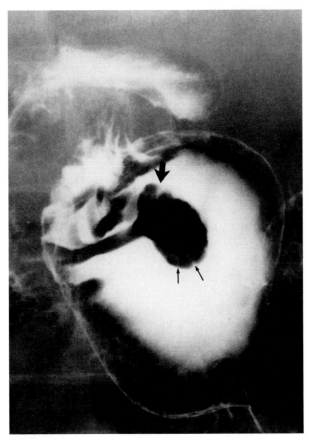

Figure 6.6 Surface pattern in a tubulovillous adenoma. The endoscopist requested an upper GI series "… to see if an antral leiomyoma was prolapsing into the duodenal bulb." The upper GI series shows a 1.5 cm polypoid lesion (large arrow) that is not prolapsing into the duodenal bulb. The barium study also shows that this is not a submucosal leiomyoma, but a tumor originating in the mucosa. The finely lobulated contour (large arrow) and barium in the interstices of the polyp (thin arrows) indicate that the tumor has a mucosal origin, most likely either a hyperplastic or adenomatous polyp.

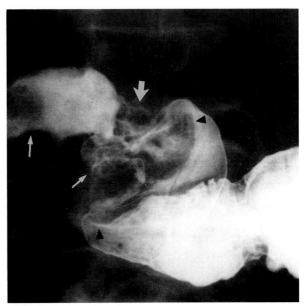

Figure 6.7 Not all biopsies are correct. Six weeks before this barium enema was performed, endoscopy revealed a stricture in the proximal colon, thought to be benign. The endoscopist could not traverse the stricture with the endoscope. A biopsy at the edge of the stricture showed chronic inflammation. The patient was discharged. The patient returned 6 weeks later with abdominal distension. A spot radiograph from a barium enema shows partial obstruction to the flow of barium and a long circumferential lesion (thin arrows) with shelf-like margins (arrowheads) and nodular mucosa (thick arrow). The radiologic diagnosis of adenocarcinoma of the transverse colon was confirmed at surgery.

contrast agent use ionic water-soluble contrast agents (e.g. ditriazoate meglumine and ditriazoate sodium – Gastroview, Malinckrodt, Inc. St Louis, MO). These agents are used because they are absorbed from the soft tissue of the neck, mediastinum, and retroperitoneum or from the pleural or intraperitoneal space. Barium will only slowly resorb if it extravasates into soft tissue or the peritoneum. A barium study is contraindicated in patients with suspected colonic perforation. Colonic perforation during barium enema can introduce feces and barium into the peritoneal space which can result in peritonitis and even death. Water-soluble contrast agents are inferior to barium, however, in the demonstration of perforations or fistulas, or any intraluminal pathology. If a water-soluble study of the pharynx or esophagus does not demonstrate a suspected perforation, it is repeated with barium because there is little risk with barium in the soft tissue of the neck or mediastinum. If a water-soluble study of the stomach, small bowel, or colon does not demonstrate a suspected perforation, a barium study is not usually performed because of risk of barium peritonitis.

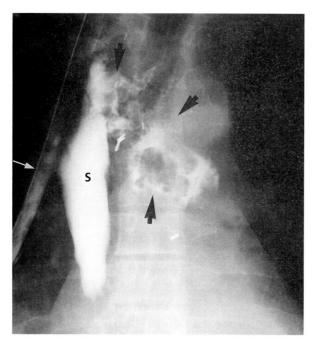

Figure 6.8 Perforation after esophagogastrectomy. Overhead radiograph of the mid-chest shows water-soluble contrast filling a 10-cm collection (black arrows) in the mediastinum medial to the stomach (S). Contrast has entered the right pleural tube (white arrow).

Single versus double contrast

Single contrast means that one contrast agent is used, double contrast means that two contrast agents are used (Figure 6.9). Biphasic examination means that both a single and a double contrast study are performed. During single contrast, the lumen of a viscus is filled with contrast agent (Figure 6.10). The radiologist looks at the size, shape, position of bowel, and the luminal contour. The radiologist looks for radiolucent filling defects in the barium pool, protrusions into the lumen that replace the contrast agent (Figures 6.11 and 6.12). The radiologist compresses the bowel to evaluate contour, pliability, and mobility of loops. Portions underneath the ribs or deep in the pelvis are difficult to compress.

During double contrast, the radiologist coats the mucosal surface with medium to high viscosity barium, then distends the lumen with a radiolucent contrast agent such as air or methylcellulose. The radiologist looks at the barium-etched mucosal surface en face, the shallow barium pool on the

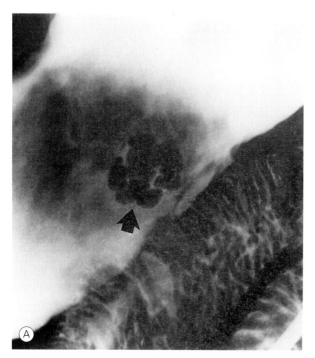

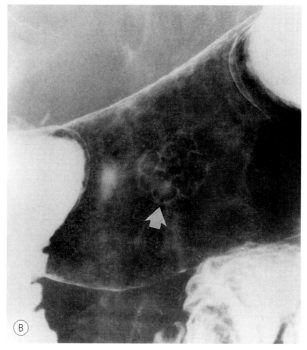

Figure 6.9 Single contrast in comparison to air contrast. (A) Spot radiograph of the barium-filled stomach obtained with compression depicts a polypoid mass (arrow) as a focal grouping of 3 to 5-mm ovoid and polygonal radiolucent nodules in the barium pool. This proved to be a tubulovillous adenoma. (B) Spot radiograph of the tubulovillous adenoma in air contrast shows a focal area of radiolucent nodules (arrow) etched in white by barium (reproduced with permission from Rubesin SE. *Principles of Performing a Double Contrast Upper Gastrointestinal Series*. Westbury, NY, E-Z-EM, 2000; 1–29: Figs 2B and 2D).

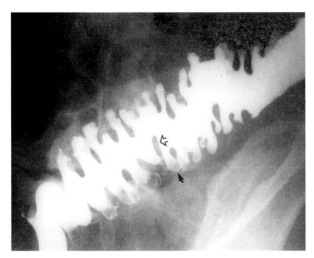

Figure 6.10 Single contrast technique. Overhead prone angled view of the colon from a single contrast barium enema shows a lumen filled with barium. Multiple barium-filled diverticula (arrow) protrude from the expected luminal contour. Circular muscle thickening is manifest as protrusions (open arrow) into the lumen.

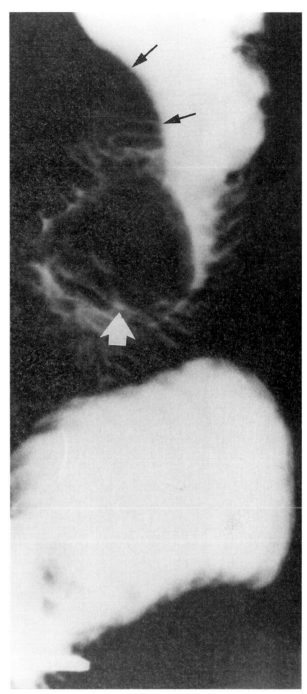

Figure 6.12 Single contrast barium-filling phase of double contrast enteroclysis shows a 1.5 cm rounded polypoid protrusion (white arrow) into the barium column. One wall of the pedicle is seen (black arrows). This was one of several hamartomas in a patient with unsuspected Peutz–Jeghers syndrome.

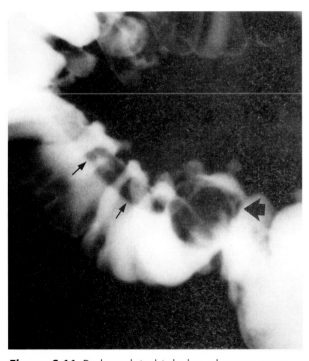

Figure 6.11 Pedunculated tubular adenoma seen during single contrast phase of double contrast barium enema. A 1.5 cm finely lobulated polyp (large arrow) is seen as a lobulated radiolucent filling defect in the barium column. The 3 cm long pedicle is depicted as a tubular radiolucent filling defect in the barium pool (small arrows).

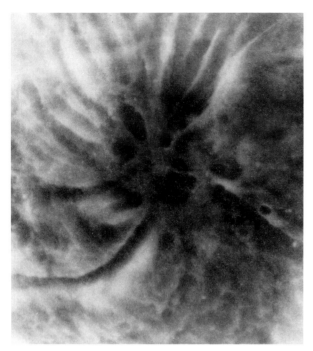

Figure 6.13 The shallow barium pool. Coned down view of the gastric fundus obtained as the radiologist flows a shallow pool of high-density barium across the mucosal surface of the gastric fundus during a double contrast upper GI series. There are many 4 to 5-mm, round to ovoid radiolucencies displacing the shallow barium pool. Folds swirl toward the area of focal mucosal nodularity. This was an early gastric cancer confined to the upper layer of the submucosa.

posterior wall (dependent surface) (Figure 6.13), and the luminal contour. The advantage of double contrast over single contrast is that a double contrast examination demonstrates the en face mucosal detail etched in white by barium, whereas in a single contrast examination, the radiologist can only look for lesions large enough to displace the barium column (about 6–10 mm in size).

Double contrast technique can only be used in patients who can stand and turn on a fluoroscopic table and patients who can understand and communicate with the radiologist. In general, single contrast examinations are used in immobile patients, in patients who are unable to understand or communicate with radiologist, during the immediate postoperative period, in any situation with suspected perforation, or when the small intestine is to be studied without an intubation technique.

Preparation for contrast studies

Preparation of both the patient and the radiologist is an often neglected portion of any examination. The radiologist should provide written instructions and a description of the examination to each referring physician, so that the referring physician's office can hand these instructions to each patient being scheduled for a radiologic examination.

The radiology referral form is a prescription for the examination. The referring physician should write on the referral form enough information so that the radiologic examination can be tailored to the clinical question that needs to be answered. The radiologist needs to be prepared with the pertinent clinical history, physical findings, and surgical history.

In general, non-emergent contrast studies performed by mouth (barium swallow, upper gastrointestinal series, small-bowel follow-through) have the following preparation:

1. nothing by mouth after 9 to 11 pm the evening before the examination
2. no (or diminished) insulin the day of the examination
3. avoid salivary stimulants (smoking, gum chewing, throat lozenges, etc.)
4. no oral medications that coat the mucosa (e.g. antacids)
5. leave dentures or other swallowing appliances in place so the patient swallows in a normal fashion.

Non-emergent colon examinations require as clean a colon as possible. Success of colonic preparation depends primarily on the patient's age, intrinsic colonic motility, underlying colonic disease, and medications that alter colonic motility. The clinician's office should be able to explain the preparation verbally as well as hand out the radiologist's instruction sheet. The referring clinician should consider a 1.5 and 2 day preparation in patients who have known or suspected colonic hypomotility, i.e. immobile or elderly patients, patients taking opiates or drugs with anticholinergic side effects, and patients with intrinsic colonic motor disorders such as diabetes, hypothyroidism, and scleroderma. The preparation varies widely from radiologist to radiologist, but at our hospital it includes the following:

1. clear liquids for breakfast, lunch, and dinner the day before the examination
2. encourage extra drinking of water or other liquids to maintain adequate hydration

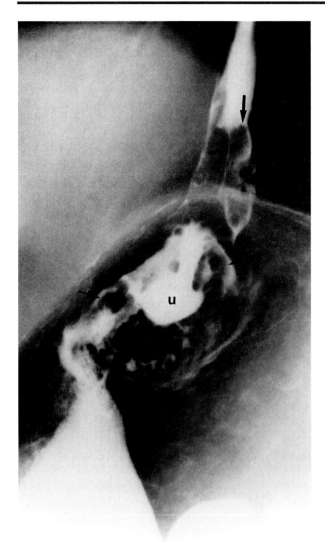

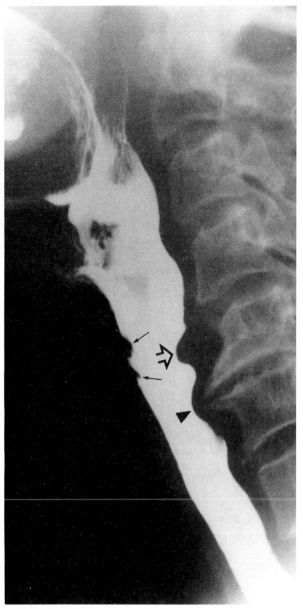

Figure 6.14 Adenocarcinoma of the gastric cardia. This 27-year-old man complained of minimal substernal discomfort. There is a large ulcerated tumor in the gastric cardia manifested as a barium-filled ulcer (u) surrounded by mucosal nodularity (thin arrows). Tumor extends into the distal esophagus, the tumor manifested as a thick nodular fold (thick arrow).

3. one bottle of magnesium citrate or two bottles of Fleets Phosphasoda at 5 pm the day before the examination
4. four 5 mg bisacodyl tablets taken with one glass water at 10 pm the day before the examination
5. a bisacodyl suppository inserted early on the morning of the examination.

Some institutions will add a 2 liter cleansing enema at least 1 hour prior to the examination.

Figure 6.15 Incomplete opening of the cricopharyngeus in a patient with neck discomfort and heartburn. Image obtained during passage of the barium bolus shows a hemispheric bar (open arrow) caused by incomplete opening of the pharyngoesophageal segment. Also note osteophytes impressing the posterior wall of the cervical esophagus (arrowhead) and redundant mucosa at the level of the cricoid cartilage, the "post-cricoid impression" (thin arrows). Gastroesophageal reflux was seen at fluoroscopy (reproduced with permission from Rubesin SE. Oral and pharyngeal dysphagia. *Gastroenterol Clin North Am* 1995; 24: 331–352, Fig. 7).

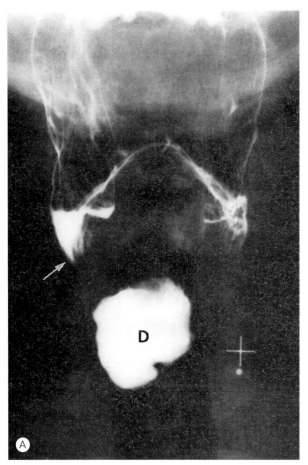 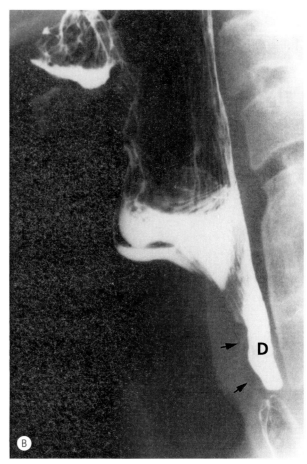

Figure 6.16 Zenker's diverticulum. (A) Frontal view of the pharyngoesophageal segment shows a 2.5 cm sac (D) midline below the tips of the piriform sinuses (right piriform sinus identified by arrow). (B) In the lateral view, the diverticulum (D) is a flat barium-filled sac behind the pharyngoesophageal segment (black arrows) (reproduced with permission from Rubesin SE. Pharynx. In Laufer I, Levine MS (eds) *Double Contrast Gastrointestinal Radiology* 2nd edn. Philadelphia, WB Saunders, 1992; 73–105: Figs 4.12B and C).

Large volume colonic lavage agents (e.g. Golytely) are not used at our hospital as they leave excessive fluid in the colon that diminishes barium coating.

Barium swallow

Swallowing begins in the cerebral cortex with the voluntary movement of a bolus toward the lips and ends at the gastric cardia. A double contrast video-pharyngoesophagram ("barium swallow") examines oral, pharyngeal, and esophageal motility and the morphology of the pharynx, esophagus, and gastric cardia. Given the fact that the bolus quickly moves from the lips to the pharyngoesophageal segment ("cricopharyngeus"), movements of various structures must be recorded by dynamic imaging of greater than 20 frames per second (such as video or digital video). Symptoms from esophageal disease are frequently referred to the neck; therefore, in a patient with suprasternal symptoms, the radiologist should examination the oral, pharyngeal, and esophageal phases of swallowing. In patients with substernal symptoms, the radiologist focuses on the esophagus and gastric cardia (Figure 6.14). Nevertheless, many esophageal diseases have associated findings in the pharynx. For example, patients with gastroesophageal reflux frequently have abnormal epiglottic tilt, incomplete opening of the cricopharyngeus (Figure 6.15), or early closure of the cricopharyngeus or upper cervical esophagus. There is also a strong association between Zenker's diverticulum (Figure 6.16) and gastroesophageal reflux.

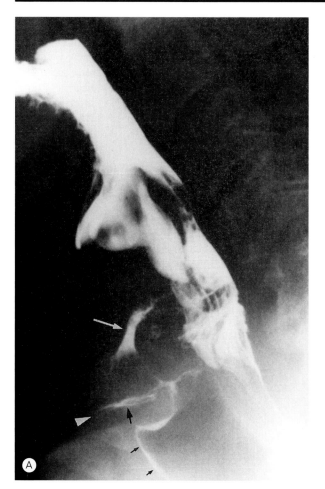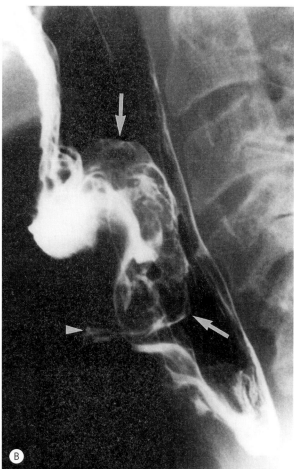

Figure 6.17 Laryngeal penetration due to epiglottic carcinoma. (A) Spot radiograph during drinking shows barium entering the laryngeal vestibule (white arrow). The laryngeal ventricle (large black arrow) and anterior commissure (arrowhead) are coated with barium. Barium coats the anterior wall of the trachea (small black arrows). (B) Spot radiograph obtained during phonation shows a large, lobulated barium-etched mass (arrows) replacing the epiglottis. The anterior commissure is identified (arrowhead). Note how the motility is better demonstrated during drinking (A) and the morphology is better demonstrated in a static image (B).

Barium studies are the best test for pharyngeal motility, especially laryngeal penetration (Figure 6.17), overflow aspiration, or abnormalities of the cricopharyngeus. Barium studies cannot be used to screen for tumors in the palatine tonsils or base of the tongue as these areas are intrinsically nodular and often protuberant because of their underlying lymphoid tissue. Barium studies, however, detect

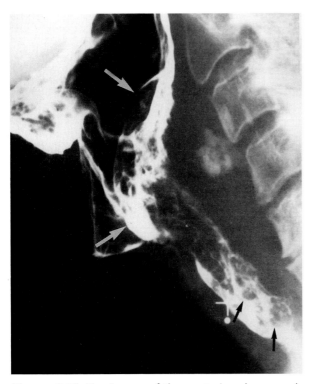

Figure 6.18 Carcinoma of the posterior pharyngeal wall extending into the pharyngoesophageal segment. The posterior contour of the pharynx is obliterated. The mass of tumor is seen protruding into the pharyngeal airspace (white arrows). There is soft tissue where the normal air space of the pharynx should be. Barium coats coarsely lobulated mucosa (black arrows). This patient had a "normal" ENT endoscopic examination 4 months prior to this study (reproduced with permission from Rubesin SE. Oral and pharyngeal dysphagia. *Gastroenterol Clin North Am* 1995; 24: 331–352, Fig. 14).

97% of structural abnormalities in the hypopharynx (Figures 6.18–6.20). They cannot, however, evaluate the vocal cords.

Barium studies are probably the first choice over both endoscopy and pH probe studies in patients with substernal dysphagia as they give a global assessment of motility (Figure 6.21), morphology (Figures 6.22–6.24), and gastroesophageal reflux. Barium studies are inferior to 24-hour pH probe studies in determining patients who have gastroesophageal reflux, as during the brief 5 minutes of fluoroscopy, gastroesophageal reflux will be detected in only 50% to 70% of all patients who reflux. Barium examinations are superior to endoscopy, however, in detecting the percentage of patients who reflux, because many of these patients

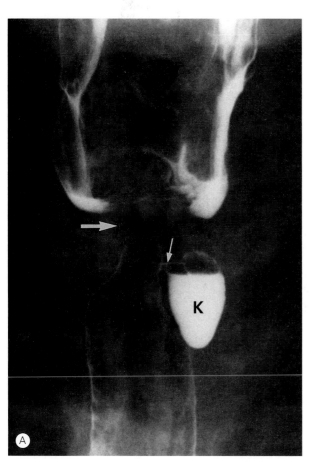
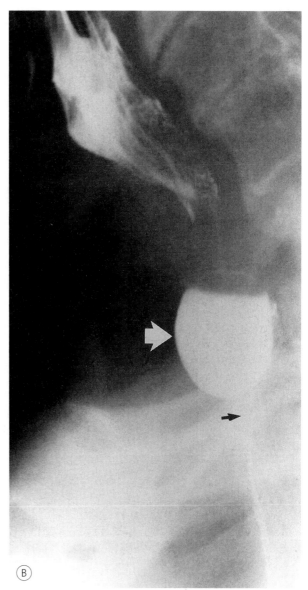

Figure 6.19 Killian–Jamieson diverticulum (lateral proximal cervical esophageal diverticulum). (A) Frontal view of the pharyngoesophageal junction shows a 2 cm barium and air-filled sac (K) lateral to the proximal cervical esophagus, just below the level of the cricopharyngeus (large arrow). The neck of the diverticulum (small arrow) is etched in white. (B) Lateral view of the pharyngoesophageal segment demonstrates that the diverticulum (white arrow) lies partly anterior to the expected course of the cervical esophagus (black arrow) (reproduced with permission from Rubesin SE. Pharynx. In: Levine MS, Rubesin SE, Laufer I (eds) *Double Contrast Gastrointestinal Radiology* 3rd edn. Philadelphia, WB Saunders, 2000; 61–89: Fig. 4.16).

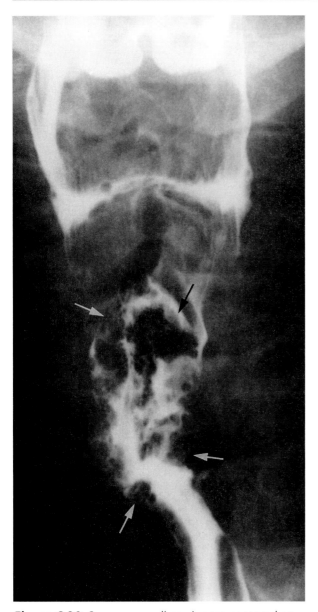

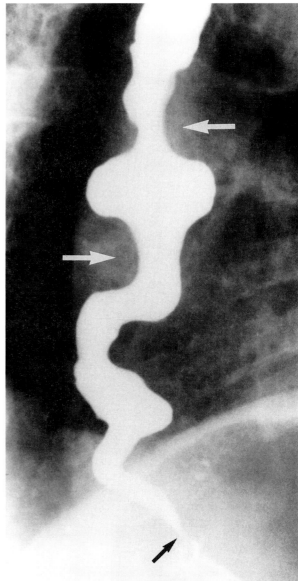

Figure 6.20 Squamous cell carcinoma centered at the pharyngoesophageal segment. This patient had undergone two "normal" ENT endoscopic examinations with 3 months of the barium swallow. The pharyngoesophageal segment and upper cervical esophagus is expanded by a nodular mass (arrows). The pharyngoesophageal segment is a difficult region to examine by both endoscopy and barium studies (reproduced with permission from Rubesin SE. Gallery of double contrast terminology. *Gastroenterol Clin North Am* 1995; 24: 259–288, Fig. 7).

Figure 6.21 Diffuse esophageal spasm with hypertensive lower esophageal sphincter. There are deep contractions (white arrows) indenting the lumen of the esophagus. The lower esophageal sphincter is tapered with a beak-like configuration (black arrow).

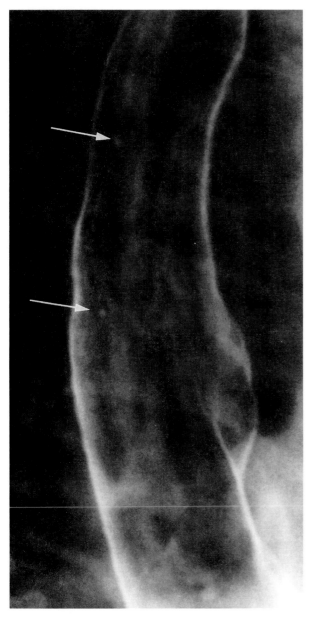

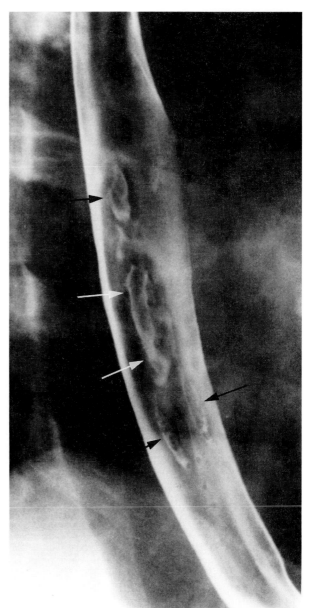

Figure 6.22 Herpes esophagitis in an immunocompetent host. A 16-year-old man with acute odynophagia. Tiny punctate barium-filled ulcers (arrows) are surrounded by radiolucent halos of edema.

Figure 6.23 Cytomegalovirus ulcers in a patient with acquired immunodeficiency syndrome (AIDS). Large, shallow, barium-filled ulcers (arrows) are surrounded by lucent rims of edema (reproduced with permission from Rubesin SE, Levine MS. Differential diagnosis of esophageal disease on esophagography. *Appl Radiol* October 2001; 1–22: Fig. 3).

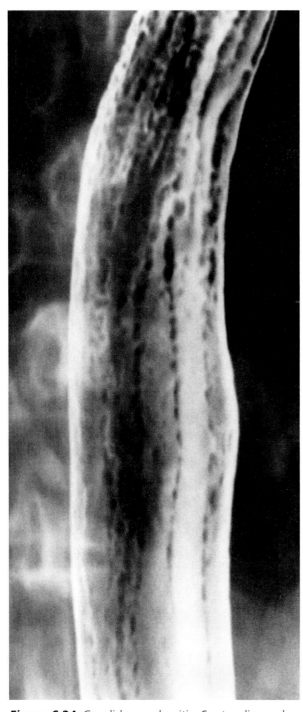

Figure 6.24 Candida esophagitis. Spot radiograph of mid-esophagus in a middle-aged woman with Crohn's disease treated by steroids. Numerous 1 to 3-mm ovoid radiolucent plaques are aligned longitudinally in rows. The intervening mucosa is smooth.

do not have endoscopically visible esophagitis. Barium studies are superior to endoscopy in detecting mild reflux-induced strictures (Figure 6.25).

In patients with long-standing gastroesophageal reflux disease, barium studies may be used as a screening examination to determine who needs endoscopy. Barium studies are clearly inferior to endoscopy in diagnosing Barrett's esophagus, given endoscopy's ability to obtain a biopsy. However, a barium study may determine who may benefit from endoscopy. Patients with Barrett's esophagus have such long-standing gastroesophageal reflux that they have morphologic changes that can be detected during a barium swallow, such as esophagitis, ulceration, or stricture formation. If a double contrast esophagram is normal, or shows only a hiatal hernia, the risk of Barrett's esophagus is less than 1%. If a double contrast esophagram shows reflux esophagitis, the risk of Barrett's esophagus is about 10% to 20%. If a study shows a

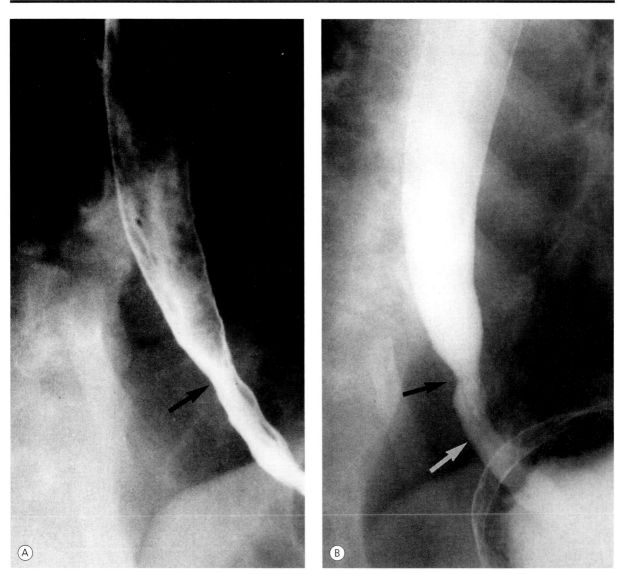

Figure 6.25 Reflux-induced stricture missed at endoscopy. A 42-year-old man complained of solid-food dysphagia. (A) An erect double contrast view shows a smooth, tapered narrowing of the distal esophagus (arrow). (B) An image obtained during prone drinking shows a mild, 7 mm in width, smooth, tapered narrowing (black arrow) of the distal esophagus above a small hiatal hernia (white arrow). A 12-mm barium tablet stuck at this site for 3 minutes. Two weeks before this picture was taken an endoscope was passed through this region and the endoscopist did not see a stricture.

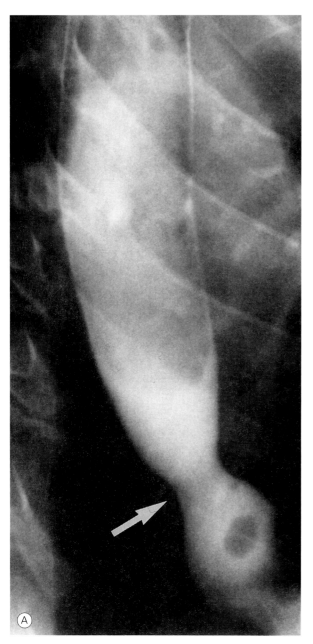

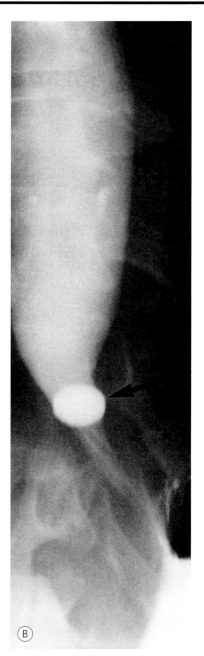

Figure 6.26 Benign esophageal stricture in a patient with dysphagia for solids. (A) Spot radiograph obtained during prone drinking shows a 1.5 cm in length, smooth, tapered stricture (arrow) of the distal esophagus (a bubble is present in the small hiatal hernia). (B) Spot radiograph obtained after the patient swallowed a 12.5 mm barium tablet and drank barium-tinged water. The tablet (arrow) stuck at the distal esophageal stricture.

benign stricture (Figure 6.26), the risk of Barrett's esophagus is about 20% to 40%. If a double contrast study shows a reticular mucosal pattern or an ulcer or stricture above the level of the left atrium, the risk of Barrett's esophagus is about 70%.

Barium studies are excellent at detecting symptomatic esophageal cancers (Figures 6.27 and 6.28). At our hospital we detected 99% of symptomatic esophageal cancers. The one lesion that was missed had a biopsy positive for adenocarcinoma, but on surgical resection no invasive adenocarcinoma was found.

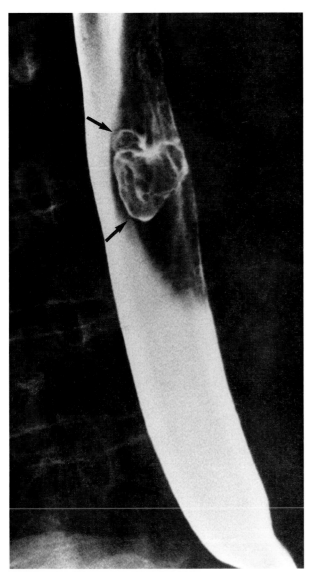

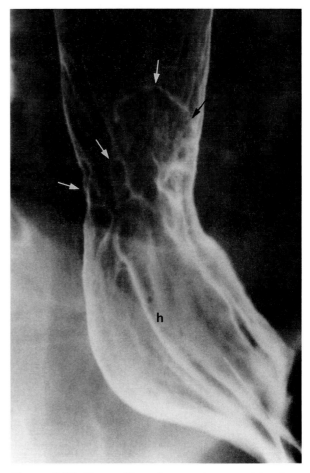

Figure 6.28 Plaque-like adenocarcinoma arising in Barrett's esophagus. Spot radiograph of the distal esophagus shows a focal area of mucosal nodularity (arrows). A large hiatal hernia (h) is seen in this erect image, indicating shortening of the esophagus.

Figure 6.27 Polypoid squamous cell carcinoma. Digital spot image of the mid-esophagus shows a 1.5-cm lobulated mass (arrows) with a nodular surface (reproduced with permission from Rubesin SE, Levine MS. Differential diagnosis of esophageal disease on esophagography. *Appl Radiol* October 2001; 1–22: Fig. 20).

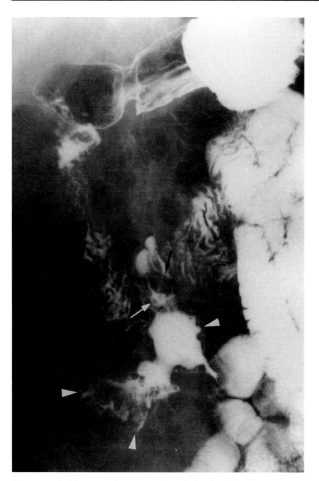

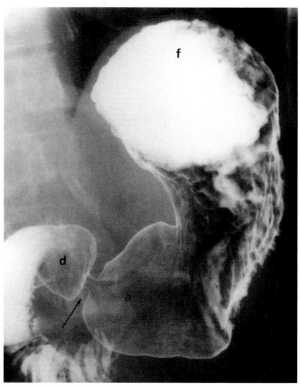

Figure 6.30 Spot radiograph of the stomach shows the gastric antrum (a), pylorus (arrow) and duodenal bulb (d) in air contrast. The gastric fundus (f) is filled and obscured by a dense pool of barium.

Figure 6.29 Lymphoma missed during both previous recent upper endoscopy and outside upper GI series. A large extraluminal cavity (arrowheads) fills with barium. A thick fold (black arrow) seen in the third portion of the duodenum surrounds a barium-filled ulcer (white arrow). An upper GI series should image the duodenal–jejunal junction.

Upper gastrointestinal series

A double contrast upper gastrointestinal series (upper GI series) is a biphasic examination employing both double contrast and single contrast techniques. During an upper GI series, the radiologist studies esophageal motility, gastric and duodenal emptying, and the morphology of the esophagus, stomach, and duodenum to the ligament of Treitz (Figure 6.29). The radiologist "paints" the mucosal surface with barium, and then distends the lumen with swallowed air and carbon dioxide generated by swallowing an effervescent agent. Fluoroscopically directed spot images are then obtained (Figures 6.30–6.33).

Endoscopy is a superior examination in patients with acute upper gastrointestinal bleeding because endoscopy may detect a Mallory–Weiss tear, arteriovenous malformations, or small bleeding esophageal varices that an upper GI series may

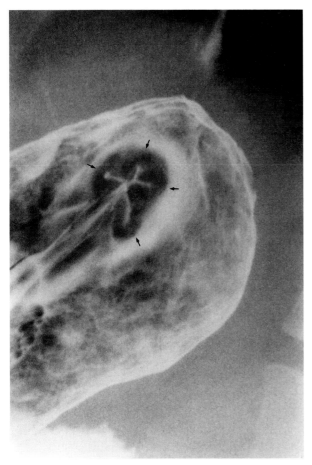

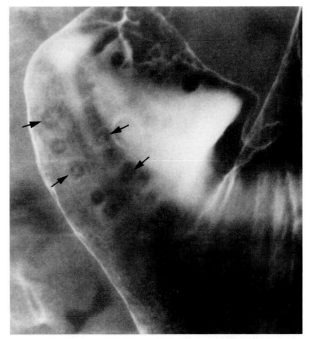

Figure 6.32 Erosive gastritis caused by aspirin. Spot radiograph of the distal gastric antrum shows numerous punctate collections of barium surrounded by radiolucent halos of edema (representative erosions are identified by arrows).

Figure 6.31 Normal gastric cardia. A "rosette" of barium-etched lines defines the gastric cardia. The esophagus is slightly protruding into the stomach, accounting for the radiolucent mass effect (arrows).

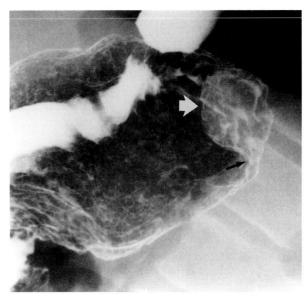

miss. Mallory–Weiss tears are linear ulcers that will be confused on barium studies with barium-etched lines arising from normal rugal folds. Arteriovenous malformations are flat lesions that are not detected on an upper GI series because they neither alter the areae gastricae pattern of the stomach nor protrude or depress the lumen. Double contrast studies are about 85% accurate in detecting duodenal ulcers (Figures 6.34 and 6.35). Barium studies will detect almost all ulcers in a duodenal bulb that is not scarred. Barium studies may, however miss an acute ulcer in a scarred, sacculated duodenal bulb.

Figure 6.33 Gastrointestinal stromal tumor. Spot radiograph of the gastric fundus shows a round, sessile mass (white arrow) protruding from the posterior wall. Abrupt margins (black arrow) with the lumen are seen. This is the typical appearance of a submucosal mass.

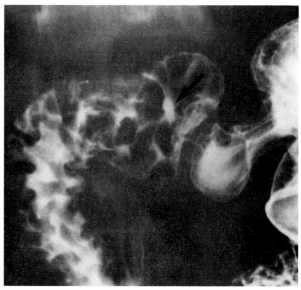

Figure 6.34 Ulcer, posterior wall of the duodenum. Spot radiograph obtained with the patient in a left posterior oblique position shows an 8-mm oblong barium collection (arrow). Thick, lobulated folds radiate toward the ulcer.

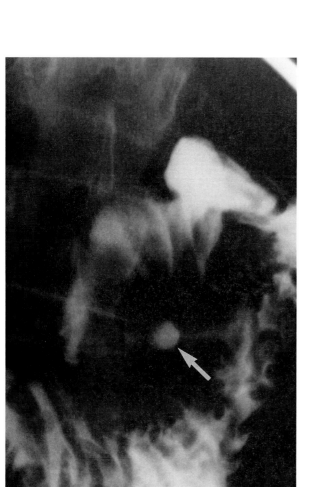

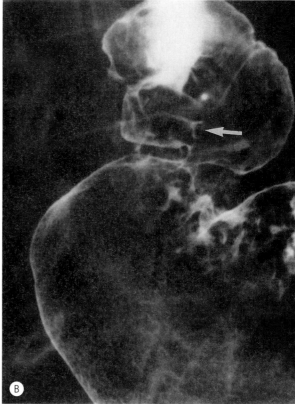

Figure 6.35 Ulcer, anterior wall of the duodenum. (A) Spot radiograph obtained with the patient in a prone right anterior oblique position (face down), results in barium filling a 5-mm niche (arrow). (B) With the patient in a left anterior oblique position (face up), the barium falls out of the ulcer leaving a barium-etched ring shadow (arrow). Note the areae gastricae pattern in the gastric antrum (reproduced with permission from Rubesin SE. *Principles of Performing a Double Contrast Upper Gastrointestinal Series*. Westbury, NY, E-Z-EM; 2000: 1–29, Fig. 32).

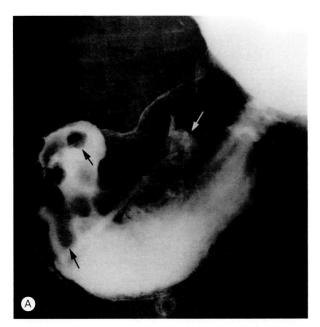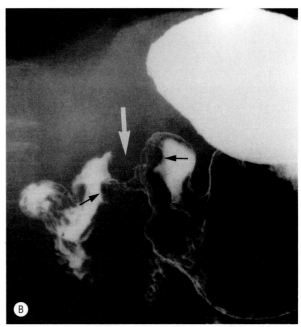

Figure 6.36 Gastric cancer missed at endoscopy. An elderly man was post-radiation therapy for pharyngeal cancer and could not swallow. This patient had a feeding gastrostomy tube (white arrow in A) placed 3 weeks before this upper GI. The barium study was performed through the gastrostomy tube. (A) Spot radiograph of the distal gastric body and proximal gastric antrum obtained with the patient in a supine position shows the gastrostomy tube. Large nodules of mucosa are seen in the proximal gastric antrum (representative nodules identified by black arrows). No gastric emptying was yet seen. (B) Spot radiograph of distal gastric antrum and duodenum obtained with the patient in the right lateral position shows a circumferentially narrowed distal antrum and pylorus (long arrow) with an irregular contour. The tumor proximal and distal to the annular narrowing has shelf-like margins (short arrows).

For chronic upper abdominal pain, however, barium studies are the equal of endoscopy in detection of gastric ulcers and the equal, if not better, in the detection of gastric cancers (Figure 6.36). The radiographic criteria for a benign gastric ulcer are a round or ovoid niche that protrudes from the lumen, with or without a smooth ulcer collar, with smooth straight folds radiating toward or to the edge of the ulcer (Figures 6.37 and 6.38). No mass effect, mucosal nodularity, or irregular, nodular, or clubbed folds are seen. These radiographic criteria for a benign ulcer are met in two thirds of patients with gastric ulcers, and in these patients endoscopy is not necessary. A follow-up examination 6 to 8 weeks after treatment may be performed to demonstrate healing and confirm the diagnosis of benign ulcer. When the radiographic criteria for a malignant ulcer are met, more than 95% of these lesions are malignant (Figure 6.39). The radiographic findings are equivocal in only about 30% of patients with gastric ulcers, and in this situation either barium or endoscopic follow-up after therapy or immediate endoscopy is required.

In Japan, early gastric cancers are detected almost equally by barium studies or by endoscopic examination (95.3% versus 95.8% respectively). In

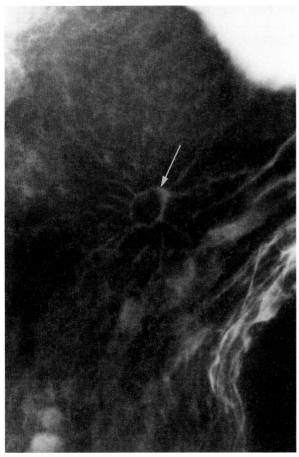

Figure 6.37 Small gastric ulcer. Barium has etched the margin of the ulcer, depicted as a ring-shadow (arrow). Smooth, straight folds radiate to the ulcer's edge (reproduced with permission from Rubesin SE, Laufer I. Pictorial glossary of double contrast radiology. In Gore RM, Levine MS, Laufer I (eds) *Textbook of Gastrointestinal Radiology*. Philadelphia, WB Saunders; 1994: 50–80, Fig. 5.26A).

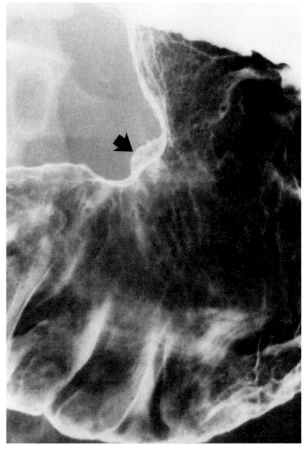

Figure 6.38 Ulcer at the incisura angularis seen in profile. A barium-etched ulcer (arrow) protrudes from the expected luminal contour at the incisura angularis (reproduced with permission from Rubesin SE, Laufer I. Pictorial glossary of double contrast radiology. In Gore RM, Levine MS, Laufer I (eds) *Textbook of Gastrointestinal Radiology*. Philadelphia, WB Saunders, 1994; 50–80: Fig. 5.15C).

the US, early gastric cancers comprise only 5% to 10% of cancers detected (see Figure 6.13), because patients are only studied when they are symptomatic. Barium studies are superior to endoscopy in evaluating patients with linitis plastica, because the majority of this type of tumor is submucosal (Figure 6.40).

There is very poor correlation between symptoms, endoscopic findings, and results of biopsy in patients with gastritis. Given the lack of consensus with what to do with patients with *Helicobacter pylori* gastritis, a combination of a barium examination with serologic testing for *H. pylori* may be a cost-effective way to study patients with chronic abdominal pain. Barium studies can only suggest a

diagnosis of *H. pylori* gastritis, based on a prominent areae gastricae pattern, enlarged lobulated folds, or a lymphoid follicular pattern. A double contrast examination will demonstrate most MALTomas (Figure 6.41).

Small-bowel studies

The small intestine is a difficult area to evaluate, either by enteroscopy or by per-oral barium studies. The length and tortuosity of the mesenteric small bowel combined with peristalsis and "telescoping" of the small intestine make endoscopy very

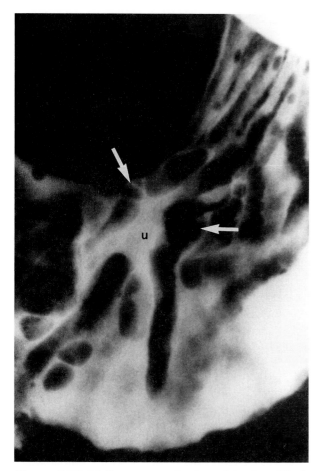

Figure 6.39 Malignant gastric ulcer. A barium-filled ulcer crater (u) is surrounded by coarsely lobulated nodules and nodular folds (arrows) (reproduced with permission from Rubesin SE, Laufer I. Pictorial glossary of double contrast radiology. In Gore RM, Levine MS, Laufer I (eds) *Textbook of Gastrointestinal Radiology*. Philadelphia, WB Saunders, 1994; 50–80: Fig. 5.26B).

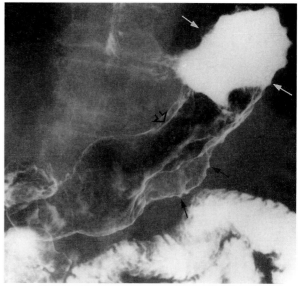

Figure 6.40 Linitis plastica. Diffuse narrowing of the gastric fundus and body is seen. The contour is slightly irregular (arrows). Despite the diffuse narrowing, the mucosa of the gastric body is smooth (open arrow), indicating the predominant submucosal nature of the tumor (reproduced with permission from Rubesin SE, Laufer I. Pictorial glossary of double contrast radiology. In Gore RM, Levine MS, Laufer I (eds) *Textbook of Gastrointestinal Radiology*. Philadelphia, WB Saunders, 1994; 50–80: Fig. 5.22).

difficult. The fluid in the small intestine creates an environment hostile to barium suspensions. High-density barium designed for use in the esophagus and stomach is not effective in evaluating overlapping small-intestinal loops. The high-density barium is too dense and pelvic loops are easily obscured by the dense barium. Therefore the radiologist cannot effectively combine a double contrast upper gastrointestinal series with a small-bowel follow-through. If the small bowel is to be effectively examined, barium designed for the small bowel should be used.

During a small-bowel follow-through, the patient drinks 500 to 1000 mL of "thin barium." Distension of the small bowel is limited by the rate of barium

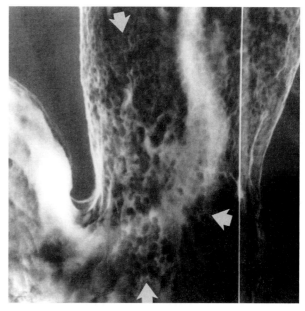

Figure 6.41 MALToma. The polygonal areae gastricae pattern of the stomach has been replaced by a 4-cm focal area of mucosal nodularity (arrows) at the incisura angularis.

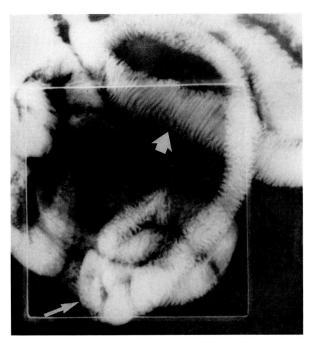

Figure 6.42 Normal small-bowel follow-through. Spot radiograph from a small-bowel follow-through examination performed with barium appropriate for the small intestine. Some loops are distended and their folds are easily seen (thick arrow). Other loops are overlapped (long arrow) and show little morphologic detail.

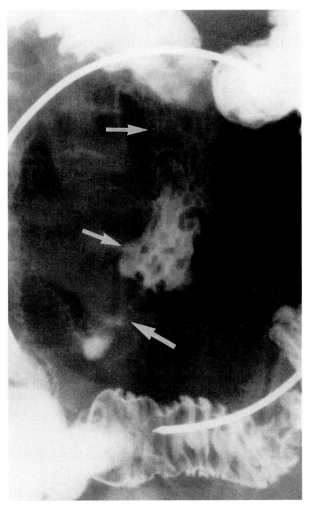

Figure 6.44 Cobblestoning (short arrows) in Crohn's disease. Spot radiograph of the lower ileum shows polygonal-shaped radiolucent nodules ("cobblestones") separated by transversely and longitudinally oriented barium-filled grooves. The barium-filled grooves are the knife-like clefts demonstrated at pathology, the cobblestones are the relatively uninflamed mucosa between the clefts. A stricture (long arrow) is seen distal to the cobblestoning.

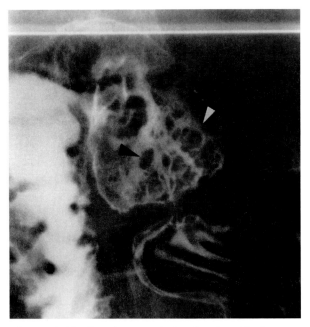

Figure 6.43 Gastric metaplasia, duodenal bulb. Spot radiograph of the duodenal bulb obtained with compression shows many polygonal radiolucent filling defects (arrowheads) in the barium pool, clumped together in the juxtapyloric duodenal bulb.

exiting from the stomach at the pylorus and the speed of small-bowel transit. Luminal distension will be poor if pyloric emptying is slow or if small-bowel transit is too fast. A small-bowel follow-through relies on fluoroscopically guided compression spot images (Figures 6.42–6.44). The radiologist splays apart the overlapping small-bowel loops by compression and palpation to evaluate for pliability of the walls, fixation of loops, and movement of filling defects (bubbles, food debris, and pills) in the barium column. Overheads

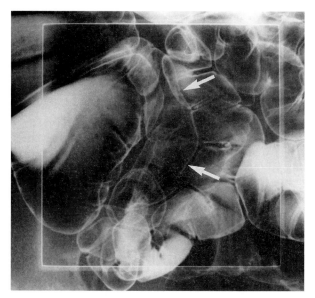

Figure 6.45 Per-oral pneumocolon. After thin barium has passed into the colon and after intravenous glucagon has been used to relax the colon and ileocecal valve, air is insufflated into the colon. Air refluxes into the terminal ileum (arrows) in 85% of patients resulting in air-contrast views of the mucosa.

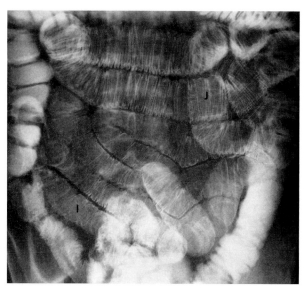

Figure 6.46 Normal enteroclysis. Overhead image obtained at the end of the study shows diffuse distension of the small intestine. The number, depth, and thickness of valvulae conniventes is greater in the jejunum (J) than in the ileum (I). The luminal diameter of the jejunum is greater than that of the ileum.

of the small bowel are of little value except to show the big picture. Spot images are of paramount importance. Air may be insufflated into the colon after barium reaches the transverse colon and an air-contrast examination of the terminal ileum may be performed (per-oral pneumocolon). This examination results in excellent visualization of the terminal ileum (Figure 6.45).

Small-bowel enema (enteroclysis) is a technique where the radiologist passes a catheter either through the nose or mouth to the first loop of the jejunum. This can be an uncomfortable procedure that many patients want to undergo only once. Therefore, the referring clinician must judiciously select patients for enteroclysis. Light sedation may be used, but the patient must be awake enough to turn on the fluoroscopic table or avoid aspiration if they vomit. Catheter passage to the jejunum is successful in about 85% of patients.

One advantage of enteroclysis over small-bowel follow-through is that the catheter bypasses the pylorus, allowing the radiologist to fully distend the small bowel with contrast agents (Figure 6.46). An unspoken advantage of enteroclysis is that the radiologist remains in the fluoroscopic suite, palpating the small intestine, following both the barium and methylcellulose columns. Enteroclysis results in superior visualization of the luminal contour and the valvulae conniventes (Figures 6.47 and 6.48).

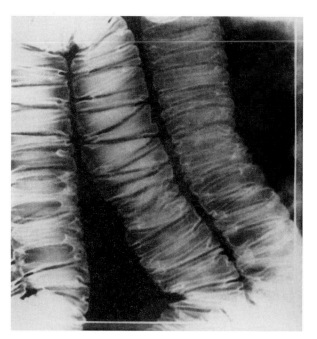

Figure 6.47 Normal small-bowel folds. The valvulae conniventes (arrows identifying two representative folds) are perpendicular or slightly angled to the longitudinal axis of the small bowel. The valvulae are thicker and taller in the jejunum than the ileum.

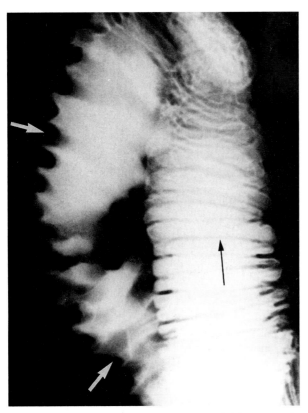

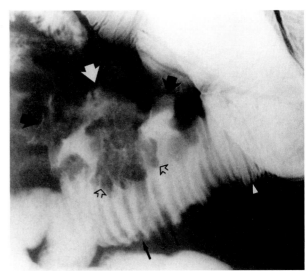

Figure 6.48 Normal versus abnormal folds. Normal mid-small-bowel folds (black arrow) are contrasted with folds enlarged by an infiltrating lymphoma (white arrows).

Figure 6.49 Cavitary lymphoma. A large barium-filled cavity is identified (thick arrows). Coarsely lobulated nodules (open arrows) of lymphoma disrupt the mesenteric border of the small bowel. Smooth thick valvulae conniventes (thin arrows) are the result of circumferential extension of the lymphoma in the submucosal space. For comparison, an arrowhead identifies a normal-sized fold (reproduced with permission from Rubesin SE, Laufer I. Pictorial glossary of double contrast radiology. In Gore RM, Levine MS, Laufer I (eds) *Textbook of Gastrointestinal Radiology*. Philadelphia, WB Saunders, 1994; 50–80: Fig. 5.24).

In some patients, enteroclysis results in better visualization of pelvic loops. In other patients, the pelvic loops and the terminal ileum are better visualized during small bowel follow-through.

Enteroclysis is superior to small-bowel follow-through in detection of short lesions, (e.g. tumors (Figures 6.49–6.51), skip lesions in Crohn's disease, and NSAID strictures) and diseases that affect mucosal folds (Figure 6.52). A small-bowel follow-through is probably adequate to evaluate patients with diseases with long segments of abnormality, for example Crohn's disease (Figure 6.53) or

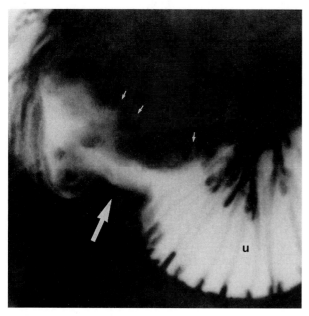

Figure 6.50 Adenocarcinoma of the distal jejunum. A 3-cm focal annular narrowing (large arrow) of the small intestine is present, with shelf-like margins and irregular mucosa. Barium tracks into the interstices of the tumor (small arrows). Low-grade obstruction is implied by dilatation of the "upstream" bowel (u) (reproduced with permission from Herlinger H, Rubesin SE. Obstruction. In: Gore RM, Levine MS, Laufer I (eds) *Textbook of Gastrointestinal Radiology*. Philadelphia, WB Saunders, 1994; 931–966: Fig. 52.41).

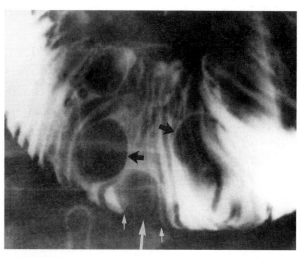

Figure 6.51 Metastatic melanoma. Many submucosal lesions are seen. En face, the tumors are well-circumscribed, round with a smooth surface (black arrows). In profile, there is focal loss of the luminal contour (large white arrow). Abrupt angles to the luminal contour (small white arrows) are seen (reproduced with permission from Rubesin SE, Laufer I. Pictorial glossary of double contrast radiology. In: Gore RM, Levine MS, Laufer I (eds) *Textbook of Gastrointestinal Radiology*. Philadelphia, WB Saunders, 1994; 50–80: Fig. 5.12).

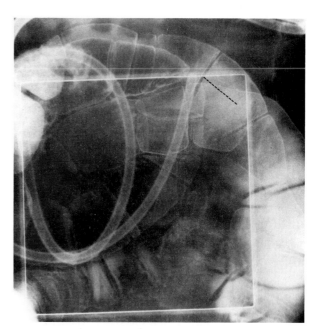

Figure 6.52 Celiac disease. Spot radiograph of the jejunum obtained during enteroclysis shows one to two normal-sized folds per inch (1 inch is demonstrated by the dashed line). Normally, the proximal jejunum has four to seven folds per inch. The loss of valvulae conniventes reflects the loss of surface area in celiac disease.

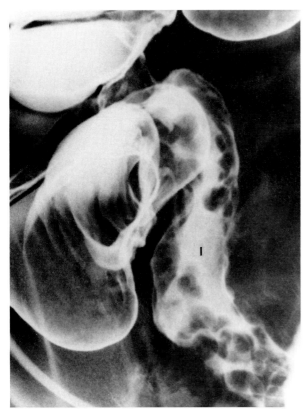

Figure 6.53 Crohn's disease demonstrated on per-oral pneumocolon. Coarsely lobulated mucosa is seen in the terminal ileum (I).

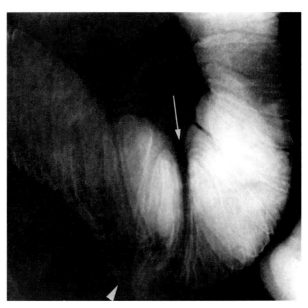

Figure 6.54 Adhesions. An adhesive band appears as a thin radiolucency (long arrow) narrowing the lumen of the ileum. Abrupt angulation of the contour of the bowel (arrowhead) and tethering of folds toward the angulation are signs indicative of adhesions.

ischemia. Clinicians should be careful when ordering enteroclysis in patients with gastrointestinal bleeding. Patients with truly unexplained chronic gastrointestinal bleeding are candidates for enteroclysis. In patients with acute gastrointestinal bleeding, debilitated patients, or patients on coumadin, the clinician should consider a small-bowel follow-through to look for large lesions or long segments of ischemia or hemorrhage before ordering an enteroclysis. This radiologist is not certain whether a small-bowel enema or follow-through is a superior test in patients with suspected adhesions (Figure 6.54). Overdistension of the small

bowel achieved during enteroclysis results in the detection of more adhesions than during small-bowel follow-through. The follow-through is more "physiologic", however, giving more reliable information if an adhesion is obstructive.

Colon studies

A double contrast barium enema is a fluoroscopically guided study that emphasizes spot images of the colon in multiple projections, with

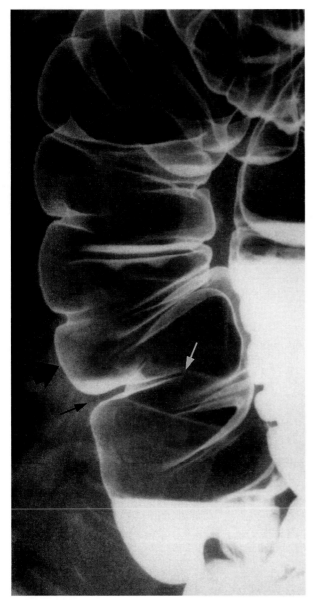

Figure 6.55 Normal colonic morphology. Spot radiograph of the ascending colon obtained with the patient in an erect position shows the haustral sacculations (representative sac identified by thick black arrow). The interhaustral folds (representative fold identified in profile by a thin black arrow and en face by a thin white arrow) do not cross the entire lumen. The colonic surface is smooth.

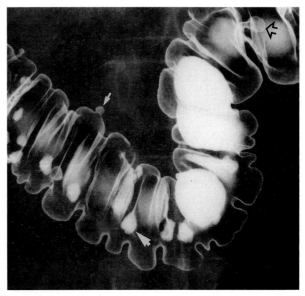

Figure 6.56 Spot radiograph of the mid-transverse colon shows many barium-filled diverticula en face (large arrow). When barium spills out and the diverticula fill with air, in profile the diverticula appear as barium-etched sacs (small arrow) and en face as ring shadows (open arrow) (reproduced with permission from Rubesin SE, Laufer I. Diverticular disease. In: Levine MS, Rubesin SE, Laufer I (eds) *Double Contrast Gastrointestinal Radiology*. Philadelphia, WB Saunders, 2000; 471–493: Fig. 14.9).

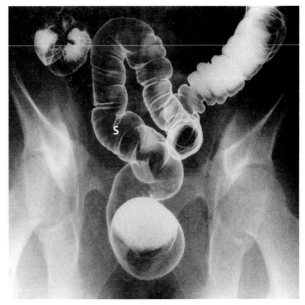

Figure 6.57 Prone angled overhead view of normal sigmoid colon. This view "opens up" the distal sigmoid colon (S) (reproduced with permission from Rubesin SE, Laufer I. Double contrast barium enema: technical aspects. In: Levine MS, Rubesin SE, Laufer I (eds) *Double Contrast Gastrointestinal Radiology*. Philadelphia, WB Saunders, 2000; 331–356; Fig. 11.25).

adequate luminal distension and barium coating (Figures 6.55 and 6.56). Overhead views are primarily of value in projections the radiologist cannot obtain (decubitus or angled views) or to show the "big picture" and the overall location and distribution of lesions (Figures 6.57 and 6.58).

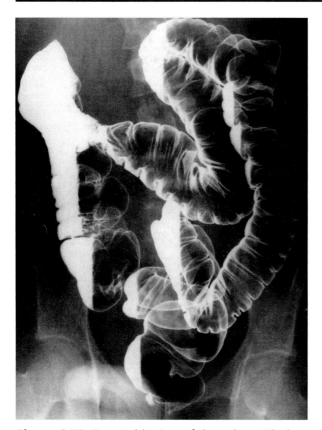

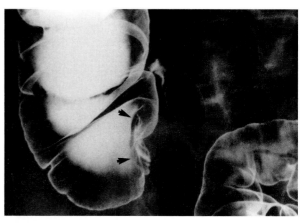

Figure 6.59 Middle-aged woman with vague abdominal complaints. Colonoscopy had demonstrated erythematous cecal mucosa. The barium enema demonstrates the value of barium studies in extrinsic diseases. Extrinsic mass impression on the medial border of the base of the cecum (arrows) is compatible with an appendiceal mass, most likely from appendicitis. An appendiceal abscess was found at surgery.

Figure 6.58 Cross table view of the colon with the patient lying with their right side down (right lateral decubitus view) (reproduced with permission from Rubesin SE, Laufer I (eds) Double contrast barium enema: technical aspects. In: Levine MS, Rubesin SE, Laufer I (eds) *Double Contrast Gastrointestinal Radiology*. Philadelphia, WB Saunders, 2000; 331–356; Fig. 11.224).

In the past several years barium enemas have been ignored in articles in major journals. The reasons for the decline of barium enema have little to do with the technique itself, but are connected with the economic and practice interests of radiologists, gastroenterologists, and internists. Radiologists have little incentive to perform quality barium enemas. All barium studies are labor intensive. Reimbursement rates for barium studies are poor. For comparison purposes, the 2002 Pennsylvania Medicare reimbursement rate of the professional fee for a contrast-enhanced CT of the abdomen and the pelvis is $129, whereas the professional fee for a double contrast barium enema is $52. A radiologist can interpret two CT scans in the time it takes to perform and interpret one double contrast barium enema. Thus, a radio-logist can generate about five times the income spending a day reading CT scans compared to the income from a day performing barium enemas. The radiologist will not have worn the 15 to 25 pound lead "apron" required in fluoroscopy nor have had to insert enema tips into patients' rectums. This lack of incentive to perform barium enemas has led to a nationwide decline in interest in performing barium enemas and a corresponding decline in the quality of studies performed.

Double contrast barium enemas are superior to endoscopy in diseases that involve the extramucosal portion of colon or the serosa (Figure 6.59). If there is a question that intraperitoneal implants (Figure 6.60) or endometriosis (Figure 6.61) involves the colon, a barium enema is a superior examination to endoscopy. A barium enema is superior in

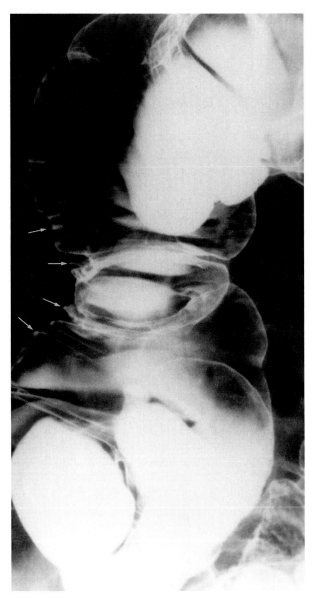

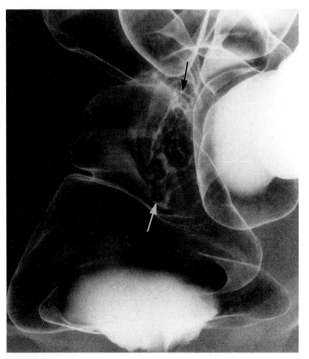

Figure 6.61 Endometriosis involving the rectosigmoid junction. The colonic mucosa is thrown into smooth, undulating (pleated) folds (arrows) when the endometrial tissue invades the serosa of the colon (reproduced with permission from Rubesin SE, Laufer I. Pictorial glossary of double contrast radiology. In: Gore RM, Levine MS, Laufer I (eds) *Textbook of Gastrointestinal Radiology*. Philadelphia, WB Saunders, 1994, 50–80, Fig. 5.38).

Figure 6.60 Ovarian carcinoma with intraperitoneal implants in the right paracolic gutter involving ascending colon. The right lateral border of the ascending colon has a spiculated contour (arrows) (reproduced with permission from Rubesin SE, Laufer I. Tumors of the colon. In: Levine MS, Rubesin SE, Laufer I (eds) *Double Contrast Gastrointestinal Radiology*. Philadelphia, WB Saunders, 2000; 357–416; Fig. 12.92F).

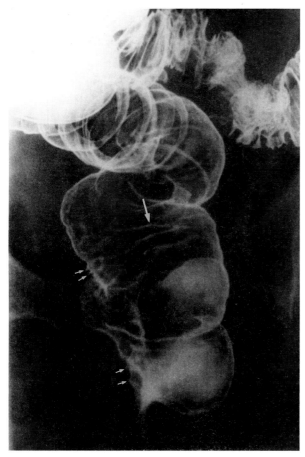

Figure 6.62 Prostatic carcinoma invading the rectum. The rectal ampulla is flattened on the right lateral wall. The contour is spiculated (short arrows). The mucosa is thrown into folds (arrow) radiating toward the desmoplastic process caused by infiltrating prostatic cancer (reproduced with permission from Rubesin SE, Levine MS, Bezzi M, *et al*. Rectal involvement by prostatic carcinoma: radiographic findings. *AJR* 1989; 152: 53–57, Fig. 1A).

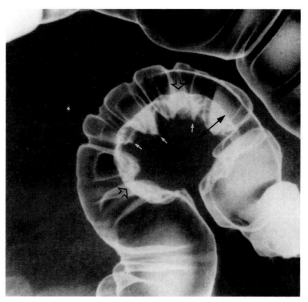

Figure 6.63 Endometrioma causing obstructive symptoms. The sigmoid colon is narrowed by a smooth-surfaced mass (open arrows) on the inferior border. The wall is thickened (double arrow) by the desmoplastic reaction and reactive muscular hyperplasia to the endometrial tissue invading the muscularis propria. Spiculation of the contour (short arrows) typical of "serosal desmoplastic disease" is present (reproduced with permission from Rubesin SE, Laufer I. Tumors of the colon. In: Levine MS, Rubesin SE, Laufer I (eds) *Double Contrast Gastrointestinal Radiology*. Philadelphia, WB Saunders, 2000; 357–416; Fig. 12.93).

demonstrating direct extension of inflammatory or neoplastic disease invading the colon (Figure 6.62). Barium enema is superior to endoscopy in evaluating patients with chronic lower abdominal pain (Figure 6.63). Computed tomography has replaced barium studies for the detection of acute diverticulitis because of the rare, but theoretic, risk of perforation and barium-induced peritonitis. Nevertheless, barium enema is excellent at showing either the pericolic abscess directly (Figure

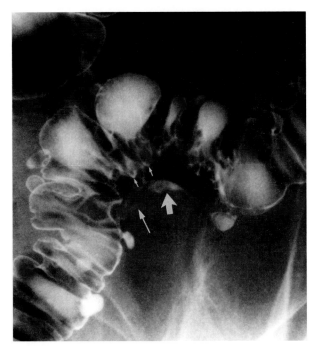

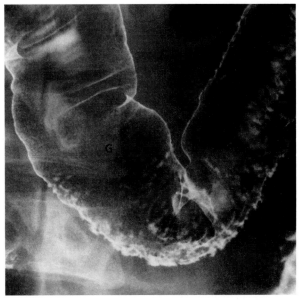

Figure 6.64 Elderly surgeon with chronic left lower quadrant pain. Spot image of the sigmoid colon shows barium enema findings typical for diverticulitis. Barium tracks outside the luminal contour forming a 1-cm flame-shaped extraluminal collection (thick arrow). One of the pericolic fistulas is identified by the long arrow. The colon adjacent to the pericolic abscess is spiculated (representative spicules identified by short arrows). The colonic mucosa is smooth, diverticula can be seen (reproduced with permission from Rubesin SE, Laufer I. Diverticular disease. In: Levine MS, Rubesin SE, Laufer I (eds) *Double Contrast Gastrointestinal Radiology*. Philadelphia, WB Saunders, 2000; 471–493; Fig. 14.24).

Figure 6.65 Ulcerative colitis with a transition zone in mid-transverse colon. The most proximal colonic surface is smooth. Granular mucosa (G) of mild ulcerative colitis is seen. Larger deep "collar button" ulcers are seen distally (representative ulcer is identified by an arrow). The deep ulcers arise on a background of granular mucosa.

6.64) or the secondary effects of the pericolic inflammatory process upon the wall of the colon. Either a barium enema or colonoscopy, however, should be performed as a follow-up, after treatment study in patients with a CT diagnosis of diverticulitis to make sure that CT has not mistaken a perforated colon cancer from diverticulitis. Barium studies are excellent in demonstrating the distribution of inflammatory bowel disease (Figure 6.65). A double contrast barium enema will

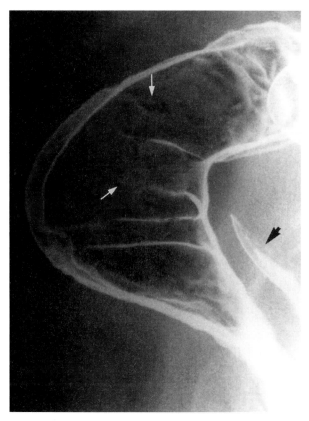

Figure 6.66 Crohn's disease. Multiple aphthoid ulcers are manifest as 1 to 4-mm punctate, ovoid and triangular barium collections surrounded by radiolucent halos of edema (representative aphthoid ulcers are identified by white arrows). Barium in the vagina (black arrow) is from an anoperineal fistula just off the film.

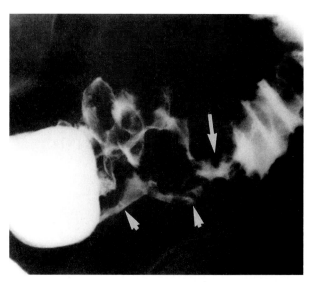

Figure 6.67 Crohn's colitis. This young woman carried an 8-year diagnosis of ulcerative colitis. No prior barium studies had been performed. An endoscope could not be passed through a stricture. A barium enema was requested to exclude a neoplasm arising in ulcerative colitis. Spot radiograph shows a colo-colic fistula (short arrows) entering the sigmoid colon in several places. A focal narrowing of the sigmoid colon is seen (long arrow). The mucosa is mildly nodular. A diagnosis of Crohn's disease was made.

demonstrate the terminal ileum in about 85% of patients. In patients with Crohn's colitis (Figure 6.66), barium studies are superior in the demonstration of fistulas and strictures. Not infrequently, a patient will have a diagnosis of inflammatory bowel disease changed by the results of a barium enema (Figure 6.67).

When radiologists are interested and trained in the performance of barium enemas, double contrast barium enema equals endoscopy in the detection of

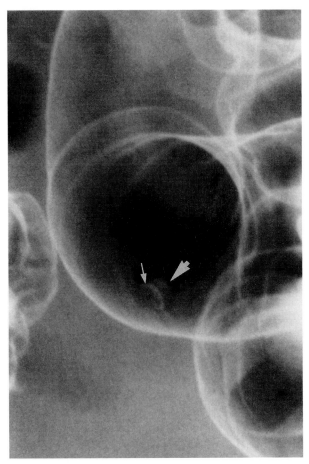

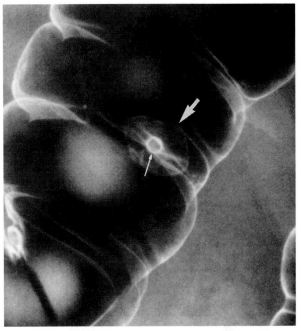

Figure 6.69 A 1-cm pedunculated tubular adenoma seen en face. The head of the polyp is seen as a barium etched line (thick arrow) surrounding a finely nodular area of increased density. The stalk of the polyp is the inner ring shadow (thin arrow) (reproduced with permission from Rubesin SE. Tumors of the colon. *Semin Colon Rectal Surg* 1993; 4: 94–111, Fig. 5).

Figure 6.68 A 5-mm tubular adenoma distal sigmoid. A "bowler hat" or "hat" sign is seen, representing a small polyp. The top of the hat (large arrow) represents the top of the polyp, the brim of the hat (small arrow) represents the base of the polyp (reproduced with permission from Rubesin SE. Tumors of the colon. *Semin Colon Rectal Surg* 1993; 4: 94–111, Fig. 2).

colon cancers and approaches endoscopy in the detection of polyps larger than 1 cm (Figures 6.68–6.75). When we performed a quality assurance study at our hospital from 1989 to 1992, using a barium preparation inferior to the one we now use, double contrast barium enemas diagnosed 93% of colon cancers and endoscopy diagnosed 92% of colon cancers, excluding regions of the colon not reached by the endoscope. Using an improved barium suspension, we have an even higher detection rate for colonic cancers today. If a study performed in Indiana is correct, however, the double

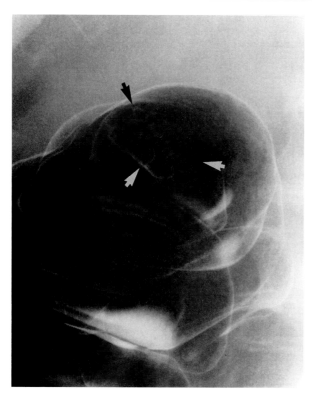

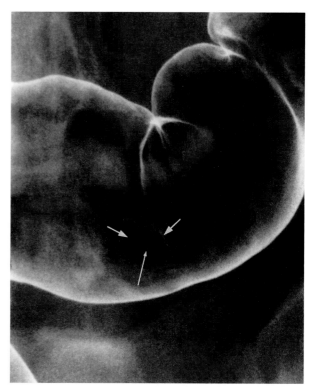

Figure 6.70 Carpet lesion of the hepatic flexure. A 1.5-cm flat lesion is manifest as a focal reticular pattern of barium-filled grooves (arrows). This was a tubulovillous adenoma (reproduced with permission from Rubesin SE. Tumors of the colon. *Semin Colon Rectal Surg* 1993; 4: 94–111, Fig. 9).

Figure 6.72 Umbilicated microinvasive colon cancer. Close-up view of the sigmoid colon demonstrates a 7-mm finely nodular lesion (short arrows) with a central umbilication (long arrow). The carcinoma just extended into the upper layer of the submucosa. This lesion was prospectively identified on barium study (reproduced with permission from Rubesin SE, Laufer I. Tumors of the colon. In: Levine MS, Rubesin SE, Laufer I (eds) *Double Contrast Gastrointestinal Radiology*. Philadelphia, WB Saunders, 2000; 357–416: Fig. 12.18).

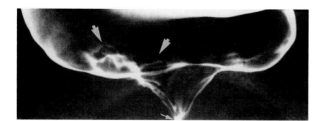

Figure 6.71 Tubulovillous adenoma missed on endoscopy. A 1.5 cm focal area of nodular mucosa (large arrows) is seen 1.5 cm proximal to the anorectal junction (small arrow). This soft lesion was not felt on digital examination and was not detected on endoscopy (reproduced with permission from Rubesin SE, Laufer I. Tumors of the colon. In: Levine MS, Rubesin SE, Laufer I (eds) *Double Contrast Gastrointestinal Radiology*. Philadelphia, WB Saunders, 2000; 357–416: Fig. 12.17C).

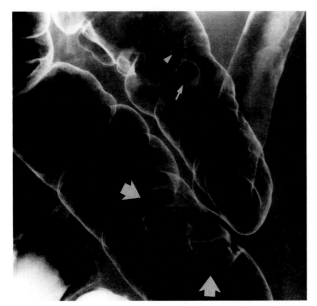

Figure 6.73 Synchronous tubular adenoma of the sigmoid colon and adenocarcinoma of the proximal rectum. A 3-cm polypoid mass with nodular mucosa is seen in the proximal rectum (large arrows). The head (small arrow) and stalk (arrowhead) of a pedunculated polyp are etched in white by barium (reproduced with permission from Rubesin SE. Tumors of the colon. *Semin Colon Rectal Surg* 1993; 4: 94–111, Fig. 11).

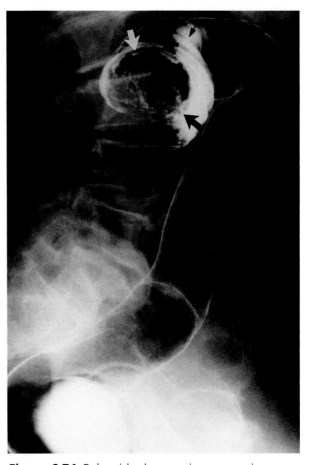

Figure 6.74 Polypoid adenocarcinoma causing intussusception. An overhead view shows a 5-cm coarsely nodular mass (large arrows). Parallel folds of the colonic mucosa (thin arrow) indicate foreshortening because of intussusception. No colon fills proximal to the tumor (reproduced with permission from Rubesin SE, Laufer I. Pictorial glossary of double contrast radiology. In Gore RM, Levine MS, Laufer I (eds) *Textbook of Gastrointestinal Radiology*. Philadelphia, WB Saunders, 1994; 50–80: Fig. 13A).

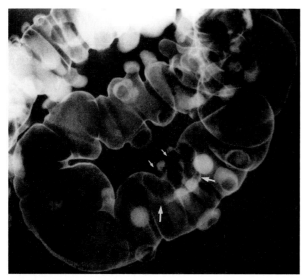

Figure 6.75 Colonic carcinoma arising in an area of diverticulosis. The contour of sigmoid colon is focally disrupted (small arrows) and a polypoid mass (large arrows) projects into the lumen (reproduced with permission from Rubesin SE, Laufer I. Diverticular disease. In: Levine MS, Rubesin SE, Laufer I (eds) *Double Contrast Gastrointestinal Radiology*. Philadelphia, WB Saunders, 2000; 471–493: Fig.14.41).

contrast detection rate for colonic cancer performed by general radiologists is about 85%. Even with this rate, barium enema is more cost effective than colonoscopy, given colonoscopy's risk of perforation and hemorrhage, and the low rate of cancer in patients without risk factors (about 1 in 400). Even with the cancer detection rate of 85%, a barium enema is still a superior test to flexible sigmoidoscopy. At our hospital 45% of colon cancers are out of reach of the flexible sigmoidoscope. Therefore, even if the flexible sigmoidoscope reached the splenic flexure in each patient, 45% of colon cancers would be missed.

Further reading

TEXTBOOKS:

Gore RM, Levine MS (eds). *Textbook of Gastrointestinal Radiology*. Philadelphia: WB Saunders; 2000:815–837

Herlinger H, Maglinte DDT, Birnbaum BA (eds). *Clinical Imaging of the small intestine*, 2nd ed. New York: Springer; 1999.

Levine MS, Rubesin SE, Laufer I (eds). *Double contrast gastrointestinal radiology*. Philadelphia, WB Saunders, 2000

Rubesin SE (ed). *Gastrointestinal Learning File*. Reston, VA: The American College of Radiology, 2002

ARTICLES:

Eddy DM. Screening for colorectal cancer. *Ann Intern Med* 1990; 113:373–384.

Glick S, Wagner JL, Johnson CD. Cost-effectiveness of double-contrast barium enema screening for colorectal cancer. *AJR* 1998; 170:629–636

Levine MS, Chu P, Furth EE, Rubesin SE, Laufer I, Herlinger H. Carcinoma of the esophagus and esophagogastric junction: sensitivity of radiographic diagnosis. *AJR* 1997; 168:1423–1426

Levine MS, Rubesin SE, Herlinger H, Laufer I: Double contrast upper gastrointestinal examination: technique and interpretation. *Radiology* 1988; 168:593–602.

Levine MS, Rubesin SE. Radiologic investigation of dysphagia. *AJR* 1990; 154:1157–1163

Low VHS, Levine MS, Rubesin SE, Laufer I, Herlinger H. Diagnosis of gastric carcinoma: sensitivity of double-contrast barium studies. *AJR* 1994; 162:329–334.

McCarthy PA, Rubesin SE, Levine MS, Langlotz CT, Laufer I, Furth EE, Herlinger H. Colonic cancer: morphology detected with barium enema examination versus histopathologic stage. Radiology 1995; 197:683–687

Moch A, Herlinger H, Kochman ML, Levine MS, Rubesin SE, Laufer I. Enteroclysis in the evaluation of obscure gastrointestinal bleeding. *AJR* 1994; 163:1381–1384

Rubesin SE, Gilchrist AM, Bronner M., Saul SH, Herlinger H, Grumbach K, Levine MS, Laufer I. Non-Hodgkin lymphoma of the small intestine. RadioGraphics 1990; 10:985–998

Rubesin SE, Jessurun J, Robertson D, Jones B, Bosma JF, Donner MW. Lines of the pharynx. RadioGraphics 1987; 7:217–237

Rubesin SE, Laufer I. Pictorial review: principles of double contrast pharyngography. Dysphagia 1991; 6:170–178

Chapter 7

Clinical Application of Magnetic Resonance Imaging in the Abdomen

Dushyant Sahani, Anil Shetty and Sanjay Saini

Introduction

Magnetic resonance imaging plays an important role in the evaluation of the abdomen and the pelvis. It delineates the anatomical morphology and, to some extent, investigates functional aspects as well. Its most important role is in the diagnostic evaluation of patients with known or suspected cancer. Compared with other imaging studies, MRI provides intrinsically higher soft-tissue contrast resolution and therefore is an attractive alternative to CT, especially when the use of iodinated contrast material is contraindicated. In addition, because MRI is devoid of ionizing radiation it can be used safely in children, young adults, and pregnant women.

Strengths of magnetic resonance imaging

The strengths of MRI include intrinsic soft-tissue contrast, multiplanar imaging capability, and high sensitivity for the presence or absence of contrast enhancement. Other important strengths of MRI include its effectiveness at demonstrating non-contour-deforming disease such as small pancreatic ductal adenocarcinomas, and its ability to delineate and characterize a variety of focal liver lesions. An important hallmark of MRI is its safety. Many patients who undergo MRI do so because they are allergic to iodine-based contrast agents and therefore are not ideal candidates for CT, or they have elevated serum creatinine, raising the fear that iodine-based contrast agents will adversely affect renal function. These two patient groups are best studied by MRI because of the safe nature of the contrast agents used in conjunction with this technique. No patient preparation is required before the procedure.

Weaknesses of magnetic resonance imaging

Magnetic resonance imaging does not show up some critical factors such as receptor binding (important in drug studies), or functional features such as blood flow or electrical activity. It has no dynamic ability (except to image structural changes which, of course, occur over weeks or years). The MRI technique can induce tissue heating from the radio-frequency field, and electrical currents in conductive tissues from the static and dynamic impressed magnetic fields (static fields induce currents because of blood flowing relative to the field).

Contraindications

Patients for whom MRI is contraindicated include those who have

1. a heart pacemaker, because of the associated risks of movement, reed switch closures, or damage
2. certain ferromagnetic implants, primarily because of the possibility of movement or dislodgment of these objects
3. metallic foreign bodies (metal silver) in their eyes
4. an aneurysm clip in their brain
5. severe claustrophobia, although more open scanners are now available and medical sedation makes the test easier to tolerate.

Currently little data exists to establish MRI risk for pregnant patients. Generally accepted procedure limits MRI use during pregnancy, especially during the first trimester, except however when the radiologist and referring physician determine that the benefit to the patient and/or fetus outweighs the potential risk. New mothers should wait 24 hours after injection of MR-contrast agents before resuming nursing.

Indications

Magnetic resonance imaging is achieving greater use in the overall evaluation of the abdomen and pelvis as radiologists and clinicians gain more experience with this technique. For example, in our practice MRI is the preferred imaging method for evaluating abdominal disease in oncology patients because of its excellent ability in detecting and characterizing liver lesions. Pelvic malignancies of all kinds are also extremely well delineated by MR, for instance gynecologic malignancies are well demonstrated using fast-scanning sequences and breath-hold imaging. In particular MRI is excellent for the evaluation of small pancreatic ductal carcinoma. It is also a very valuable investigative tool in patients who cannot tolerate iodine contrasts and who have deranged renal functions or are in renal failure.

Techniques

Magnetic resonance imaging techniques useful for examination of the abdomen

The difference between the signal intensities of diseased tissues and background tissue has to be maximized to make the disease tissues more conspicuous. For diseased tissues situated within or adjacent to fat, this is achieved by manipulating the signal intensity of fat, which can be low to high in signal intensity on both T1-weighted and T2-weighted images. Conversely, diseased tissues which are moderate to high in signal intensity, such as subacute blood or proteinaceous fluid, are more conspicuous if fat is rendered low in signal intensity with the use of fat-suppression techniques. On T2-weighted images, diseased tissues, which are low in signal intensity, such as fibrous tissue, are most conspicuous on sequences in which background fat is high in signal intensity, such as echo train spin-echo sequences. Extracellular MRI contrast agents such as gadolinium chelate may be routinely employed since they provide at least two further imaging parameters that are able to detect and characterize disease, specifically the pattern of blood delivery (i.e. capillary enhancement) and the size and/or rapidity of drainage of the interstitial fluid (interstitial enhancement).

Magnetic resonance angiography

One of the most important recent developments in body MRI has been magnetic resonance angiography. Gadolinium-enhanced three-dimensional gradient echo with effective slice thickness of less than 2 mm and 22-second data acquisition allows high-quality, non-invasive, vascular imaging.

Magnetic resonance cholangiopancreatography

The techniques used to perform MRCP are the same techniques that can be used to perform magnetic resonance urography, magnetic resonance myelography, or magnetic resonance bowel studies. Bile-duct imaging exploits the long T2 times of fluid. Hence, heavily T2-weighted fast spin-echo techniques are used. This can be done in a variety of methods including thin section 2D or 3D with MIP, or thick slab 2D without MIP in a breath-hold or non-breath-hold. The test is relatively short in duration and, if needed, can be supplemented with magnetic resonance evaluation of the liver and pancreas. By combining sequences that evaluate tissue parenchyma with magnetic resonance cholangiography, MRI is also able to provide comprehensive information of biliary tract disease, including the level of biliary obstruction, cause of obstruction, and extent of the disease process.

Applications

Liver

Computed tomography has been widely used for evaluating both focal and diffuse hepatic diseases. More recently, however, MRI has proved to be effective in detecting and characterizing hepatic abnormalities. Development of tissue-specific magnetic resonance contrast agents has further improved the accuracy of hepatic MRI. Liver evaluation is commonly undertaken in patients in whom, because of tumor type, symptoms, or serum markers, liver metastases are suspected. Live MRI is used when iodinated contrast media cannot be administered, for example when the patient has had a prior contrast reaction, or has renal insufficiency. In addition, since liver lesion detection with CT or ultrasonography is compromised in patients with fatty infiltration, MRI serves as an effective supplementary test. Ultrasound and CT remain the primary imaging studies for the liver, but MRI is often used to diagnose atypical presentations of liver lesions. Metastatic disease is a common indication for primary MRI hepatic

imaging. In fact, MRI may eventually replace CT as the first-line imaging study in metastatic disease. One reason for this is the recent approval of multiple hepatic imaging agents that allow concentrated uptake in the hepatocytes or reticuloendothelial system, thus accentuating the normal liver parenchyma and increasing the visibility of metastatic lesions.

The main goals of liver MRI are the detection and characterization of liver lesions detected on CT or ultrasound. For patients undergoing surgical therapy, hepatic vascular mapping is also undertaken to help plan liver resection or transplantation.

Benign hepatic tumors

Hemangioma Hemangioma is the most common benign liver tumor, they are often found incidentally. Hemagiomas are more common in women than in men (8:1). Typically, hemagiomas are asymtomatic with no malignant potential. Magnetic resonance imaging is useful in differentiating hemangiomas from other benign and malignant hepatic neoplasms, based on very long T2 relaxation of hemangiomas compared with other hepatic masses. Other characteristic MRI features include a sharp margin and internal homogeneity. Typical early hyperintense peripheral nodular enhancement with complete fill-in on delayed images on dynamic gadolinium-enhanced MRI of hemangiomas help in diagnosis. For possible hemangiomas less than 1.0 cm in size, the sensitivity of single photon emission computed tomography (SPECT) has been reported to range from 0% to 20%. Since small size often prohibits diagnostic characterization on MRI, biopsy or follow-up imaging to document stability are recommended. Overall sensitivity and specificity of MRI in characterizing liver hemagiomas is 90% to 95%.

Focal nodular hyperplasia The most common benign hepatocellular tumor of the liver is focal nodular hyperplasia with an incidence of 1 in 100 individuals, it is more common in women compared to men (12:1). Like hemangiomas, focal nodular hyperplasia is an asymtomatic tumor, often incidentally discovered on imaging. Unlike hepatocellular adenomas, there is no risk for malignant transformation or intraperitoneal bleeding with focal nodular hyperplasia. On unenhanced MRI, focal nodular hyperplasia often has signal intensity characteristics similar to that of the hepatic parenchyma. The central scar is hypointense on T1-weighted images and hyperintense on T2-weighted images. Gadolinium-enhanced MRI

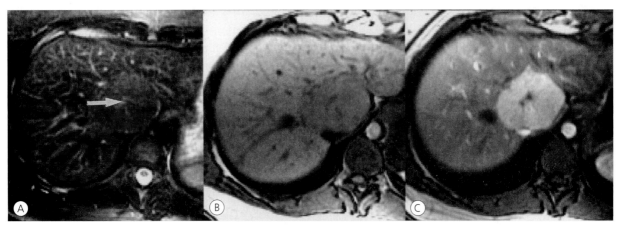

Figure 7.1 Focal nodular hyperplasia. A large, well-defined mass in the liver, which on T2-weighted image (A), shows a bright central scar (arrow). Compared to the precontrast T1 image (B), this lesion shows intense enhancement after gadolinium contrast administration.

reveals homogenous enhancement, similar to that observed with contrast-enhanced CT (Figure 7.1) with delayed enhancement of the central scar. Unlike adenomas and hepatocellular carcinoma, focal nodular hyperplasia lacks presence of capsule. Liver specific contrast agents may be helpful in further characterizing focal nodular hyperplasia. Typically, after administration of mangafodipir trisodium (Mn-DPDP), there is homogenous enhancement of the tumor, similar or slightly more than the surrounding liver parenchyma. Focal nodular hyperplasia shows significant decrease in signal intensity on ferumoxides – enhanced T2-weighted images. This aids in the differentiation of focal nodular hyperplasia from other focal hepatic lesions. Magnetic resonance imaging has been shown to possess an overall sensitivity of 70% and specificity of 100% in characterizing focal nodular hyperplasia.

Hepatocellular adenomas Hepatocellular adenomas are uncommon benign hepatic neoplasms with non-specific ultrasound findings of a well-defined benign lesion or a malignant lesion. On MRI, most lesions are heterogeneous in signal intensity with the majority being hyperintense on T1-weighted images and isointense or hyperintense on T2-weighted images. Between 50% and 60% of the adenomas are hyperintense on T1-weighted images because of the presence of intracellular fat or hemorrhage within the tumor. On dynamic contrast-enhanced gradient echo imaging, adenomas usually appear hyperintense to hepatic parenchyma. The tumor capsule, if present, is dark on T2-weighted image and is better delineated on the equilibrium-phase images. Like focal nodular hyperplasia,

hepatic adenomas may show enhancement after Mn-DPDP contrast administration and signal loss after administration of SPIO contrast.

Simple hepatic cysts On MRI examination, simple hepatic cysts are well-defined, homogenous lesions that are hypointense on T1-weighted images and markedly hyperintense on heavily T2-weighted images, with a lack of enhancement after contrast administration. Abscesses, hydatid cysts, intrahepatic bilomas, and cystic neoplasms may be distinguished from simple cysts by virtue of features such as a thick irregular wall, mural nodules, internal septations, or density more than 20 HU on CT.

Liver abcesses Pyogenic abscesses in the liver can result from infection from various routes such as biliary, arterial, portal venous, local extension, and penetrating or blunt trauma. On MRI, hepatic abscesses are hypointense relative to liver parenchyma on T1-weighted images, and are markedly hyperintense on T2-weighted images, often surrounded by a local area of slight T2 hyperintensity representing peri-lesional edema. Rim enhancement is seen in most cases. With MRI, the lesions amoebic liver abcesses are hypointense on T1-weighted images and heterogeneously hyperintense on T2-weighted images. On CT scan, involvement of liver tissue by *Echinococcus granulosus* appears as uni- or multiloculated cysts with thin or thick walls, usually with daughter cysts seen as smaller cysts with septations at the margin of the mother cyst. On MRI, the presence of a hypointense rim on T1- and T2-weighted images, and a multiloculated appearance are considered to be important diagnostic features.

Benign lipomatous tumors Benign lipomatous tumors of the liver include lipoma, angiomyolipoma, myelolipoma, and angiomyelolipoma. Their appearance on CT and MRI depends on the amount of fat present. This should be interpreted with caution if significant soft-tissue components are present, because hepatocellular carcinoma can contain fat. The CT and MRI appearance of hepatic myelolipoma is indistinguishable from that of lipoma and angiomyolipoma. The appearance of mesenchymal hamartoma on CT and MRI varies from that of a solid mass containing multiple small cysts to a multilocular cystic mass with septations and enhancing solid portions. Imaging features of other rare benign hepatic tumors such as hemangio-endothelioma, lymphangioma, leiomyoma, fibroma, and biliary adenoma have also been reported.

Malignant liver lesions

Liver metastases Accurate assessment of the liver is of immense importance in the clinical evaluation of most oncologic patients. On MRI metastases are usually hypointense on T1-weighted images and hyperintense on T2-weighted images. Some lesions may have a central area of hyperintensity, the "target" sign, on T2-weighted images,

which corresponds to central necrosis. Metastases from colorectal carcinoma may reveal low signal intensity central areas relative to the higher intensity tumor edge on T2-weighted images, the "halo" sign. On dynamic contrast-enhanced MRI, metastases demonstrate enhancement characteristics similar to those described for CT (Figures 7.2, 7.3). Hypovascular lesions are seen as hypointense masses that may show rim enhancement during the hepatic arterial phase. Hypervascular lesions usually are seen as hyperintense masses during the hepatic arterial phase, but may become isointense and thus imperceptible during the redistribution phase. Metastases may demonstrate a hypointense rim compared with the center of the lesion on delayed images, the "peripheral washout" sign. Most recent studies have shown MRI to be more sensitive than contrast-enhanced CT for the detection of hepatic metastases. Development of tissue-specific contrast agents such as ferrumoxides, mangafodipir trisodium, gadolinium ethoxybenzyl diethylenetriaminepentaacetic acid (Gd-EOB-DTPA) and gadobenate dimeglumine have further improved the detection and characterization of the focal hepatic lesions in patients with a known malignancy. These agents improve the tumor detection by virtue of their liver-specific contrast uptake. Tumors lacking

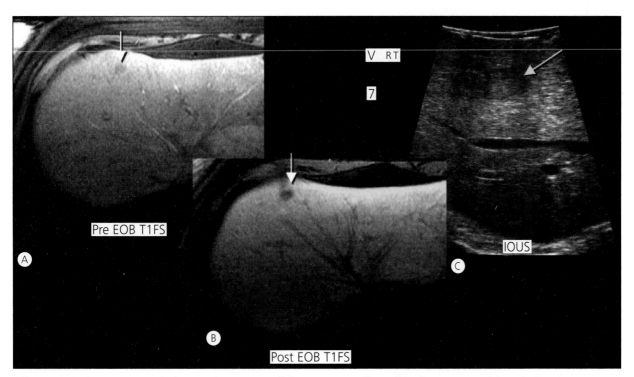

Figure 7.2 Liver metastasis from colon cancer. (A) Precontrast liver MRI shows a suspicious lesion in segment IV (arrow), which is more obvious (B) on the post-hepatobiliary contrast enhanced MRI (arrow), this was a confirmed metastasis on (C) an intraoperative sonography and surgery.

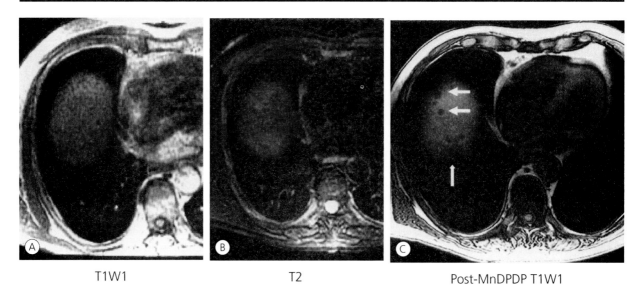

T1W1   T2   Post-MnDPDP T1W1

Figure 7.3 Liver metastasis from colon cancer. (A) Precontrast T1-weighted and (B) T2-weighted MRI images show a subtle area of signal abnormality in the dome of the right lobe of the liver. (C) On the post-hepatobiliary specific contrast (mangafodipir trisodium) enhanced MRI, multiple discrete liver lesions are identified in the right lobe (arrows).

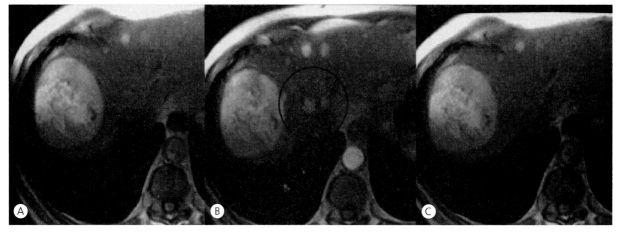

Figure 7.4 Melanoma metastasis. (A) Precontrast MRI in a patient with melanoma shows multiple T1 bright lesions in the liver. (B) After gadolinium administration, additional metastases are evident (circle) in the arterial phase, which are less conspicuous in (C) the portal venous phase.

normal liver tissue are therefore more confidently identified. Additionally the agent provides a prolonged window (few hours) for imaging the liver, therefore high resolution, thin-slice imaging of the liver can be performed. Recent studies have shown MRI to be superior to contrast-enhanced CT for the detection of hepatic metastases (Figure 7.4).

Intrahepatic cholangiocarcinoma Arises from the epithelium of small intrahepatic bile ducts. Cholangiocarcinomas have T1 and T2 characteristics similar to those of other malignant liver masses such as metastases. Typically, they are hypointense relative to liver parenchyma on T1-weighted images and have mixed signal on T2-weighted images. On dynamic scanning they have been reported to show hyperintese enhancement more centrally within the tumor on the equilibrium-phase images mimicking the delayed enhancement of hemangiomas. This effect is

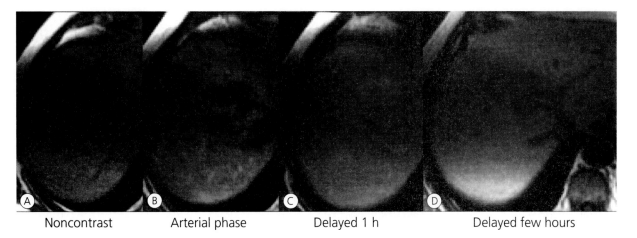

| Noncontrast | Arterial phase | Delayed 1 h | Delayed few hours |

Figure 7.5 Cholangiocarcinoma. (A) A lobulated mass in the dome of the liver involving segments IV and VIII. (B) This lesion shows progressive enhancement from periphery to center in the arterial phase and (C) subsequent delayed phase images obtained at an hour post-injection. (D) On the image obtained a few hours post-injection there is washout of contrast from the periphery of the tumor with persistent enhancement in the center.

probably due to the exuberant desmoplastic reaction (fibrosis) induced by the tumor, which retains the contrast centrally within the tumor on the delayed phase (Figure 7.5). Additionally there may be retraction of the liver capsule (Figure 7.6) and segmental biliary dilatation distally within the liver.

Hepatocellular carcinoma Consists of abnormal hepatocytes arranged in a typical trabecular, sinusoidal pattern. Typical MRI findings include a capsule, central scar, intramural septa, daughter nodules, and tumor thrombus. Almost 90% of hepatocellular carcinomas are hyperintense on T2-weighted images, with the remainder being isointense. On T1-weighted images hepatocellular carcinoma has variable signal intensity relative to hepatic parenchyma (Figure 7.7). A tumor capsule (Figure 7.7) may be seen on T1-weighted images. Hepatocellular carcinomas characteristically show early peak contrast enhancement, and absent or minimal delayed enhancement (Figures 7.7, 7.8). These enhancement features are useful in differentiating hepatocellular carcinoma from hemangioma, which generally shows early peripheral enhancement, marked peak enhancement more than 2 minutes after injection, and marked delayed enhancement at 10 to 12 minutes. Hepatocellular carcinoma may show enhancement on delayed images after mangafodipir. However, such enhancement is not specific for hepatocellular carcinoma and can be seen with other primary hepatocellular tumors, such as focal nodular hyper-

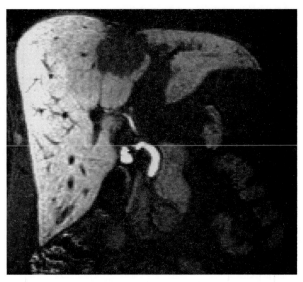

Figure 7.6 Cholangiocarcinoma in the dome of the liver is well delineated on hepatobiliary contrast-enhanced T1 MRI. Note uniform enhancement of the background liver parenchyma and T1 bright contrast excreted in bile duct.

plasia and adenoma, and uncommonly with hepatic metastases (carcinoid). Dynamic contrast-enhanced MRI is slightly superior to helical CT for detecting hepatocellular carcinoma in patients with chronic liver disease as MRI has superior soft tissue resolution and contrast sensitivity than CT. Recent

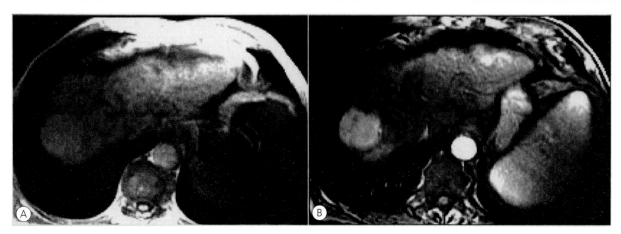

Figure 7.7 Hepatocellular carcinoma. (A) Precontrast T1-weighted and (B) post-contrast T1-weighted image demonstrates a well-defined, capsulated mass in the left lobe, which enhances strongly in the arterial phase of the contrast administration (arrow).

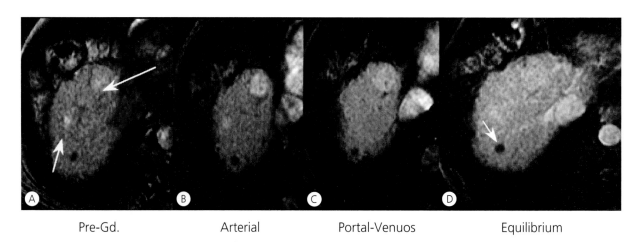

| Pre-Gd. | Arterial | Portal-Venuos | Equilibrium |

Figure 7.8 Hepatocellular carcinoma. (A) Precontrast T1-weighted image demonstrates a slightly T1 bright lesion in the dome of the liver (arrows) which enhances in (B, C) the arterial phase images of the contrast MRI. (D) Note non-enhancing lesions in the liver consistent with a liver cyst (small arrow).

publications in the radiology literature have described the value of iron oxide contrast agents in detection and characterization of hepatocellular carcinoma. In one of the studies accuracy of ferumoxides-enhanced MRI and combined CT during arterial portography and CT hepatic arteriography was reported to be 0.964 and 0.948 respectively. The mean specificity of MRI was 99% in comparison to combined CT during arterial portography and CT hepatic arteriography at 94%.

Fibrolamellar hepatocellular carcinoma Is a less aggressive tumor with a better prognosis. On MRI it appears hypointense on T1-weighted images and hyperintense on T2-weighted images, with the central scar being hypointense on both sequences. The scar in focal nodular hyperplasia is hyperintense on T2-weighted images and shows delayed enhancement (Figure 7.1), whereas that in fibrolamellar hepatocellular carcinoma has been reported to be hypointense on T2-weighted images with no delayed enhancement.

Biliary cystadenocarcinomas Are uncommon cystic, septated neoplasms. On MRI, they have variable signal intensity depending on their protein content and the presence or absence of hemorrhage. Generally, biliary cystadenoma and cystadenocarcinoma cannot be distinguished reliably on imaging studies.

Epithelioid hemangioendotheliomas Appear as hypodense multiple masses with occasional calcification on unenhanced CT. After contrast administration, the tumor enhances peripherally. The tumor is hypointense relative to hepatic parenchyma on T1-weighted MRI and heterogeneously hyperintense on T2-weighted images.

Diffuse liver disease

Hepatic steatosis (fatty metamorphosis) may be associated with a variety of clinical disorders. Ultrasound shows a diffuse or focal increase in the echogenicity of liver. Magnetic resonance imaging is extremely useful in providing a definite diagnosis when a CT scan is equivocal. Proton chemical shift imaging techniques can readily diagnose focal and diffuse fatty infiltration. Computed tomography and MRI can give a non-invasive diagnosis of liver iron overload. Patients with moderate or marked hepatic iron overload reveal increased density on unenhanced CT images. Hepatic attenuation of 70 HU or more are characteristically seen in patients with iron overload. However, high hepatic attenuation values are not specific for iron overload and can be seen in conditions such as glycogen storage disease and Wilson's disease. Magnetic resonance imaging is accurate for detecting significant iron overload and shows a dramatic reduction in the hepatic signal intensity in patients with excess iron deposition. The hypointensity seen on MRI is more specific for the diagnosis of iron overload than the high attenuation revealed by CT. The role of imaging in cirrhosis is to identify the effects of portal hypertension and to detect the presence of hepatocellular carcinoma. Regenerative nodules are better appreciated on MRI than on CT and are generally hypointense on both T1-weighted and T2-weighted images because of their hemosiderin content. As the uptake of the hepatobiliary contrast agents in cirrhosis is not uniform, Gd-DTPA-enhanced MRI is the imaging modality of choice for the early detection of heaptocellular carcinoma. Extrahepatic imaging features of cirrhosis are ascites, splenomegaly, and portosystemic colateral vessels.

Vascular imaging

On MRI, intralumenal signals that cannot be attributed to flow-related artifacts suggest thrombus. Patients with suspected thrombus must be imaged with flow-sensitive gradient echo sequences. Associated findings such as perfusion abnormalities and portosystemic colaterals can also be delineated with MRI. The status of the hepatic veins, liver, and portal hypertension in Budd–Chiari syndrome can be assessed non-invasively with Doppler ultrasound, CT, and MRI. Magnetic resonance imaging is the only modality capable of comprehensive preoperative assessment of the liver parenchyma of the liver donor, which involves assessment of the vascular (hepatic arteries, portal vein, and hepatic veins) and biliary anatomy (Figure 7.9). A relatively high percentage of variant anatomy (40%–50%) in the liver makes accurate vascular road mapping an important surgical prerequisite. A combination of three-dimensional volumetric MRI using a breath-hold technique along with MRCP sequences is used to accomplish the surgical goal. Magnetic resonance imaging is equally effective in assessing biliary and vascular complications after liver-transplant surgery.

Biliary tract

Choledocholithiasis and malignant bile-duct obstruction are the most clinically important common diseases involving the bile tree. Magnetic resonance imaging is the ideal procedure to diagnose these conditions. Preoperative MRI is also useful to study the anatomy and check for any anatomical variants. It permits evaluation of ducts following intervention to help define therapy results (Figure 7.10). Postoperative biliary complications such as biliary leaks and bile-duct injuries can be detected. If the index of suspicion is high for an obstruction ERCP is used to visualize the biliary tree. Significant advantages are that it provides unparalleled resolution and allows implementation of therapeutic measures at the time of the initial diagnosis. It is associated with morbidity and mortality rates of 7% and 1% respectively. Magnetic resonance cholangiopancreatography is preferred because it is non-invasive and does not require the administration of contrast medium.

Magnetic resonance cholangiopancreatography uses the relatively stationary nature of bile (compared with blood) to delineate the intrahepatic and extrahepatic biliary system. This procedure may be performed in patients in whom ERCP has

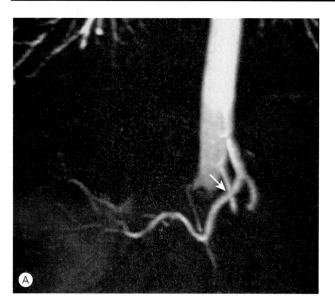 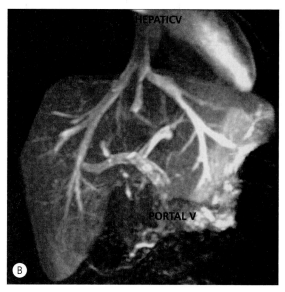

Figure 7.9 Contrast-enhanced three dimensional magnetic resonance angiography demonstrating normal vascular anatomy of the liver in a living donor. (A) Three-dimensional volume reconstruction image of the hepatic artery (arrow) and (B) hepatic and portal veins.

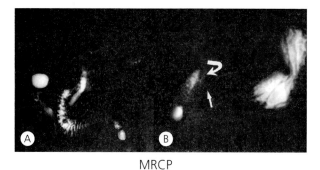

MRCP

Figure 7.10 Single-shot fast spin-echo magnetic resonance cholangiopancreatography. (A, B) These images depict the biliary and pancreatic ductal anatomy – pancreatic duct (small arrow), common bile duct (curved arrow).

failed or who are unsuitable for that procedure. It has been found that MRCP is especially useful in postsurgical patients and patients with anomalous biliary systems. Retained gallstones, recurrent choledocholithiasis, strictures, biliary and pancreatic neoplasms, and chronic pancreatitis may all be assessed by this non-invasive method. Magnetic resonance cholangiopancreatography may be helpful in patients with an otherwise low probability of a biliary abnormality, who would ordinarily undergo

the more invasive ERCP to rule out the abnormality. Typical sequences use rapid and breath-hold techniques to minimize the time a patient must spend in the scanner. Both thin-slice and thick-slab images are obtained in multiple planes that are typically centered on the common bile. At MRI common duct stones appear hypointense (Figures 7.11, 7.12) and sizes as small as 3 mm can be detected. Smaller stones are not as significant clinically and may pass on their own.

Biliary strictures are evaluated with the same approach as that used for X-ray cholangiography, with malignant strictures having an abrupt cut-off or rat-tail appearance, and benign strictures having a smooth, long, and tapering appearance.

Sclerosing cholangitis Primary cholangitis may occur in isolation, but many cases are associated with inflammatory bowel disease. Secondary sclerosing cholangitis is seen in the context of pre-existing biliary disease such as prior surgery, biliary stones, infection, and chemotherapy. The abnormalities of the bile-duct caliber can be diagnosed with magnetic resonance cholangiographic sequences, but the accuracy of the technique has not been established. The best visualization of the duct wall has been with breath-hold fat-suppressed spoiled gradient echo images acquired 1 minute after gadolinium administration.

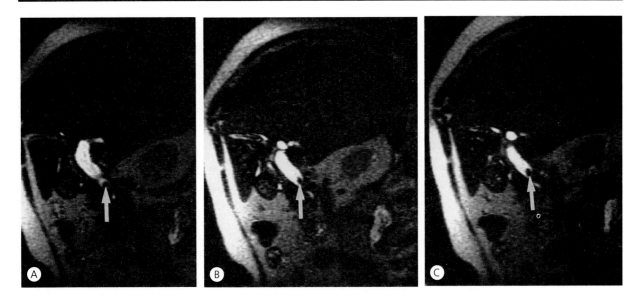

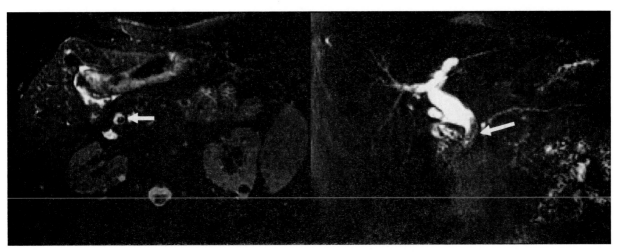

FSE T2 Axial   SSFSE T2 Coronal MRCP

Figure 7.11 and 7.12 Choledocholithiasis. T2-magnetic resonance cholangiopancreatography images demonstrate dilated intra- and extrahepatic bile ducts with a presence of T2 dark calculus in the CBD (arrow).

Limitations of magnetic resonance cholangiopancreatography Magnetic resonance cholangiopancreatography is in the process of continuous development. It provides limited spatial resolution, therefore, unlike ERCP or a cholangiogram, it may be impossible to tell the difference between benign and malignant strictures, and subtle cholangitis might elude detection. One limitation of MRCP is that air can hide stones. If there is air in the duct it will turn the duct black and a stone will not be visible on MRCP. Another limitation is flow artifacts.

Pancreas

Magnetic resonance imaging is an extremely good technique for examining the pancreas. However its use is limited because of the excellent performance of CT and ultrasound and the paucity of pancreas-directed clinical signs and symptoms. Nevertheless, the test is useful in confirmation of

1. normal pancreas in whom diffuse or focal pancreatic enlargement is detected incidentally by ultrasound or CT

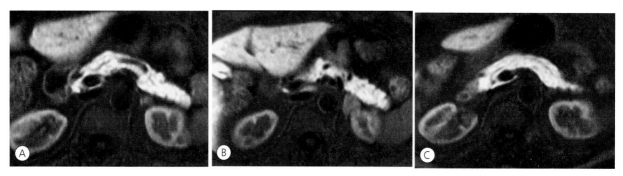

Figure 7.13 Contrast-enhanced MRI of the normal pancreas. Uniform enhancement of the entire pancreas is evident because of avid uptake of mangafodipir trisodium contrast by the functioning pancreatic parenchyma.

2. evaluation of unexplained recurrent pancreatitis or persistent peripancreatic fluid collections
3. efficient staging of pancreatic carcinoma
4. localization of pancreatic islet cell tumors
5. detection of exclusion of iron overload involving the pancreas, spleen, and/or other abdominal organs.

Techniques

To examine the pancreas, standard liver and/or bile-duct techniques are supplemented with high-resolution fat-saturation T1-weighted images. Multiphase dynamic scanning is advocated for the detection of islet cell tumors. In addition, for vascular staging of non-neuroendocrine pancreatic tumors, dynamic extracellular Gd-chelate-enhanced imaging should be used. Since the hepatocyte- directed magnetic resonance contrast agent Teslascan also enhances the pancreas, in selected cases tissue-specific contrast-enhanced T1-weighted fat-saturation pancreatic evaluation may be performed (Figure 7.11).

In addition, MRCP is being rapidly accepted as a non-invasive and accurate method of imaging the pancreatic duct and is now considered to be the primary imaging technique for the diagnosis of chronic pancreatitis.

Normal anatomy and variants

The pancreas is usually divided into head, neck, body, and tail regions for descriptive purpose. On MRI, the normal pancreas has a signal intensity similar to that of the liver on most MRI sequences (Figure 7.13). It has a relatively high signal intensity in comparison to liver on in-phase T1-weighted images. The head and neck regions of the pancreas

reveal lateral contour anomalies in up to 35% of individuals, the most common of which is discrete lobulation of pancreatic tissue lateral to the gastroduodenal or the anterior superior pancreaticoduodenal artery. In annular pancreas, MRI shows apparent thickening of the posterior, anterior, and lateral wall of the descending duodenum caused by tissue having a signal intensity and enhancement pattern similar to the pancreatic parenchyma. In addition, MRCP demonstrates the aberrant pancreatic duct encircling and extending lateral to the duodenum. The anomalous union of the pancreatic and bile ducts has been postulated to allow reflux of pancreatic enzymes into the bile duct, thus weakening the bile duct wall.

Acute pancreatitis

Acute pancreatitis is an acute inflammatory process of the pancreas that may include suppuration, necrosis, and hemorrhage of pancreatic tissue with variable involvement of other regional and remote tissues. Computed tomography is the imaging modality of choice for the diagnosis and staging of suspected acute pancreatitis, for follow-up, and to provide guidance for percutaneous and surgical intervention. Other complications associated with pancreatitis include arterial pseudoaneurysms, aneurysms, or thrombosis of the splenic, mesenteric or portal veins that can be readily demonstrated with MSCT. The severity of acute pancreatitis can be readily assessed with contrast-enhanced CT. Recent reports have raised concerns about possible aggravation of pancreatic injury with the iodinated contrast agents in both experimental and human studies. In these circumstances, MRI with gadolinium offers a safer alternative and excludes the radiation burden associated with CT. The T2-weighted images and gadolinium-enhanced fat-suppressed T1-weighted sequences with MRCP may help in defining therapeutic planning and demonstrate the size, location, and possible communication of a pseudocyst with the pancreatic duct, possible choledocholithiasis, presence of ductal distention, or disruption of the pancreatic duct. It has been recommended that pre-drainage MRI should be performed in patients with pancreatic collections in order to differentiate a pancreatic abscess from pancreatic necrosis.

Chronic pancreatitis

Chronic pancreatitis is an irreversible inflammatory disease of the pancreas characterized by replacement of glandular acini, ducts, and blood vessels by fibrous tissue causing ductal strictures, obstruction, and dilatation leading to parenchymal atrophy and complications from stone formation. Both MRI and MRCP have been widely accepted as the primary imaging modality in the diagnosis of chronic pancreatitis. Magnetic resonance findings include atrophy of the gland, changes in signal intensity of pancreatic parenchyma, irregular dilatation of the pancreatic duct, pancreatic calcification, and chronic pseudocysts (Figure 7.14). Magnetic resonance cholangiopancreatography demonstrates pseudocysts in or near the pancreas, as well as ductal abnormalities, including segmental dilatation, narrowing, and ductal-filling defects representing calculi or mucinous casts in pancreatic ducts. In some instances, the ductal communication of pseudocysts can be demonstrated with MRCP (this can frequently be difficult with ERCP). Focal pancreatitis has been reported to occur in 20% of cases and typically involves the pancreatic head. Magnetic resonance cholangiopancreatography following secretin may help to demonstrate an associated stricture of the pancreatic duct and the altered filling dynamics of pancreatic fluid that is generally absent in pancreatic malignancy. A positive duct-penetrating sign on MRCP seen as a smoothly stenotic or normal main pancreatic duct penetrating through the apparent tumor may be useful in the distinction from pancreatic malignancies.

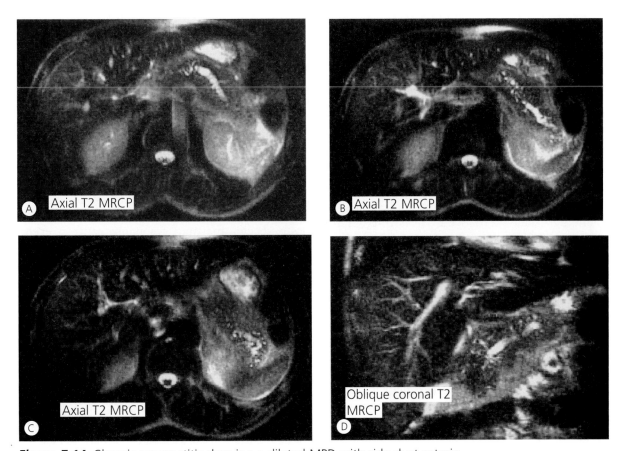

Figure 7.14 Chronic pancreatitis showing a dilated MPD with side-duct ectasia.

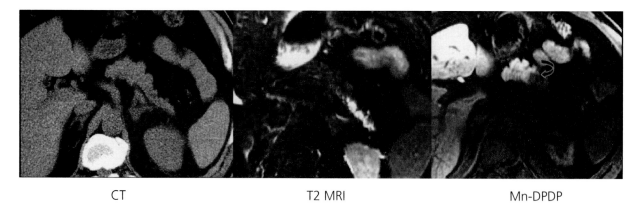

CT   T2 MRI   Mn-DPDP

Figure 7.15 Lesion detection after mangafodipir trisodium administration. (A) CT and T2-weighted MRI image shows atropic distal body tail with dilated pancreatic duct with no obvious mass. Post-mangafodipir trisodium MRI shows a well-demarcated tumor in the distal body of the pancreas (arrow) causing pancreatic duct obstruction.

Autoimmune pancreatitis is defined as a special form of chronic pancreatitis caused by an auto-immune mechanism or associated with autoimmune and related diseases such as primary sclerosing cholangitis and ulcerative colitis. Typical magnetic resonance characteristics include focal or diffuse pancreatic enlargement, the absence of parenchymal atrophy, and significant pancreatic-duct dilatation proximal to the site of stenosis, the absence of peripancreatic spread, the clear demarcation of the lesion, and the presence of a peripancreatic rim enhancement on contrast examination.

Pancreatic trauma

In some instances, MRCP may show the duct disruption as well as associated fluid collections. It also offers a useful alternative to invasive ERCP in assessing delayed complications secondary to pancreatic-duct injury.

Pancreatic neoplasms

Pancreatic adenocarcinoma Pancreatic adeno-carcinoma is one of the leading causes of cancer death in the western world. About 90% of pancreatic tumors are ductal adenocarcinomas. Neuroendocrine tumors and acinar cell carcinomas constitute about 2% to 5% of all pancreatic tumors. With regard to MRI, T1-weighted spin-echo images with and without fat suppression and immediate post-gadolinium spoiled gradient echo images have been found to be superior to spiral CT imaging for detecting small lesions. Because of their scirrhous character from dense fibrotic tissue, pancreatic adenocarcinomas are generally slightly hypointense relative to pancreatic tissue on T2-weighted images but are difficult to visualize unless there is substantial necrosis. Being relatively hypovascular, the ductal adenocarcinomas enhance to a lesser extent than normal pancreatic tissue on early post-contrast images. Hence, they appear distinctly hypointense to the maximally enhanced pancreas during the arterial phase of dynamic contrast enhancement.

However, a thin rim of greater enhancing pancreatic tissue is commonly observed in pancreatic cancers and this may help to establish the focal nature of the disease process. Normal pancreatic tissue becomes hyperintense on T1-weighted images after intravenous administration of the tissue-specific magnetic resonance contrast agent, mangafodipir trisodium (Figures 7.13, 7.16).

As pancreatic adenocarcinomas do not take up manganese, they are well delineated in the background of enhanced normal pancreatic parenchyma (Figure 7.15) on T1-weighted fat-suppressed images. T1-weighted spin-echo imaging has been reported to be superior to dynamic contrast-enhanced CT imaging for the determination of vascular encasement. Gadolinium-enhanced T1-weighted spoiled gradient echo is extremely useful for evaluating arterial and venous patency (Figure 7.17).

Three-dimensional contrast-enhanced dynamic magnetic resonance angiography with fat suppression exquisitely delineates vascular encasement or

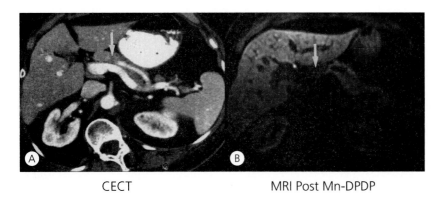

CECT   MRI Post Mn-DPDP

Figure 7.16 Intrapancreatic versus extrapancreatic – CECT (A) shows a mass in the pancreatic neck. Mangafodipir trisodium-enhanced MRI clearly shows the lesion to be extrapancreatic lymph node.

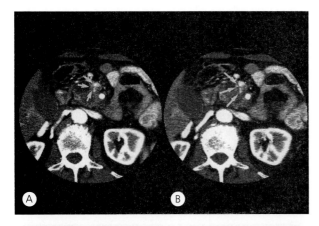

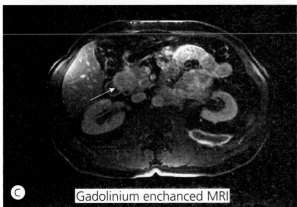

Gadolinium enchanced MRI

Figure 7.17 Pancreatic head cancer staging with CT and MRI. (A and B) CT and (C) gadolinium-enhanced MRI correlation of a mass in the head of the pancreas, encasing the superior mesenteric artery and vein (arrow).

occlusion for the determination of non-resectability as well as regional vascular anatomy (Figure 7.17).

Pancreatic neuroendocrine tumors Pancreatic neuroendocrine tumors or islet cell tumors are believed to originate from the neuroendocrine cells of the pancreas. On T1-weighted fat-suppressed images, these lesions are hypointense to pancreatic parenchyma. The T1 and T2 relaxation times of these tumors are long relative to the normal pancreas. Because of the longer relaxation time, these tumors exhibit high signal intensity relative to the normal pancreas on T2-weighted images, facilitating the detection of small tumors. Being hypervascular, these tumors frequently demonstrate homogenous or ring enhancement during the arterial phase of GD-DTPA-enhanced dynamic MRI.

Cystic pancreatic neoplasms Cystic lesions of the pancreas are frequently encountered in clinical practice. Pseudocysts, usually secondary to pancreatitis and trauma, comprise approximately 75% of the cystic pancreatic lesions. Cystic neoplasms constitute 10% of the pancreatic cysts. Early differentiation of primary cystic neoplasms from adenocarcinomas and other pancreatic malignancies is important because asymptomatic microcystic adenomas do not require surgical excision whereas macrocystic cystadenomas or cystadenocarcinomas may require surgery. Pre-operative attempts to definitively diagnose cystic tumors as serous or mucinous using invasive and non-invasive techniques have had limited success. Although CT has remained the primary imaging technique for evaluation of the pancreas, MRI and sonography are often useful in revealing and characterizing pancreatic lesions of all types but have not been successful at differentiating subtypes of cystic pancreatic masses.

Magnetic resonance cholangiopancreatography has made it possible to non-invasively visualize the pancreatic and bile ducts without the use of contrast material. Gadolinium enhancement is often helpful in further characterizing pancreatic neoplasms.

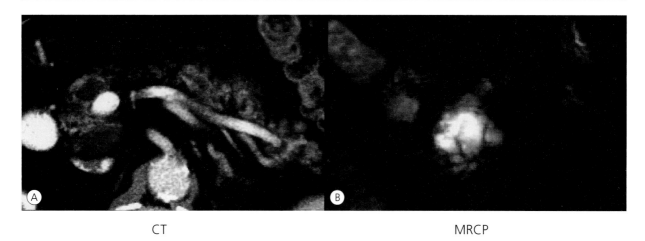

CT   MRCP

Figure 7.18 Intraductal papillary mucinous tumor. (A) CT and (B) magnetic resonance cholangiopancreatography correlation of a patient with mixed main duct and collateral duct intraductal papillary mucinous tumor. Note the clustering of cysts in the head/uncinate process with gross MPD dilatation.

Primary cystic pancreatic neoplasms In the strictest sense, cystic neoplasms of the pancreas consist of serous microcystic neoplasms and mucinous macrocystic neoplasms.

Serous cystadenoma (microcystic/glycogen rich cystadenoma) is considered to be a benign cystic pancreatic neoplasm. Radiologically, most lesions appear as solitary, large, multiseptated cystic masses with small individual cysts that range in size from 1 to 20 mm. At MRI they appear hypointense on T1-weighted images and hyperintense on T2-weighted images. Septae are better demonstrated at MRI and are seen as T2-dark thin strands. The central scar is hypointense on T1-weighted images with variable enhancement secondary to fibrosis. Dynamic gadolinium-enhanced MRI with delayed images can be helpful in demonstrating the enhancement within the central scar. Malignant serous cystadenocarcinomas are distinctly rare.

Mucinous cystic tumor (macrocystic cystadenoma and cystadenocarcinoma) are potentially malignant cystic tumors that occur almost exclusively in women during the fifth to sixth decades. The majority of tumors occur in the pancreatic body and tail. They appear as encapsulated, multilocular cysts lined by tall mucin-synthesizing cells and have a characteristic cellular, ovarian-type stroma. Magnetic resonance imaging demonstrates a T2 bright cystic lesion that displaces or compresses the adjacent pancreatic duct. On T1-weighted images, they may have a variegated appearance depending on the protein content of the fluid or antecedent hemorrhage. The MRI appearance of intracystic hemorrhage may also have a variable signal

intensity depending on the evolutionary stage of blood-breakdown products. Septae and mural nodules seen are also better demonstrated at MRI. On T2-weighted images, mural nodules are typically seen as filling defects in a T2 bright cyst. The appearance of a unilocular tumor can be indistinguishable from that of a pseudocyst, but the clinical history can help to make this distinction. Differentiation of the mucinous cystic tumors from the serous counterpart is often difficult because of overlap in the imaging features. The presence and location of tumor calcification is an important characteristic that can be helpful in arriving at an accurate diagnosis. Typically, more than 25% of the mucinous tumors show peripheral calcifications which is a rare finding in serous neoplasms. Additionally, central calcification, when present, are a feature of serous tumors.

Intraductal papillary mucinous tumors are uncommon pancreatic neoplasms characterized by papillary proliferation of ductal epithelium associated with ductal dilatation and variable mucin production.

Computed tomography is often the initial modality with which intraductal papillary mucinous tumors are suspected or diagnosed, although the clinical and imaging findings of chronic pancreatitis may obscure the correct diagnosis. In main duct-type tumors, MRCP shows moderate to marked, and usually diffuse, dilatation of the main pancreatic duct. Branch duct-type tumors show grapelike clusters of cysts with mild or absent dilatation of the main pancreatic duct (Figure 7.18). Sometimes mural nodules are seen as filling defects within the main pancreatic duct or the cystic lesion. These imaging findings are relatively specific to intraductal papillary mucinous tumors of the pancreas, and diagnosis can usually be established using MRCP, although it is often difficult to differentiate a main duct-type intraductal papillary mucinous tumor from chronic pancreatitis and a branch duct-type intraductal papillary mucinous tumor from a pancreatic pseudocyst with ductal communication. However, ERCP is mandatory for the diagnosis of an intraductal papillary mucinous tumor of the pancreas, although it does have some drawbacks

- acute pancreatitis occurs in 5% of patients after the examination
- technical failure is possible
- false-negative tissue sampling.

In several recent reports investigators compared MRCP and ERCP in evaluating mucin-producing tumors of the pancreas. Most of these investigators reported the superiority of MRCP to ERCP in evaluating intraductal papillary mucinous tumors of the pancreas and concluded that MRCP is the first and best choice among imaging techniques in assessing these lesions. The reason MRCP is better than ERCP at depicting the dilated main pancreatic duct and cystic lesions is that mucinous fluid produced by the tumor, or the tumor itself inhibits adequate inflow of the contrast material into the main pancreatic duct or the cystic dilated branches.

Papillary and solid epithelial neoplasm is a low-grade malignant neoplasm that typically affects young women. A fluid–fluid level secondary to hemorrhage may be seen within the tumors and is shown to better advantage with MRI.

Primarily solid pancreatic neoplasms with secondary cystic changes

Ductal adenocarcinoma is the commonest malignant pancreatic tumor that comprises approximately 85% of pancreatic neoplasms. Lymph node metastases are frequently present at presentation. Cystic degeneration in ductal adenocarcinomas is extremely uncommon. Large tumors may have partially cystic cavities because of areas of hemorrhage or necrosis.

Rare cystic pancreatic neoplasms

Acinar cell adenocarcinoma is a rare cystic variant of acinar cell carcinoma. Radio-pathologic findings of these tumors are indistinguishable to those of serous cystadenomas.

Lymphoma Pancreatic lymphoma is almost invariably of the non-Hodgkin's B cell type and may be associated with concomitant infection with a retrovirus or Ebstein–Barr virus (Burkitt's lymphoma). Magnetic resonance imaging demonstrates diffuse or focal pancreatic enlargement that is isointense to normal pancreatic parenchyma on both T1 and T2 images. Contrary to the post-mangafodipir enhancement of the normal pancreas, these lesions do not show any uptake of mangafodipir.

Pancreatic metastases The most common primary tumors that metastasize to the pancreas are from the lung, breast, kidney and melanomas. On MRI, they appear hypointense on T1-weighted images and hyperintense on T2-weighted images. The majority of metastases are hypointense to a background of high signal pancreas on T1-weighted fat-suppressed images. Contrast-enhanced CT and MRI may be useful in the evaluation of pancreatic metastases by showing features such as increased vascularity in the presence of a hypervascular primary malignancy.

Kidney

Renal mass characterization

Atypical renal masses often are found incidentally on ultrasound or CT. These masses often have primarily cystic components but may have septa, nodularity, and questionable enhancement. Magnetic resonance imaging is helpful in assessing these lesions and classifying them as either mildly atypical cysts or cystic neoplasms (Figure 7.19).

Atypical renal masses are scanned before and after administration of gadolinium using breath-hold T1-weighted sequences in the axial and coronal planes, the sagittal plane is added if further delineation is needed. Mildly atypical cysts may have one or two thin septa but no enhancement; otherwise they have signal characteristics of a simple cyst and may be safely followed. More complex lesions have multiple thick septa, mural nodules, and enhancement; they are considered neoplastic until proven otherwise.

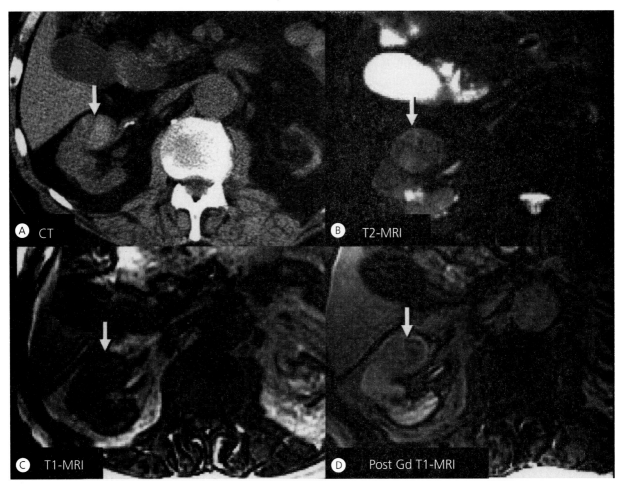

Figure 7.19 Renal cell carcinoma characterization in a patient with poor renal function. (A) Non-contrast CT shows a hyperdense lesion in LK. (B and C) MRI image has better characterization showing a lesion (a solid mass) which (D) enhances after Gd-DTPA administration.

Tumor staging

Renal MRI helps to establish the presence and extent of a tumor thrombus in renal cell carcinoma. Because artifacts often occur on contrast-enhanced CT as the renal veins enter the inferior vena cava, MRI is useful in assessing this area. Typically, axial, coronal, and saggittal T1-weighted sequences are performed. The typical appearance is an irregular mass with ill-defined margins. Tumors are generally slightly hypointense on T1-weighted images and slightly hyperintense on T2-weighted images relative to the renal cortex. Following gadolinium administration, heterogeneous enhancement is apparent on immediate post-gadolinium images, and enhancement diminishes on delayed post-contrast images (Figure 7.20).

Adrenal gland

Magnetic resonance imaging of the adrenal glands is performed primarily to distinguish an adrenal adenoma from a metastatic lesion. Adrenal adenomas are often incidentally noted on CT scans, and characteristics may be equivocal or the patient may have no known primary neoplasm. These masses typically are unilateral and less than 3 cm in diameter. Because adrenal adenomas contain intracellular lipids, opposed-phase or chemical-shift MRI scanning is used to distinguish these lesions from non-lipid-containing metastatic lesions. A lesion signal that decreases on the opposed-phase image is characteristic of an adenoma. Other benign fat-containing lesions of the adrenal system, such as myelolipoma or

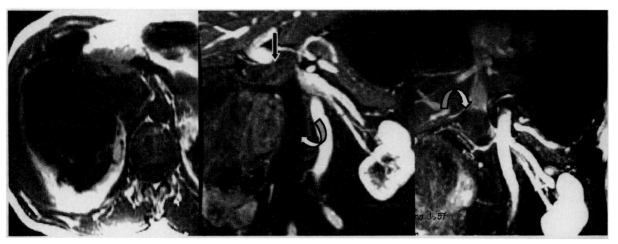

T1-MRI   Post 3D Gd T1-MRI

Figure 7.20 Pre-operative staging of renal cell carcinoma. Contrast-enhanced MRI demonstrates a large mass replacing the right renal parenchyma with tumor extension in the right renal vein (curved arrow) and IVC (open arrow).

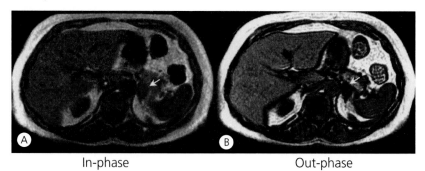

In-phase   Out-phase

Figure 7.21 Adrenal adenoma in a patient with colon cancer. (A) In-phase MRI image shows a nodule in the left adrenal gland, which (B) loses its lipid-rich T1 signal on the out-phase MRI image (arrow).

lipoma, also may lose signal on the opposed-phase image. However, these lesions usually have focal collections of fat that are readily visible on CT and do not present the same diagnostic challenge. Metastatic lesions maintain a similar appearance on the in-phase and opposed-phase images, a characteristic that distinguishes them from adenomas.

Benign masses

Adrenal cyst Pseudocysts are the most common clinically detected cysts, and usually arise from hemorrhage into a normal adrenal gland. The majority of the adrenal cysts are low in signal intensity on T1-weighted images and high in intensity on T2-weighted images. Adrenal cysts are sharply marginated and do not enhance on gadolinium-enhanced images.

Adrenal hemorrhage Adrenal hemorrhage occurs secondary to bleeding diathesis, severe stress,

and blood loss, causing hypotension or trauma. Magnetic resonance imaging is very sensitive for the detection of adrenal hemorrhage and is superior to CT imaging. Subacute hemorrhage is high in signal intensity on T1-weighted images and the high signal intensity is more conspicuous on T1-weighted fat-suppressed images.

Non-hyperfunctioning adenomas Benign non-functioning adrenal adenomas are usually an incidental finding identified in approximately 1% of the adult population. Most adrenal adenomas appear slightly hypointense or isointense to the liver on T1-weighted images and slightly hyperintense or isointense on T2-weighted images. Contrast enhancement on enhancement of the entire lesion on immediate post-gadolinium capillary-phase images is common for adenomas and rare for other entities. On chemical shift opposed phase images, lipid-rich adenomas lose their signal intensity compared to the liver and spleen (Figure 7.21).

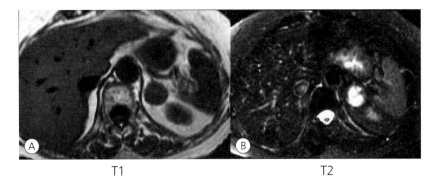

T1   T2

Figure 7.22 Adrenal pheochromocytoma. Left adrenal tumor seen with (A) low signal intensity on T1-weighted image and (B) a very bright signal on T2-weighted image.

Myelolipomas These are rare, benign tumors of the adrenal gland, composed of variable amounts of fat and myeloid tissue. Diagnosis of a myelolipoma is based on the identification of macroscopic fat within the lesion on CT or MRI. Fat-saturated MRI may be performed to prove the fatty content if needed.

Malignant masses

Metastases Metastases are the most common malignant lesions to involve the adrenal glands. The deposits vary in size from microscopic involvement to large tumor masses. On T2-weighted images, metastases are frequently high in signal intensity. Metastases have irregular margins and enhance, in a heterogeneous fashion, features which are well shown on gadolinium-enhanced T1-weighted fat-suppressed images. On chemical shift imaging, metastasis maintains its signal intensity. If an adrenal mass cannot be characterized as an adenoma in a patient with known cancer, biopsy of the adrenal mass is recommended to confirm that it is metastasis.

Pheochromocytoma These and other paragangliomas classically have a "lightbulb" (very intense) appearance on T2-weighted images (Figure 7.22). Pheochromocytoma has been listed as one of the contraindications for administration of iodinated contrast material, but the abdomen can be scanned with MRI for evidence of adrenal masses, or in typical locations for paragangliomas such as the organ of Zuckerkandl and the sympathetic chain.

Imaging with indium-111 (^{111}In) and pentetreotide (OctreoScan) or iobenguane sulfate-131 (^{131}I) typically is used if the patient is hypertensive and has biochemical evidence of pheochromocytoma but the MRI shows no evidence of adrenal or other abdominal masses.

Neuroblastoma Neuroblastoma is one of the most common solid tumors of children younger than 5 years of age. Tumors arise from the neural crest and sympathetic ganglia. They are generally high in signal intensity on T2-weighted images and enhance with gadolinium. Magnetic resonance imaging is effective at evaluating both the primary tumor and metastases in these patients, who are predominantly pediatric, because of the high intrinsic soft-tissue contrast resolution which is beneficial in patients with minimal body fat.

Gastrointestinal tract

While gastrointestinal tract MRI is still an evolving technology, several clinical applications have already emerged. Magnetic resonance imaging performs well at evaluating intrinsic bowel disease and concurrent metastatic evaluations, this is especially true in patients with rectal carcinoma. With current techniques, assessment of the primary tumor, as well as a metastatic survey to include a search for hepatic metastases is both feasible and reproducible. Other indications for gastrointestinal MRI include the evaluation of inflammatory conditions. Specifically, multiplanar imaging combined with intravenous contrast and fat suppression make MRI a robust technique for the identification of enteric fistulas. Magnetic resonance imaging has also proved useful for the diagnosis of Crohn's disease and ulcerative colitis; it can often distinguish between the two in addition to assessing the severity of disease. Magnetic resonance enteroclysis, a combined functional and morphologic imaging method, has only recently been performed in clinical practice with adequate image quality and sufficient small-bowel distention.

Crohn's disease

Crohn's disease is the most common inflammatory small-bowel disease in North America. It is well examined by MRI. Severe disease is characterized by walls more than 1 cm thick and a length of involvement of more than 15 cm. Single-shot fast spin-echo and gadolinium-enhanced T1-weighted fat-suppressed spoiled gradient echo images demonstrate characteristic findings, i.e. transmural involvement, skip lesions, and mesenteric inflammatory changes. Magnetic resonance imaging may be the modality of choice to examine for the presence of Crohn's disease in patients with a contraindication to barium examinations or CT imaging. It is an inflammatory mucosal disease that affects the large bowel and will be discussed later in this chapter. Small-bowel involvement is the sequelae of pancolonic disease.

Congenital anomalies

These occur in association with other congenital abnormalities. Magnetic resonance imaging has been successful in evaluating these conditions because it directly demonstrates the rectal pouch and sphincter muscles in multiple planes.

Colo-rectal cancer

Advances in the treatment of rectal carcinoma have increased the importance of accurate preoperative staging. Knowledge of the depth of tumor spread through and beyond the bowel wall influences the selection of patients who will benefit from preoperative adjuvant therapy. Computed tomography is the primary modality to assess lymph nodes and distant metastases. Endorectal coil MRI can be used as a focused study to evaluate the tumor extent within the muscle layers to differentiate the T2 and T3 lesions and to detect involvement of the anal sphincter of levator ani muscle by rectal cancer.

On T1-weighted spin-echo images, rectosigmoid tumors appear as a wall thickening with a signal intensity similar to, or slightly higher than, that of skeletal muscle (Figure 7.23). Extension of the tumor beyond the bowel wall into perirectal fat (T3) can be well delineated on these T1-weighted images, as the infiltrating tumor is of intermediate signal against the high signal of perirectal fat. Coronal plane MRI is useful to establish the involvement of levator ani muscle and anal sphincter. Involvement of adjacent organs can be identified on axial and coronal planes. Tumor recurrence is the presence of more than 40% contrast enhancement.

Bladder

Magnetic resonance imaging is appropriate for anatomic staging of previously detected and diagnosed bladder neoplasms, for planning radiation therapy, and for serial evaluations of the therapeutic response. In the instance of large pelvic masses, the multiplanar capability of MRI is useful to demonstrate the organ of origin of the mass, and the structures involved. Magnetic resonance imaging provides a non-invasive and atraumatic method of delineating congenital anomalies of the bladder and urethra including the evaluation of bladder

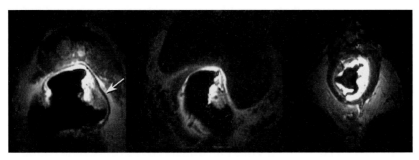

Figure 7.23 Rectal cancer: Endorectal coil MRI shows a polypoid intraluminal tumor limited to the rectal wall as the peripheral dark stripe of the muscularis propria is intact.

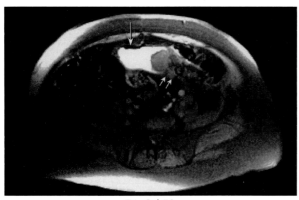

T1-Gd FS

Figure 7.24 Bladder cancer. Post-contrast T1-weighted fat-saturated image demonstrates a lobulated mass in the bladder with contiguous extension into the sigmoid colon (small arrows). Presence of air in the bladder (large arrow) is indicative of a colovesicle fistula.

exstrophy, epispadias, diverticula, and urachal anomalies. Some investigators have used MRI to complement conventional radiography in the evaluation of traumatic injury to the urethra and bladder neck (Figure 7.24).

In the evaluation of the female urethra, MRI is indicated for the evaluation and staging of carcinoma of the urethra, and for the detection and characterization of urethral diverticula. Magnetic resonance imaging is superior to CT for staging bladder cancer because of its ability to allow better imaging of trigone, prostate, and seminal vesicles. The reported accuracy of MRI for staging bladder cancers varies from 73% to 96%. It is important to differentiate postsurgical fibrosis or granulation tissue from recurrence. T2-weighted images show a high signal if it is tumor recurrence or a low signal if it is fibrosis.

Prostate gland and seminal vesicles

The most common indication for MRI is preoperative staging of patients with biopsy-proven prostatic carcinoma. The accuracy of TRUS and body coil MRI for local staging of prostate cancer is similar at 60% to 70%. Localized proton spectroscopy of the prostate, performed as part of an endorectal MRI examination, shows promise as an accurate, non-invasive means of identifying prostatic carci-

noma. Prostatic carcinoma appears in the peripheral zone as a low-signal area in the background of a normal high-signal peripheral zone on T2-weighted images. Seminal vesicle invasion is suggested by the low signal within the seminal vesicle. However, this should be differentiated from post-biopsy hemorrhage. T1-weighted images help to make this distinction by demonstrating high signal or susceptibility effect in the presence of blood products. Coronal or sagittal images are the best for evaluating the hyperplasia and prostatic carcinoma. Magnetic resonance imaging is used as a supplemental imaging technique for tumor detection because of its multiplanar ability and excellent soft-tissue contrast.

Retroperitoneum

Accurate depiction of tumor involvement of the peritoneum is critical to the diagnosis and management of cancer patients. Unfortunately, the small size of peritoneal tumor implants renders them difficult to image by helical CT and non-enhanced MR. It has been shown that gadolinium-enhanced MRI with fat-suppressed, spoiled gradient-recalled-echo sequences is exquisitely sensitive for depicting peritoneal tumors. Malignant involvement of the peritoneum may occur as a result of intraperitoneal seeding of tumor cells from primary malignancies of the ovary and gastrointestinal tract. These tumor cells will then spread according to the pathways of ascitic flow, as shown by Myers. Eventually, dissemination of intraperitoneal tumor may involve all of the peritoneal surfaces of the abdomen and pelvis, including the free peritoneal surfaces, the bowel serosa, perihepatic and perisplenic ligaments, mesentery, and omentum.

Magnetic resonance imaging examination for patients with peritoneal disease includes breath-hold, fat-suppressed T2-weighted imaging and fat-suppressed gadolinium-enhanced spoiled gradient echo imaging of the abdomen and pelvis in the axial and coronal planes. For the fat-suppressed T2-weighted imaging, the examiner may use a single-shot rapid acquisition relaxation-enhanced technique, such as single-shot fast spin-echo or half-Fourier acquired single-shot turbo spin-echo, to rapidly acquire T2-weighted images. Since each image is acquired independently, there is minimal or no motion artifact. Both single-shot fast spin-echo and half-Fourier acquired single-shot turbo spin-echo acquisitions use half-Fourier techniques, which reduce the signal-to-noise ratio. The addition of fat suppression brings a further reduction in signal, making these images less useful for body coil imaging. For body coil imaging of the abdomen and pelvis, we prefer a fat-suppressed, breath-hold fast spin-echo acquisition. The time of breath holding is 25 seconds for each of the twelve slices. These images have better SNR than the fat-suppressed single-shot fast spin-echo images but exhibit more artifact from bowel peristalsis.

Lymph node imaging

Lymph node imaging is commonly performed for staging lymphoma or metastatic disease. Magnetic resonance imaging and CT perform equally well in detecting lymph nodes. Magnetic resonance imaging is reserved for a focused examination (e.g. for the evaluation of pelvic nodes in prostatic or cervical malignancies) or in problem-solving situations. Size criteria are commonly utilized: usually lymph nodes over 10 mm in size are considered pathological, except for axillary, groin, and jugulodigastric nodes, which can be as large as 15 to 20 mm in normal patients. The presence of bright signal and heterogeneity in the lymph nodes on T2-weighted images are indicators of metastatic disease. Recent clinical trials conducted with reticuloendothelial system-specific contrast agents such as iron oxide have shown the ability to differentiate a benign from a malignant lymph node. This is because lymph nodes replaced by tumor, in contrast to normal tumors, lack reticuloendothelial cells.

Further reading

Bankman I. *Handbook of Medical Imaging: Processing and Analysis*. Academic Press, 2000.

Dawson P, Cosgrove DO, Grainger RG. *Textbook of Contrast Media*. Isis Medical Media, San Francisco CA, 1999.

Hashemi HR, Bradley GW. *MRI the Basics*. Lippincott, Williams & Wilkins, 1997.

Higgins CB, Hricak H, Helms CA. *Magnetic Resonance Imaging of the Body*. Lippincot Raven, 1997.

Mitchell DG. *MRI* Principles. Saunders, Philadelphia PA, 1999.

Pennsylvania College of Technology http://curie.pct.edu/courses/evavra/PCWM/at/DPlou/Plourde.htm

Pettersson H, Allison D, von Schulthess GK, Smith H-J (eds). *The Encyclopaedia of Medical Imaging, vol. 1, Physics, Techniques and Procedures*. NICER Institute/ISIS Medical Media, Lund, Sweden, 1998.

Pomeranz S. *MRI Total Body Atlas*. MRI Education Foundation, 1992.

Postgraduate Medicine Online http://www/postgradmed.com/issues/2001/06_01/schnitker.htm

Radiology Infonet http://www/radinfonet.com/cme/semelka/semlk_01.htm

Semelka RC, Archer SM, Reinhold C. *MRI of the Abdomen-A Text Atlas*. Wiley –Liss, 1999.

Smith RC, Lange RC. *Understanding Magnetic Resonance Imaging*. CRC, Boca Raton FL, 1997.

Sprawls P. *Magnetic Resonance Imaging: Principles, Methods, and Techniques*. Madison WI, Medical Physics Publishing, 2000.

Vlaardingerbroek MT, den Boer JA. *Magnetic Resonance Imaging: Theory and Practice* 2nd edn. New York NY, Springer-Verlag, 1999.

Westbrook C, Kaut C, *MRI in Practice* 2nd edn. Blackwell Science, 1998.

Chapter 8

Percutaneous Management of Biliary Obstruction

Michael C. Soulen

Introduction

Interventional radiologists in most settings are able to provide a wide variety of diagnostic and therapeutic procedures to aid in the evaluation and management of patients with gastrointestinal disease. In addition to biliary interventions, which are the main focus of this chapter, most units are prepared to handle interventions centered on bleeding episodes of variceal and non-variceal etiology. Transjugular intrahepatic portosystemic shunt procedures are being more frequently performed and the indications are expanding, although a high-volume unit appears to have the lowest overall morbidity for this service. Various procedures for nutritional access, including PIC lines and direct G-tubes, and J-tubes are performed at the majority of centers.

Biliary strictures are among the most challenging clinical problems facing interventional radiologists. The diagnosis can be difficult to make definitively, and the therapeutic procedures performed are the most morbid radiological procedures both in terms of acute and long-term complications. Over 90% of strictures that present to the Interventional Radiology service are malignant. The majority of these are pancreatic carcinoma, the fourth leading cause of cancer death in this country. Less commonly biliary obstruction is caused by cholangiocarcinoma, gallbladder carcinoma, metastatic disease to the porta, or primary hepatoma.

Roughly 10% of strictures are benign. The majority of these are iatrogenic: injuries to the bile duct during surgery, anastomotic strictures, and strictures induced by radiation or chemotherapy. Non-iatrogenic benign strictures are usually caused by stones or inflammatory diseases such as infectious cholangitis, sclerosing cholangitis, and oriental cholangiohepatitis. Infrequent causes include pancreatitis, trauma, benign cystic and neoplastic disorders, and cystic fibrosis.

Diagnosis

It is generally not difficult to determine the presence of a biliary obstruction. Patients typically present with painless jaundice and usually an increased alkaline phosphatase when caused by malignancy.

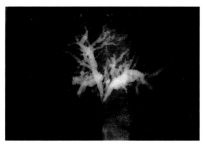

Figure 8.1 Percutaneous transhepatic cholangiogram performed after unsuccessful endoscopic cannulation. The common hepatic duct is obstructed because of cholangiocarcinoma.

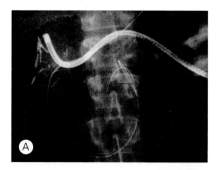

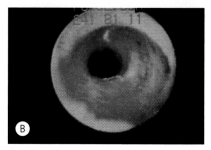

Figure 8.2 Sclerosing cholangitis with dominant strictures suspicious for cholangiocarcinoma. A) Cholangioscope inserted in to the right hepatic duct via left-duct percutaneous access. B) Cholangioscopic image of a stricture (Courtesy A. Venbruso).

Patients with superimposed cholangitis may exhibit Charcot's triad of jaundice, fever, and pain. Serologic markers for autoimmune disorders or tumors such as cholangiocarcinoma, hepatoma, or metastases may be present. Cross-sectional imaging studies demonstrate dilated duct in more than 90% of cases. Dynamically enhanced multi-detector CT will identify the etiology in 70% to 80% of cases.

Complete staging of the obstructive process may require imaging of the bile ducts. This is routinely performed non-invasively with MRCP. Magnetic resonance cholangiopancreatography is 80% to 100% sensitive for detection of bile-duct stones. Perhaps, more importantly, it has a negative predictive value of 94% to 100%, making it particularly useful to exclude stones and obviate the need for invasive procedures in these patients.

When MRCP is inconclusive, invasive imaging of the bile duct may be performed with ERCP or percutaneous transhepatic cholangiography (PTC). Adjunctive modalities include cholangioscopy and endoluminal ultrasound during the ERCP or via a percutaneous track. Cytologic diagnosis is critical for appropriate patient management.

Endoscopic retrograde cholangiopancreatography has a technical success rate of 85% to 95% and is highly operator dependent. It carries a morbidity of 4% to 8%. Complications include cholangitis, pancreatitis, bleeding, and perforation. Percutaneous transhepatic cholangiography has a technical success rate of 95% to 100% for dilated ducts and 85% to 95% for non-dilated systems. Morbidity and mortality are similar to those for ERCP.

The major advantage of ERCP is that if cannulation is successful, as it is 95% of the time in experienced hands, then diagnostic cholangiography can be followed by therapy including sphincterotomy, retrieval of stones, or stenting of strictures. Disadvantages of ERCP include its relatively high failure rate compared to PTC, and

often poorer assessment of the intrahepatic ducts, particularly in patients with hilar lesions. If contrast is injected above a stricture and not drained, urgent percutaneous drainage may be required to prevent cholangitis.

Percutaneous transhepatic cholangiography has the advantages of a high technical success rate and better delineation of intrahepatic ductal anatomy (Figure 8.1). Drainage can be achieved if necessary even if the obstruction cannot be crossed. The major disadvantages of the percutaneous approach are the higher morbidity associated with subsequent interventions during the in-patient hospital stay and limited application in patients with bleeding diatheses or parenchymal liver lesions.

Cholangioscopy has proved to be a useful adjunct for percutaneous stone removal and for evaluation of intraluminal filling defects. Unfortunately, visual inspection does not appear to distinguish benign from malignant strictures (Figure 8.2). Cholangioscopy does permit biopsy under direct vision, but it is not clear that the diagnostic yield is greater than that achieved with fluoroscopic techniques.

Endoluminal ultrasound with catheter-sized transducers is capable of imaging intraluminal calculi, stents, other filling defects, duct-wall

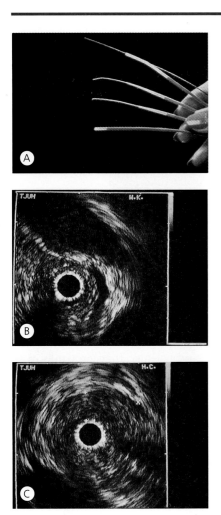

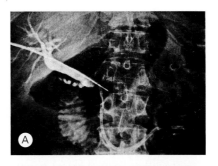

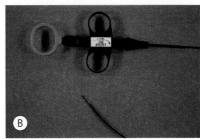

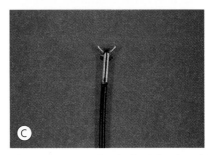

Figure 8.3 A) Catheter systems for endobiliary ultrasound. B) Endoluminal ultrasound of a normal bile duct. Note the normal wall thickness, adjacent hepatic artery and portal vein. C) Endoluminal ultrasound of bile-duct stricture. Note the thickened wall.

Figure 8.4 Methods for bile duct biopsy. A) Needle aspiration biopsy through a percutaneous biliary drain (reproduced from Cope C, Burke DR, et al. *Atlas of Interventional Radiology*. New York, Gower Medical Publishing; 1990). B and C) Forceps catheter for endobiliary biopsy.

thickness, and periductal structures (Figure 8.3). It has not proved useful in distinguishing benign from malignant disease, though it can be useful in measuring the extent of a lesion for planning radiotherapy.

Obtaining a cytological diagnosis is one of the most critical and most frustrating tasks in patients who do not present with a known cause for their stricture. Both benign and primary malignant strictures of the bile duct are scirrhous and fibrotic. The yield from bile cytology and brushings is low, though the positive and negative predictive value improves with repeated brushings. Needle aspiration biopsy is somewhat better, but still misses a significant minority of malignancies (Figure 8.4A). Use of a flexible biopsy forceps can provide specimens large enough for histologic rather than cytologic analysis, and may improve diagnostic accuracy (Figures 8.4B, 8.4C). An alternative and more expensive technique is to use an atherectomy device to cut out a portion of the stricture. This serves the dual purpose of obtaining a tissue sample that is large enough for histopathology and of opening up the strictured segment. Surgical exploration may miss 30% of cholangiocarcinomas because of the lack of associated mass and the desmoplastic reaction around the tumor cells.

Drainage of malignant obstruction

Therapy of malignant biliary obstructions can be approached in a variety of ways. Surgical resection offers the possibility for cure, but unfortunately is only possible in 10% to 15% of cases. Palliation can be achieved by surgical bypass or by endoscopic or percutaneous stenting combined with adjuvant radiation and/or chemotherapy. Comparative trials have shown no advantage between surgical versus non-surgical palliation of the obstruction in morbidity and survival. Patients undergoing laparotomy in the hopes of resecting the tumor may have palliative bypass performed at that time. Patients who are clearly unresectable can be treated endoscopically or percutaneously. Some surgeons prefer that all patients undergo preoperative biliary drainage, though a clear benefit from preoperative drainage has not been proven. Palliative management of malignant biliary obstruction may improve the quality of life.

Endoscopic therapy requires performance of a sphincterotomy and placement of a plastic or metal endoprosthesis. If a successful diagnostic ERCP has been performed, then the technical success rate for performing a sphincterotomy is very high. For low strictures such as pancreatic carcinoma, stent placement is successful 95% of the time, with a morbidity of 10% and a mortality of 2%. Success rates for hilar strictures decline significantly to around 60%, and complications increase to 17% with 8% mortality. Higher success rates can be obtained using a rendezvous procedure, in which an interventional radiologist passes a guidewire percutaneously down through the biliary tree into the duodenum, where it can be retrieved and pulled out through the mouth, or ERCP cannulation may take place next to the wire. With this through-and-through approach, an endoprosthesis can be passed retrograde without creating a large transhepatic track. Use of the rendezvous technique increases the success rate for retrograde stenting of hilar strictures to 89%.

Percutaneous biliary drainage has a high success rate, but suffers from an acute, serious complication rate of 15%. These life-threatening complications include sepsis in 11% and bleeding in 4% of cases. Once internal drainage has been achieved, conversion to an internal stent is almost always possible with little added morbidity.

Advantages of retrograde endoscopic stenting are its lower morbidity and the ability to change an endoprosthesis if it becomes clogged. On the downside, endoscopically placed stents may be smaller

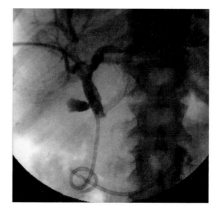

Figure 8.5 Pancreatic cancer obstructing the common bile duct. A percutaneous internal–external drain has been placed across the obstruction. Note the expelled endoscopic stent in the duodenum.

than those placed percutaneously. Because of the smaller diameter, and because they protrude in to the duodenum and so are exposed to food debris and cannot be flushed clear, the occlusion rate for these stents is higher. It is not possible to administer intracavitary radiation without percutaneous access. Conversely, percutaneous internal–external drainage allows for larger tubes which can be changed easily (Figure 8.5). Access is maintained for brachytherapy or for later interventions as the disease progresses. Unfortunately, long-term complications occur in up to 48% of patients with chronic percutaneous biliary drains, including cholangitis, skin infection, bleeding, leakage of bile and ascites, rib erosion and osteomyelitis, catheter fracture or dislodgement, and seeding of tumor cells along the track. The tubes require regular flushing and dressing, which is difficult for ill or incompetent patients. Even with optimal care, routine tube change is necessary at intervals of 8 to 12 weeks to avoid occlusion, with a cumulative cost and morbidity associated with repeated tube changes. Insertion of an internal stent avoids many of the complications of having a chronic percutaneous catheter, but repeat drainage may be required if the stent obstructs.

Stenting of malignant biliary obstructions

Patency rates for biliary endoprostheses are difficult to measure because of the high mortality in this population, but they appear to run from 68% to 94% at a follow-up of 4 to 5 months. Later series employing longer stents made from newer materials

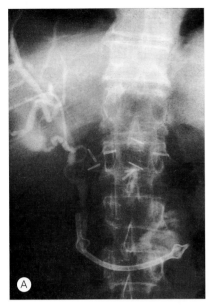
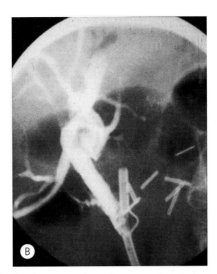

Figure 8.6 Complications of biliary endoprosthesis. A) Plastic stent placed across distal common bile duct stricture due to pancreatic carcinoma. B) Six months later, obstruction recurs due to proximal migration of the stent with perforation of the common duct.

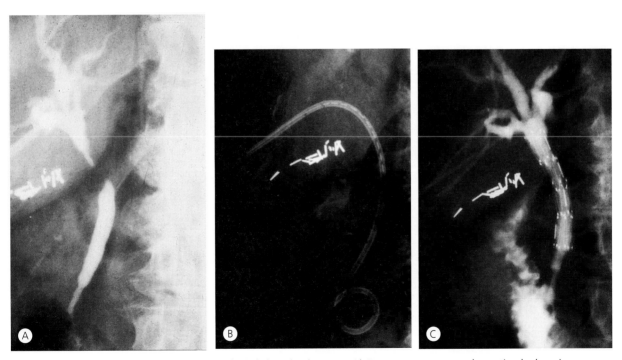

Figure 8.7 Cholangiocarcinoma treated with brachytherapy. A) Percutaneous transhepatic cholangiogram shows distal common hepatic duct stricture. B) Brachytherapy seeds placed through percutaneous biliary drain. C) Z stents placed after brachytherapy.

show patencies at the higher end of this range, with median patencies of about 6.5 months. Long-term complications are frequent, with cholangitis in 20% of cases and an average occlusion rate of 11%. Stents fracture or dislodge in 3% to 6% of cases (Figure 8.6). Despite these poor statistics most patients are reasonably well served. The average survival is only 3 to 5 months, so most patients die of their disease with the stent remaining patent. The stent palliates the symptoms of biliary

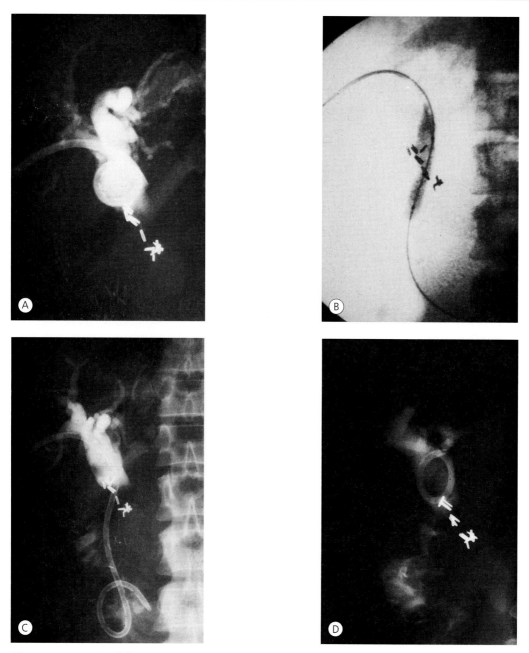

Figure 8.8 Benign biliary stricture. A) External percutaneous biliary drainage of obstructed choledochojejunostomy anastomosis. B) Balloon dilation of anastomotic stricture. C) Tube stenting of anastomotic stricture. D) Final cholangiogram after clinical trial with tube above the anastomosis demonstrating patency.

obstruction without prolonging survival. In the subset of patients with more indolent cholangio-carcinomas, stent placement may significantly increase survival to a mean of 8 months. Late complications are more of a problem in these longer-living patients.

Metal stents for biliary strictures provide a luminal diameter of 8 to 12 mm, two to three times larger than that of a plastic endoprosthesis. These stents can be delivered through a 6 F to 8 F sheath. A prospective randomized trial showed improved patency (mean 272 days versus 96 days), 30-day survival (90% versus 76%), and in a composite end-point of death or stent occlusion (121 days versus 81 days) with 10 mm Wallstents versus 12 F plastic stents. Occlusion of plastic stents occurs because of

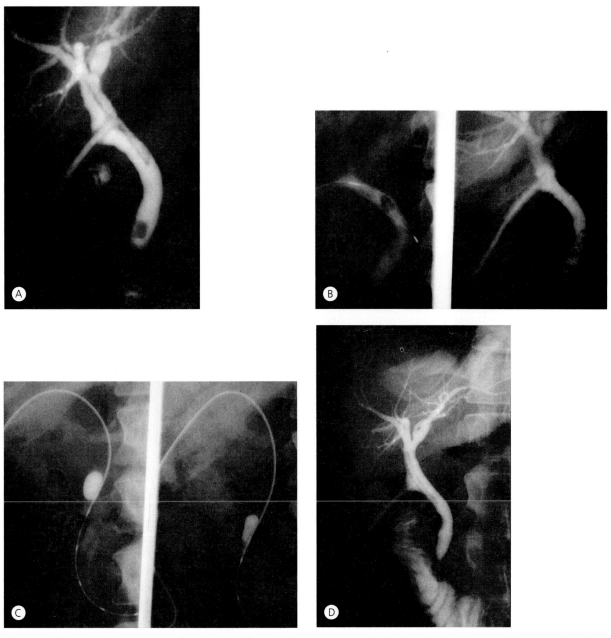

Figure 8.9 Retained common duct stone after cholecystectomy. A) T-tube cholangiogram shows retained stone in common bile duct. B) Attempted basket retrieval of stone through T-tube tract causes fragmentation. C) Fragments are pushed into the duodenum with an over-wire occlusion balloon. D) Final cholangiogram shows clearance of stones.

a sequence of bacterial adherence, glycoprotein deposition, and encrustation with bile salts. Tumor overgrowth occurs infrequently if the stent is long enough to extend well beyond the tumor margin. Conversely, the struts of metal stents epithelialize rapidly and so do not encrust with bile. However, the wide interstices between struts permit in growth of tumor and/or hyperplastic reactive epithelium. One advantage of the metal stents over plastic stents is that the metal does not fracture and rarely migrates. The cost of metal stents is much higher, ranging from $300 to $1000 each.

Use of metal stents may prove to be advantageous in patients with cholangiocarcinoma when intra-ductal radiation is administered via an iridium-192 wire prior to stent placement (Figure 8.7). This delivers 2000 to 3000 rads within a 1-cm radius. This is supplemented by external beam therapy and chemotherapy with 5-FU. The high local dose prevents tissue ingrowth through the stent without systemic morbidity. Intraductal brachytherapy followed by metal stenting improves stent patency and prolongs median survival from 8 months to 18 months with a mean stent patency of 19.5 months.

Care of the patient with percutaneous biliary drains

Because of the high frequency of complications associated with chronic biliary drainage, daily maintenance and regular catheter exchanges are essential. Catheters should be flushed thrice weekly to maintain patency, whether capped or draining externally. Exit-site cleansing and dressing changes should be done every 3 days. Elective catheter exchange should be performed every 10 to 12 weeks to prevent occlusion and cholangitis.

Symptoms such as pain, fever, or leakage of bile are indicators of catheter occlusion or migration. Patients should place capped tubes to external bag drainage, initiate antibiotics, and be seen by their interventional radiologist within 24 hours.

Patients undergoing chronic external drainage should be monitored for electrolyte and bicarbonate depletion. These can be corrected by oral supplements or reingestion of the bile.

Treatment of benign biliary strictures

Tubes and stents are unattractive options for treatment of benign strictures because of their poor long-term patency. Surgical bypass can provide definitive repair in operative candidates, with 80% technical success, 8% mortality, and a restenosis rate of about 15% to 20%. Since most benign strictures are a consequence of a previous operation, repeat surgery can be a formidable undertaking with increased risk.

Balloon dilation of bile-duct strictures can be performed with a technical success rate of 95%, with less morbidity and mortality than surgery. Because these strictures are fibrotic and prone to recoil and restenosis, prolonged stenting with large-bore (16 F to 18 F) catheters for 6 to 12 months is usually required to achieve durable patency (Figure 8.8). The cumulative morbidity of prolonged intubation and need for frequent hospital visits makes the long-term cost and complication rate similar to that of surgical repair. Patency is also not quite as good when compared to that for surgery, with 5-year patency of 65% for surgery and 55% for balloon dilation in one comparative series. Other series have reported patency after balloon dilation of 65% to 75% at 2 to 3 years.

Attempts have been made to improve upon the patency of balloon dilation by using metal stents in benign strictures. Long-term patency is not significantly improved with bare or polyurethane-coated stents. Recent work with PTFE-coated stents suggests that patency may be improved, but more investigation is necessary.

Stones

Biliary stones can be approached surgically, endoscopically, or percutaneously. Three to four percent of patients with a T-tube placed after cholecystectomy will have retained stones on subsequent cholangiography. These can usually be extracted under fluoroscopic guidance with baskets or balloons placed via the T-tube tract (Figure 8.9). Patients with biliary stones without surgical access to the ducts are usually approached endoscopically. Most common-duct stones under 1 cm in diameter can be extracted via a sphincterotomy. The transhepatic route is reserved for patients who cannot be managed by one of the above means.

Stones under 1 cm in size can usually be extracted with baskets, either out through the access tract or by pushing them into the duodenum after balloon sphincteroplasty. Larger stones may require fragmentation or dissolution. Dissolution can be performed with monooctanoin, an oily solvent that dissolves the cholesterol component of the stones. More rapid fragmentation can be performed mechanically with crushing baskets or lithotripsy using electrical or laser energy. Choledochoscopy is essential for safe and successful lithotripsy within the bile ducts. Extracorporeal shockwave lithotripsy can be performed if the stones can be targeted by ultrasound or fluoroscopy.

Further reading

Ballinger AB, McHugh M, Catnach SM, Alstead EM, Clark ML. Symptom relief and quality of life after stenting for malignant biliary obstruction. *Gut* 1994; 35(4): 467.

Coons H. Metallic stents for the treatment of biliary obstruction: a report of 100 cases. *Cardiovasc Intervent Radiol* 1992; 15(6): 367.

Eschelman DJ, Shapiro MJ, Bonn J *et al*. Malignant biliary duct obstruction: long-term experience with Gianturco stents and combined-modality radiation therapy. *Radiology* 1996; 220: 717.

Fulcher AS, Turner MA, Capps GW. MR cholangiography: technical advances and clinical applications. *Radiographics* 1999; 19: 25–41.

Gobien RP, Stanley JH, Soucek CD, Anderson MC, Vujic I, Gobien BS. Routine preoperative biliary drainage: effect on managment of obstructive jaundice. *Radiology* 1984; 152: 353–356.

Han JK, Choi BI, Kim TK, *et al*. Hilar cholangiovarcinoma: thin-section spiral CT findings with cholangiographic correlation. *Radiographics* 1997; 17: 1475–1485.

Kerlan Jr RK, Ring EJ, Pogany AC, Jeffrey Jr RB. Biliary endoprosthesis insertion using a combined peroral–transhepatic method. *Radiology* 1984; 150: 828–830.

Lammer J, Hauseger KA, Fluckiger F *et al*. Common bile duct obstruction due to malignancy: treatment with plastic versus metal stents. *Radiology* 1996; 201: 167–172.

Lichtenstein DR, Carr-Locke DL. Endoscopic palliation for unresectable pancreatic carcinoma. *Surg Clin North Am* 1995; 75(5): 969.

Mueller PR, van Sonnenberg E, Ferrucci Jr JT *et al*. Biliary stricture dilation: multicenter review of clinical management in 73 patients. *Radiology* 1986; 160: 17–22.

Nelsen KM, Kastan DJ, Shetty PC, Burke MW, Sharma RP, Venugopal C. Utilization pattern and efficacy of nonsurgical techniques to establish drainage for high biliary obstruction. *JVIR* 1996; 7: 751–756.

Nicholson AA, Royston CM. Palliation of inoperable biliary obstruction with self-expanding metal endoprostheses: a review of 77 patients. *Clin Radiol* 1993; 47(4): 245.

Pereira-Lima JC, Jakobs R, Maier M, Benz C, Kohler B, Reimann JF. Endoscopic biliary stenting for palliation of pancreatic cancer: results, survival predictive factor, and complication of 10-French with 11.5-French gauge stents. *Am J Gastroenterol* 1996; 9: 2179.

Smith AC, Dowsett JF, Russell RCG, Hatfield ARW, Cotton PB. Randomised trial of endoscopic stenting versus surgical bypass in malignant low bile duct obstruction. *Lancet* 1994; 344: 1655–1660.

Venbrux AC, Robbins KV, Savader SJ, Mitchell SE, Widlus DM, Osterman FA. Endoscopy as an adjuvant to biliary radiologic intervention. *Radiology* 1991; 180: 355–361.

Chapter 9

Computed Tomography and Ultrasound of the Abdomen and Gastrointestinal Tract

Nadia J. Khati, Michael C. Hill and Robert K. Zeman

Introduction

There have been dramatic technical advances in CT and ultrasound imaging of the abdomen. Similar advances that impact the evaluation of the patient with suspected gastrointestinal disease have occurred in MRI and nuclear medicine. While this chapter will focus on CT and ultrasound imaging findings, the relative merits of these techniques versus other non-invasive and invasive methods will also be highlighted.

Technical aspects of computed tomography and ultrasound imaging

Computed tomography

Technical refinements in CT equipment during the last 10 years have dramatically improved our ability to suppress motion and misregistration artifacts, and to visualize small structures and abnormalities with less volume averaging or blurring. This has occurred largely because of the rapid scanning, thinner sections, and the dose efficiency associated with slip-ring gantries that allow continuous X-ray tube rotation and solid state detectors found in newer helical (spiral) CT scanners.

The quality of the CT examination is greatly dependent on the quality and speed of the CT instrument and the radiologist's imaging protocol. While conventional CT scans performed with 10-millimeter thick slices and in 10-millimeter increments allow crude assessment of the biliary tract and pancreas, for example, this is suboptimal compared to images performed helically with thinner collimation of 5-millimeters or less. Conventional scanners also use a "stop and go" approach to imaging; the X-ray beam is turned on, an individual section is acquired, the X-ray beam is turned off, and then the table is advanced so that the next section may be acquired. This may result in anatomic misregistration and gaps in image coverage because of inconsistencies in breath holding. Conventional scanners may take 3 minutes or more to acquire a scan of the abdomen, resulting in low levels of contrast and poor parenchymal opacification.

A helical or spiral scan is acquired very differently. The table is advanced while the X-ray exposure and acquisition of CT data is occurring. This results in a helically shaped volumetric data set. Scanners come in single-row and multi-row detector configurations. Multi-row helical scanners (that have multiple rows of parallel detectors) are faster because they allow up to sixteen slices to be obtained at once. This results in the upper abdomen being scanned in only several seconds. A single-row scanner is slower, but can still scan the abdomen in 30 seconds or less. Multi-row data can be reconstructed as thinner sections (1.25 mm) or as overlapping sections even after the scan has been acquired (Figure 9.1). This is a major breakthrough for evaluating small lesions. These thinner overlapping data sets may be generated without additional radiation exposure to the patient, and be used to generate three-dimensional models or sections through alternative imaging planes. A similar approach is used to generate the "fly-through" views that some centers use for virtual colonoscopy.

While multi-row detector scanners inherently require a higher X-ray dose than single-row detector scanners, other steps have been taken such as better alignment of the X-ray beam and detectors which result in doses similar to that of single-row scanners.

Regardless if a single-row or multi-row scanner is used, the entire liver, biliary tract, and pancreas may be scanned while the circulating level of intravenous contrast material is at its peak. This is absolutely essential for the detection of neoplasms and for determining whether tumor spread and vascular invasion is present. The speed of helical scanning also allows adequate craniocaudal (from head to toe) coverage to be achieved, even while using 5-millimeter collimation for single-slice scanners and 1.25 to 2.5-millimeter collimation for multi-slice scanners. This type of thin collimation is rapidly being embraced as the standard for the evaluation of pancreatobiliary abnormalities and other small structures and lesions. For pancreatobiliary and dedicated hepatic CT, there

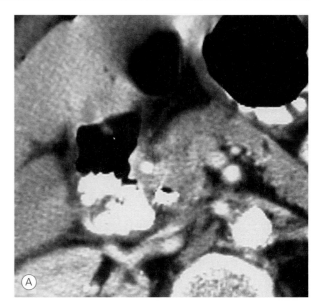

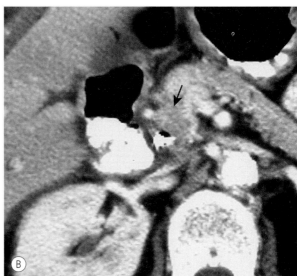

Figure 9.1 Improved ability to see a pancreatic mass by shifting slice location. A) Heterogeneous attenuation of the pancreatic head is seen with a non-specific appearance. B) By having the computer shift the slice location by 3 mm, the mass is better seen and its reduced attenuation is more apparent (arrow). The histology of the mass turned out to be infiltrative cholangiocarcinoma. A stent is present in the distal bile duct.

must be a commitment to inject contrast material using a mechanical injector at a rate of at least 3 to 4 mL/sec or higher to optimize the detection of small neoplasms. Routine abdominal scans are generally done with a slower injection rate of 2.0 to 2.5 mL/sec.

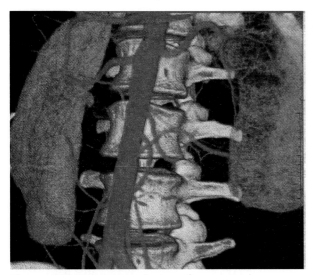

Figure 9.2 Volume rendering of computed tomography data demonstrates the aorta and its major branches.

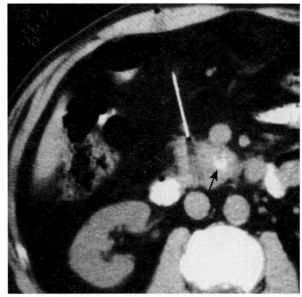

Figure 9.3 Skinny needle and core biopsies of the focally enlarged pancreas may be safely performed. This patient proved to have only chronic fibrosis. A pancreatic calcification is also seen (arrow) indicative of chronic pancreatitis.

In interpreting thin-section helical scans, one must carefully follow the various structures from section to section to look for subtle caliber or contour changes. This is especially true for tubular structures that cross from section to section such as the bile duct, splanchnic vessels, and hollow gastrointestinal tract. While this type of analysis is always part of the radiologist's three-dimensional thought process, there are now work stations that may also help, and can display multiplanar-reformatted coronal and sagittal sections as well as volume-rendered three-dimensional models for surgical planning (Figure 9.2). Even if a sophisticated graphics work station is not used, just reviewing the images on a computer monitor that allows interactively paging or scrolling between sections seems to be of benefit in understanding the anatomic relationships.

Computed tomography is used for screening and further characterizing pancreatobiliary disease, hepatic pathology, appendicitis, diverticulitis, ischemic bowel disease, complications of inflammatory bowel disease, the acute abdomen, and a whole range of suspected neoplasms and compartmental inflammatory processes. Computed tomography provides the most effective means for guiding deep biopsies of the liver, mesentery, pancreas, and adjacent lymph nodes (Figure 9.3). Since the advent of real-time monitoring of needle placement using CT fluoroscopy or with rapid acquisition and reconstruction of helical scans, procedures are safer and can be done much more quickly. While in many instances the imaging

appearance of abnormalities is not specific, the judicious use of percutaneous biopsy has proven safe and efficacious in thousands of patients.

Histologic biopsies using 18 to 20-gauge needles or biopsy guns are relatively safe, but usually not necessary if a good cytologist is available. There is no clear consensus on whether histology or cytology is better, but obtaining enough material to make a diagnosis is now far safer and easier because of improved guidance. If the stomach or intestine must be breached, a 22-gauge "skinny" needle will be used for cytology only. In our own experience, even when evaluation is limited to cytology, the diagnosis may be made in approximately 90% of patients who subsequently prove to have malignancy, provided that multiple "passes" are performed. Seeding of the biopsy tract with tumor is extremely unlikely with skinny needles, but is theoretically possible with larger needles and biopsy guns.

Ultrasound

Like CT, ultrasonography has been progressively refined since its introduction in the 1970s. Real-time ultrasonography, use of higher frequency transducers, and technical advances in transducer design and image processing, such as harmonic imaging, have improved the ability to depict subtle abnormalities, especially those that affect the echotexture of solid organs. Color flow and power Doppler are important adjunctive techniques. They are extremely sensitive to vascular flow and allow detection of slow flow in vessels, tumor vascularity, and hyperemia from inflammatory processes. Pharmacologic enhancement, such as imaging after secretin or cholecystokinin stimulation may be used for specific scenarios. In the future, use of ultrasound contrast agents will become more widespread.

Biliary ultrasonography is most frequently used in screening patients with suspected gallstones, chronic cholecystitis, acute cholecystitis, or hepatic lesions. While these diagnoses may be straightforward, they are, at times, quite challenging. In many centers, ultrasound is also used as the initial screening technique in patients who have suspected biliary obstruction. Ideally the gallbladder and biliary tract are examined in the fasting state. In most patients a 5.0-MHz transducer will be used. In obese patients, a lower frequency 3.5-MHz transducer will be necessary. Use of a lower frequency reduces the spatial resolution but allows better depth of sound penetration in heavier patients. Color and power Doppler ultrasound should be available if it proves difficult to distinguish bile ducts from vascular structures, to assess vascularity of hepatic lesions, and to evaluate the gallbladder.

Because the biliary tract and liver are evaluated using a free-hand technique, there are relatively few standardized views, but the major biliary and vascular structures must all be seen. The complex anatomic relationships in the right upper quadrant will be described in the sections on Gallbladder Imaging and Biliary Imaging in this chapter. Similarly, the liver is viewed in the axial and sagittal planes, but with many "off-axis" views to show the relationship of the various vessels and fissures to pathologic lesions. These relationships to intrahepatic anatomic structures are extremely important in localizing disease processes to a particular segment or lobe. This will be discussed further in the section on Liver Imaging.

Ultrasound may be used to guide biopsies using a special biopsy-guide transducer. Some radiologists, however, prefer to use a free-hand technique viewing the needle tangentially at a distance from the needle insertion site. Generally, ultrasound is used for more superficial biopsies than CT with the possible exception of deep hepatic lesions high within the liver. These may be targeted more successfully with ultrasound because a "creative" needle path may be

found which avoids the pleural space and can take into account patient breathing. The preferences of the radiologist will usually determine the best means of guidance for biopsy. Fluid collections are easily assessed and aspirated under ultrasound guidance. If the collection is large, a drainage catheter may be placed in it during a combined ultrasound/ fluoroscopic procedure. Some radiologists prefer CT for draining collections, but again there is a broad range of preferences.

Ultrasound is also used to assess the appendix and other inflammatory processes in the pelvis. It is typically successful in thin patients, where the compressibility of the appendix may be determined. Young women with pelvic pain may be challenging, and differentiation of gastrointestinal from gynecologic diseases frequently requires both transabdominal and transvaginal scans. Certainly pelvic inflammatory disease, ovarian torsion, appendicitis, and inflammatory bowel disease may share similar clinical and imaging features.

Evaluation of specific organs and disease processes

Liver imaging

Normal anatomy and technique

Understanding hepatic anatomy is crucial for localizing hepatic lesions, surgical planning, not mistaking normal anatomic structures for pathology, and determining whether neoplasms are potentially resectable. While the sonographic technique for examining the liver is straightforward and based on optimizing anatomic visualization, CT technique offers many different variations of contrast administration that must be carefully tailored for the type of pathology that is being considered.

Hepatic anatomy The liver is composed of the right, left, and caudate lobes. The right lobe is dominant and lies typically more posterior and inferior than the left lobe. When examined by either ultrasound or CT, the major hepatic landmarks are vascular structures (the portal and hepatic veins) and fissures. These vessels and fissures define the segmental anatomy of the liver. On ultrasound the vessels appear as tubular sonolucent structures. On CT they will show contrast enhancement. Fissures usually contain fat and appear echogenic

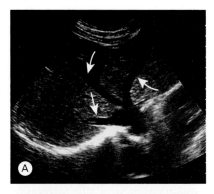

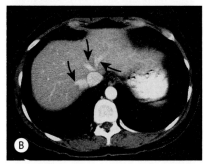

Figure 9.4 The hepatic veins are normally seen converging on the inferior vena cava. A) On ultrasound they appear as sonolucent tubular structures (arrows). B) On computed tomography they also appear tubular and of high attenuation because of contrast enhancement (arrows).

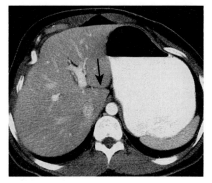

Figure 9.5 The fissure of the ligamentum venosum (arrow) is normally seen at the level of the left portal vein. It represents the boundary separating the caudate lobe from the lateral segment of the left lobe. It generally points to the esophagogastric junction.

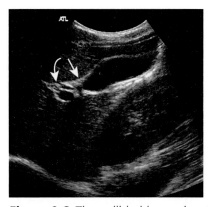

Figure 9.6 The gallbladder neck extends up into the porta hepatis. The major fissure (arrow) is usually seen extending from the gallbladder to the common hepatic duct (curved arrow) and right portal vein.

on ultrasound and of low attenuation on CT. The hepatic veins typically lie between hepatic segments or lobes and the portal veins course deeply into the central portions of segments and lobes. Hepatic veins, therefore, act as good boundaries between hepatic segments while the portal veins do not (Figure 9.4). Transverse or axial sections through the upper liver will usually reveal the right, middle, and left hepatic veins converging on the inferior vena cava. The right hepatic vein separates the anterior from the posterior segment of the right lobe. The middle hepatic vein separates the right lobe from the left lobe. The left hepatic vein separates the medial from the lateral segments of the left lobe.

More inferiorly, the hepatic veins can also be used as markers of segmental anatomy, but they become smaller and run perpendicular to the axial plane in the more caudad portions of the liver. The left portal vein is often seen crossing from the medial to the lateral segment of the left lobe. There may be a variable amount of fat in the intersegmental fissure between the left medial and lateral segments. The fissure of the ligamentum venosum is also seen in this region, separating the lateral segment of the left lobe from the caudate lobe and "pointing" to the esophagogastric junction. It represents the remnant of the fetal ductus venosus (Figure 9.5).

At a lower level still, one sees the right portal vein bifurcation intimately associated with the major fissure and the neck of the gallbladder (Figure 9.6). Both of these structures separate the right from the left lobe. In the left lobe, the intersegmental fissure will often blend into the falciform ligament and contain the remnant of the fetal umbilical vein as a small high-density bull's eye. The umbilical vein may be seen to recanalize in patients with portal hypertension. It is important not to mistake the fat-filled falciform ligament for an echogenic (on ultrasound) or low attenuation (on CT) mass.

Contrast administration strategy and computed tomography techniques

The CT technique used varies greatly depending on the patient's clinical history. Most abdominal screening studies would not be adequate for detection and characterization of small primary neoplasms (benign and malignant) in the liver. Even when screening for metastatic disease, the contrast strategy is significantly influenced by the histology of the original primary tumor.

For most routine abdominal studies, contrast will be administered using a power injector at 2 mL/sec and scans will be obtained in the portal venous phase about 70 seconds after the commencement of the contrast injection. Narrow liver windows are reviewed to bring out subtle pathology. Most practices do not perform pre- or non-contrast scans. In patients with suspected metastatic disease to the liver, pre-contrast, arterial, and portal venous phase scans will be performed for those patients whose underlying primary tumor typically is hypervascular. Many radiologists include metastatic breast cancer in this category because of its propensity to be isodense in the portal venous phase. When dealing with a potentially hypervascular lesion, contrast will typically be injected faster, at 3 to 4 mL/sec. The arterial phase occurs approximately 25 to 30 seconds after the start of the contrast injection. Most primary neoplasms of the liver are hypervascular, so a similar contrast injection strategy for the detection of hepatocellular carcinoma and for lesions such as hepatic adenoma and focal nodular hyperplasia is used.

Regardless of whether the liver is scanned in one phase or during pre-contrast, arterial, and portal venous phases, it is important to never use less than about 125 to 140 mL of 300 mI/mL non-ionic contrast. Lesser amounts of iodine will result in suboptimal enhancement of either the hepatic parenchyma or suspected tumors.

Primary benign tumors

In patients with suspected hepatic lesions or "incidentalomas" seen on ultrasound, most will be further evaluated using CT. Usually we will work-up lesions that are not simple cysts and exceed approximately 1.5 centimeters in size. In patients without a prior history of malignancy, lesions smaller than this are rarely significant. In symptomatic patients where hemorrhage has spontaneously occurred our size threshold may theoretically be less, but it is unusual for small lesions to bleed or be detected accurately in the presence of blood.

Certainly, larger lesions are accurately seen even when blood is present.

It should not be surprising that scanning with high levels of contrast and understanding CT patterns of enhancement has greatly improved our ability to detect and characterize hypervascular primary tumors of the liver. Unfortunately, lesions that contain hepatocytes, such as hepatocellular carcinoma, fibrolamellar hepatocellular carcinoma, hepatic adenoma, and focal nodular hyperplasia may look quite similar. Optimizing the scan technique based on the clinical history and correlation of ultrasound, CT, and MRI findings (with nuclear medicine occasionally) is crucial when evaluating these types of hepatic lesions. For most hypervascular or potentially hypervascular lesions, triphasic scanning is best, i.e. scanning before contrast, during the arterial phase, and during the portal venous phase.

Hepatic adenoma

Hepatic adenoma is a benign neoplasm of hepatocellular origin that most commonly occurs in young women. The lesions contain hepatocytes and Kupffer cells, but do not usually contain biliary ductules. Historically, adenoma has been linked to oral contraceptive use, but other risk factors include glycogen storage disease and anabolic steroid use. Spontaneous hemorrhage is known to occur, especially when the lesion is near the surface of the liver and subject to trauma. These tumors may be solitary or multiple and may contain fat, hemorrhage, or calcification. Most lesions are well demarcated (Figure 9.7) with a minority of patients exhibiting a true capsule around the lesion.

On ultrasound the echo pattern of hepatic adenomas is variable, but they are usually not as echogenic as hemangioma. On CT they show

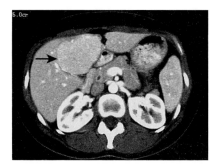

Figure 9.7 A hepatic mass (arrow) with homogenous increased attenuation and well-defined margins is seen on this arterial-phase computed tomography scan. The findings are consistent with hepatic adenoma.

homogenous enhancement in the arterial phase, (Figure 9.7) but fade and become almost isodense and barely visible in the portal venous phase. They do not demonstrate a central scar, an important feature on CT that distinguishes adenoma from fibrolamellar hepatocellular carcinoma and focal nodular hyperplasia. Whenever solitary or multiple solid hepatic masses are incidentally discovered in a young patient, performance of arterial phase scans is essential to detect adenomas and to differentiate them from other hypervascular primary hepatic lesions. If only portal phase scans are performed, a significant number of adenomas will be missed. If a known adenoma shows rapid growth on CT, malignant degeneration may be present.

Focal nodular hyperplasia

Focal nodular hyperplasia represents hepatocellular hyperplasia rather than a true neoplasm. They contain hepatocytes, biliary ductules, and a variable amount of Kupffer cells. Focal nodular hyperplasia occurs as an incidental finding in young women. It is usually solitary but rarely can be multiple. As with adenoma, focal nodular hyperplasia varies in echogenicity on ultrasound, usually appearing uniformly hypoechoic. Power Doppler may reveal low-level flow within the central scar. Focal nodular hyperplasia has a distinctive CT pattern of enhancement. It is of iso- or hypo-attenuation compared to liver on pre-contrast and portal venous phase scans. During the arterial phase, focal nodular hyperplasia brightly and homogenously enhances and will show a fine hypodense central scar or septae (Figure 9.8).

Delayed scans may show late enhancement of the central scar, a finding which is also present in fibrolamellar hepatocellular carcinoma. Focal nodular hyperplasia typically enhances more brightly in the arterial phase than adenoma. Most focal nodular hyperplasia lesions will be far more homogenous than fibrolamellar hepatocellular carcinoma, less likely to have calcification, and have less distinct margins. A valuable problem solver is a ^{99m}Tc IDA scan as three quarters or more of focal nodular hyperplasia lesions will demonstrate uptake of this biliary agent. Since they also contain Kupffer cells they also may show variable increased uptake of ^{99m}Tc sulfur colloid.

Hemangioma

Hemangiomas are one of the most common incidental hepatic lesions regardless of age. They occur more commonly in women than men and may co-exist with other benign or malignant lesions. Calcification may be present rarely. On ultrasound, most small hemangiomas are a uniformly echogenic mass (Figure 9.9). Giant hemangiomas, which exceed 10 centimeters in diameter may also occur, but they tend to have mixed echogenicity. Hemorrhage is unusual except in giant lesions abutting the hepatic surface.

Computed tomography has proven to be very good over the years in specifically diagnosing hemangioma when typical findings are present. In up to half of patients the enhancement pattern may have atypical features related to the inherent structure of the lesion, its size, or inadequate scan technique. Because of this, secondary techniques such as MRI or technetium-labeled red blood cell scanning may be necessary. On CT the hallmark of hemangioma is nodular enhancement of the lesion, which is usually peripheral and matches that of the

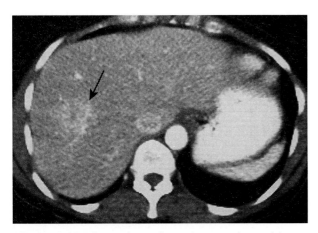

Figure 9.8 A hyperdense hepatic mass (arrow) is present within the right lobe. It is heterogeneous, has irregular margins, and contains a central scar. It is approximately 3 centimeters in diameter. The lesion was invisible and isodense in the portal venous phase. The lesion proved to be focal nodular hyperplasia.

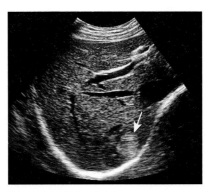

Figure 9.9 Sagittal sonogram reveals an echogenic mass (arrow) in the posterior right lobe consistent with hemangioma.

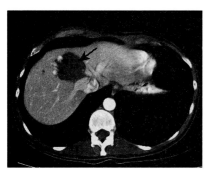

Figure 9.10 A contrast-enhanced computed tomography scan demonstrates hemangioma (arrow) within the anterior segment of the right lobe. "Puddles" of contrast are seen at the periphery of the lesion, which are very suggestive of hemangioma.

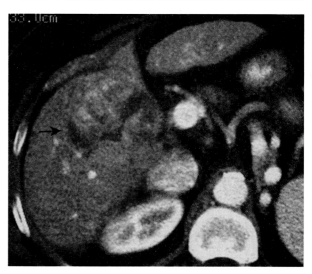

Figure 9.12 A large, heterogenous, hyperdense mass (arrow) is present in this patient with a history of cirrhosis. In this setting focal nodular hyperplasia cannot be entirely excluded, but the findings are most consistent with hepatocellular carcinoma.

Hepatocellular carcinoma and fibrolamellar hepatocellular carcinoma

Hepatocellular carcinoma remains a difficult diagnosis given that many lesions occur against a backdrop of complex structural changes due to hepatitis and cirrhosis. In addition, they vary in their vascularity, and mimic other lesions such as adenoma, focal nodular hyperplasia, and nodular regenerative hyperplasia. Fifty per cent of lesions are solitary. On ultrasound their echo pattern varies and most will show areas of increased flow on power Doppler. Most hepatomas are hypervascular and, on CT, are best seen during the hepatic arterial phase of contrast (Figure 9.12). A capsule is present in about one fifth of lesions. Early hepatocellular carcinoma usually has well-defined margins, but these may become less distinct as the tumor spreads or when vascular compromise is present. Hemorrhage and fat may occur. A central scar is usually absent. Hepatocellular carcinoma cannot be readily distinguished from dysplastic nodules of the cirrhotic liver on CT or ultrasound. Regenerative nodules are usually smaller and may contain iron, making them dense on pre-contrast scans.

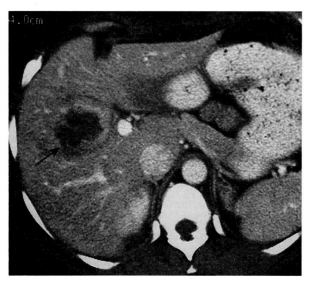

Figure 9.11 A rim-enhancing lesion (arrow) due to metastatic breast cancer is identified. Peripheral enhancement which is not nodular is suggestive of neoplasm.

blood pool (Figure 9.10). Peripheral nodular "puddles" of contrast on CT (representing the so-called "cotton-wool" staining seen on angiography) is a very specific finding suggestive of hemangioma. A ring of peripheral enhancement should not be confused with nodular enhancement. The former is more commonly seen in malignancy (Figure 9.11). Hemangiomas will often not be uniform in density, but areas of enhancement should match the enhancement of the vessels seen during that phase of contrast enhancement. Delayed scans may show centripetal "fill-in" of the lesion with contrast.

In patients with large hepatocellular carcinomas, tumor spread frequently occurs. Hepatocellular carcinoma has a propensity to invade the portal vein and bile ducts (Figure 9.13). When tumor thrombus is present in the portal vein, it frequently expands the vessel and may have arterial "feeders"

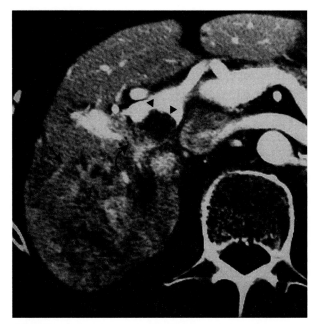

Figure 9.13 A large, heterogenous, hyperdense mass (arrow) is present in this patient with a history of cirrhosis. The lesion proved to be hepatocellular carcinoma. A low-attenuation defect is seen within the portal vein (arrowheads) This probably represents bland thrombus. An area of slightly greater attenuation (curved arrow) is also seen within the portal vein. This represents direct extension of tumor thrombus.

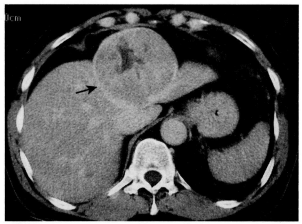

Figure 9.14 A large, encapsulated lesion (arrow) is seen replacing the medial segment of the left lobe. A low-attenuation central scar is present. The appearance suggests the fibrolamellar variant of hepatocellular carcinoma.

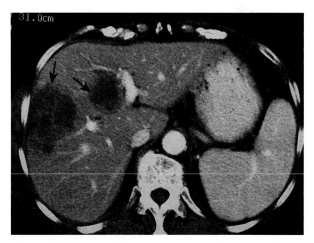

Figure 9.15 Two low-attenuation soft-tissue lesions (arrows) are present within the liver. Low-attenuation lesions are usually hypovascular in nature, in this case due to colorectal cancer.

producing dramatic enhancement in the hepatic arterial phase. Hepatocellular carcinoma may also invade or encase the bile ducts. Metastatic lymphadenopathy commonly occurs in the porta hepatis and cardiophrenic regions. Distant metastases to the lungs, bones, and peritoneum are relatively common.

Fibrolamellar hepatocellular carcinoma is a subtype of hepatocellular carcinoma that is not associated with hepatitis or cirrhosis and tends to occur in young to middle-aged females and males. The lesions are usually large and solitary. They are well defined, and 80% contain a central scar (Figure 9.14). Most will also have calcification. Fat is rare. As for conventional hepatocellular carcinoma, many fibrolamellar hepatocellular carcinoma lesions will be hypervascular during the hepatic arterial phase. Unfortunately, their enhancement pattern is quite variable and lesions show great heterogeneity. Because of the presence of a central scar, fibrolamellar hepatocellular carcinoma may be similar in appearance to focal nodular hyperplasia. Fibrolamellar hepatocellular carcinoma, however, is usually larger, more heterogeneous, and with

better defined margins than focal nodular hyperplasia. Like hepatocellular carcinoma, metastatic adenopathy, vascular encasement, and biliary obstruction may occur with advanced disease, but in general fibrolamellar hepatocellular carcinoma has a better prognosis than hepatocellular carcinoma.

Hepatic metastatic disease

Hepatic metastases may be hypo- or hypervascular depending on the underlying histology of the primary tumor. Metastatic colorectal cancer and pancreatic cancer are usually hypovascular (Figure 9.15).

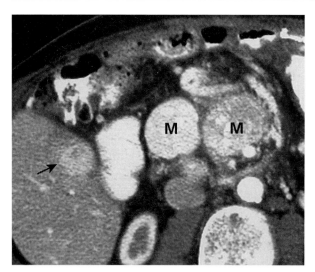

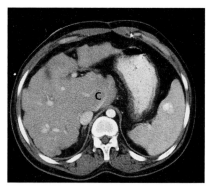

Figure 9.17 A scarred nodular liver with caudate-lobe enlargement (C) is seen in this patient with cirrhosis.

Figure 9.16 Two hypervascular pancreatic masses (M) are present on this arterial-phase scan. Note the high-attenuation liver metastasis enhancing greater than liver parenchyma (arrow). This is typical of hypervascular metastases. The lesion was barely visible on portal venous phase scans.

Hypervascular metastases include metastatic carcinoid, islet-cell carcinoma, renal-cell carcinoma, and thyroid cancer, among others (Figure 9.16). As described earlier, most centers will only perform portal venous phase imaging when looking for hypovascular metastases. Computed tomography images taken during both the arterial and portal venous phase are vital to optimize lesion detection of hypervascular metastases. Some centers add pre-contrast images also. All these refinements have resulted in an overall accuracy of lesion detection in the 80% to 85% range. While this is similar to MRI, it is at least 10% lower than would be expected for intraoperative ultrasound. Computed tomography is relatively insensitive to microscopic disease, but most patients will have lesions of variable size, not just sub-centimeter lesions.

Hypovascular metastases will typically appear hypodense on portal phase images. They enhance less than the enhanced hepatic parenchyma and therefore are of lower attenuation (Figure 9.15). They are not of water density as would be seen with a hepatic cyst, but range from 20 to 60 HU. There may be a variable halo of rim enhancement seen. Hypervascular metastases appear hyperdense during the arterial phase, i.e. they enhance more than the liver parenchyma (Figure 9.16). This occurs because they derive their blood supply from the arterial circulation, while the liver enhances much later because of its predominantly portal venous supply. During the portal phase, the liver enhances and hypervascular metastases fade. These metastases may become isodense as compared to the liver or even slightly hypodense. When they become isodense, they may be nearly invisible, even when displayed at a high-contrast, narrow-window setting.

Cirrhosis

Computed tomography and ultrasound are seldom used to detect early cirrhosis or determine its severity. In advanced disease, nodularity of the liver, distortion of the lobar architecture, and enlargement of the caudate lobe are frequent (Figure 9.17). Imaging does play a role in assessing complications of cirrhosis such as hepatocellular carcinoma and identifying vascular abnormalities that may represent a relative contraindication to shunt placement. The latter category includes partial or complete portal vein thrombosis or Budd–Chiari syndrome. The decision to shunt is obviously a clinical one, but will also depend on the anatomy and availability of patent vascular branches. Many patients with significant portal hypertension will show cavernous transformation of the portal vein, with clot and fibrosis in the main portal vein. This would preclude shunting as would tumor in the portal vein. As with MRI, CT and ultrasound may also be used to map the extent of varices and understand the vascular physiology. This is often not of clinical value, but it is surprising how often mesenteric or intramural varices are present that are not endoscopically visible in typical areas such as the esophagogastric junction.

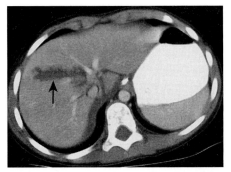

Figure 9.18 Liver lacerations appear as irregular linear areas of low attenuation (arrow). If contrast extravasation or major vessel disruption is present, embolization or surgery may be needed.

Trauma

The liver may be injured by blunt or penetrating trauma. While most penetrating trauma requires surgical exploration, blunt trauma is usually assessed non-invasively. Ultrasound is often used to determine if there is free fluid suggesting organ or visceral injury. In our experience, regardless of the result, CT is often used to look for significant injury. Within the liver, simple hematomas or small lacerations are common. These typically will be hyperdense as compared to liver on pre-contrast scans and hypodense after contrast (Figure 9.18). If active bleeding is occurring, extravasated contrast may be seen. The latter suggests the need for emergency angiography to embolize the bleeding vessel, which is usually arterial. If a broad stellate fracture is seen extending to the capsule or a laceration extending to the inferior vena cava, emergent surgery is usually necessary.

Gallbladder imaging

Cholelithiasis

Ultrasound is the main technique used to detect cholelithiasis. Sonography should be performed with a linear or curved-array transducer, ideally at 5 MHz. Its depth of penetration, however, may be inadequate in some obese patients who will have to be imaged at a lower frequency. The focal zone (narrowest part of the ultrasound beam) must be matched to the location of a suspected stone to best image shadowing. Failure to do this may not result in the detection of a shadow, one of the most important criteria in stone detection. While

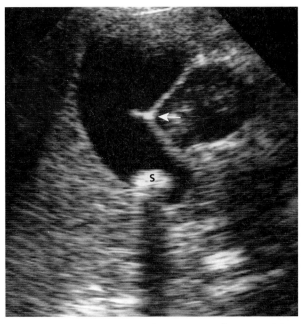

Figure 9.19 Ultrasound of Phrygian cap gallbladder exhibits an infolding of the fundus, which mimics a septum (arrow). A stone (S) is also present in this patient.

shadowing is best seen with a high-frequency transducer over the stone, a high gain setting should not be used as this may "fill-in" the shadow. The gallbladder examination is ideally conducted in the supine and left lateral decubitus position with the patient fasting for at least 8 hours to achieve sufficient gallbladder distension.

The entire gallbladder is examined axially and sagittally along its long and short axes. If a Phrygian cap anomaly is present it is important not to overlook the redundant portion of the fundus where stones may hide (Figure 9.19). The ampullary portion of the gallbladder (between the cystic duct and gallbladder neck) is another common hiding place for stones. To avoid missing stones in this region the gallbladder neck must be traced completely up to the right portal vein where it lies in the major hepatic fissure (which divides the right from the left lobes of the liver). Multiple examination positions (including the left lateral decubitus position) are used to prove that suspected stones seek gravitational dependency, and do not represent fixed anatomic lesions such as tumors or adenomyomas.

The diagnosis of cholelithiasis rests on a suspected stone exhibiting three criteria. It must:

1. be an echogenic opacity
2. cast a discrete acoustic shadow
3. seek gravitational dependency (Figure 9.20).

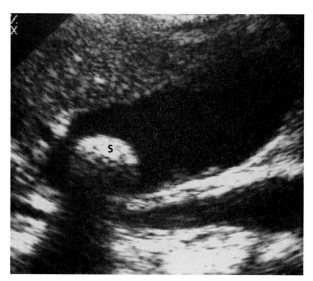

Figure 9.20 A large stone (S) is seen which seeks gravitational dependency and casts a discrete acoustic shadow.

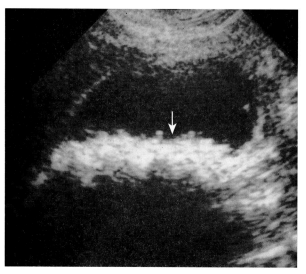

Figure 9.21 Gravel appears echogenic (arrow) and seeks dependency on sonographic examinations. Gravel casts a confluent shadow, but the individual concretions may not be separable or shadow because of their small size.

Stone size may vary and stones may be solitary or multiple. They may be surrounded by plentiful bile or reside in a confusing scarred, contracted gallbladder. Very small stones (1 to 2 mm) cast a shadow in phantom studies, but may not in clinical practice. If multiple small stones (i.e. "gravel") occupy the dependent portion of the gallbladder, they may cast a confluent shadow (Figure 9.21). In some patients with significant scarring of the gallbladder due to chronic cholecystitis, the gall-

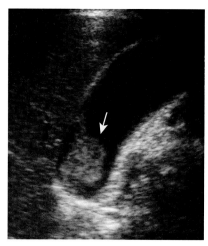

Figure 9.22 Tumefactive sludge (arrow) may clump and mimic a polyp or tumor of the gallbladder on ultrasound.

bladder may give rise to a "double-arc" appearance, which has also been called the wall-echo-shadow (or WES) complex. The anterior arc represents a thickened, scarred, hyper-reflective gallbladder wall with the more posterior arc representing a stone or stones.

Gallbladder sludge is a sonographic diagnosis that differs in appearance from "gravel"; it is echogenic but does not cast an acoustic shadow. Sludge is viscous material that seeks gravitational dependency, but not as rapidly as gravel. Sludge may form a rounded collection within the gallbladder and mimic a gallbladder polyp or tumor (so-called "tumefactive sludge") (Figure 9.22). While the significance of sludge has been debated, it is now clear that it represents lithogenic bile containing cholesterol monohydrate crystals, bilirubin granules, and a mucus glycoprotein gel, all important ingredients in stone formation. Sludge is commonly identified in patients with biliary stasis due to biliary-outflow obstruction, prolonged fasting, or the use of intravenous hyperalimentation. When sludge is seen, it will usually be reported by the radiologist since the patient is at risk for formation of macroscopic gallstones.

Acute cholecystitis

Rationale for imaging acute cholecystitis
When a patient presents with symptoms of acute cholecystitis, the physical examination is often impressive but may lack the specificity needed to differentiate the various causes of right upper

quadrant pain. Before the modern imaging era, one fifth to one quarter of patients explored for acute cholecystitis did not end up having acute cholecystitis. While many of these patients did have gallbladder disease, this rate of negative emergency exploration is no longer acceptable. Furthermore, imaging can predict which patients have complications of acute cholecystitis that may require a different management approach such as open versus laparoscopic cholecystectomy.

Laparoscopic cholecystectomy has become increasingly popular not only for elective cholecystectomy, but also in the setting of acute cholecystitis. An increasing majority of surgeons advocate early laparoscopic cholecystectomy prior to the development of post-inflammatory adhesions in the right upper quadrant. A small number of surgeons are more conservative and treat the patient with antibiotics and anti-inflammatory agents, performing an elective cholecystectomy at a later time. The latter surgeons believe once inflammation has subsided, the likelihood of injuring the bile duct is less. Regardless of which camp is correct, removal of the acutely inflamed gallbladder is being performed with an acceptable complication rate.

For the radiologist it is important to be able to determine the severity of the inflammation and identify complications (described below) that may alter the surgical approach. A perforated gallbladder is likely to require an open cholecystectomy, possibly with preoperative biloma drainage. The surgeon needs to be made aware of this kind of information before surgery; he or she will often inform the patient that there is a significant likelihood that laparoscopic cholecystectomy may be inappropriate or be a prelude to conversion to an open cholecystectomy.

Imaging findings in uncomplicated acute cholecystitis

Both sonography and cholescintigraphy are highly sensitive and specific in the diagnosis of acute cholecystitis. While a broad range of sensitivities and specificities have been reported in the literature, one can expect approximately 95% sensitivity and 85% to 90% specificity for both sonography and cholescintigraphy. The choice of which test to perform largely depends on radiologist preferences and emergency availability. Ultrasound has a slight edge in this regard, and can demonstrate other pathology outside the gallbladder, but both techniques are quite good.

On ultrasound the diagnosis of acute cholecystitis is made by looking for a triad of findings consisting

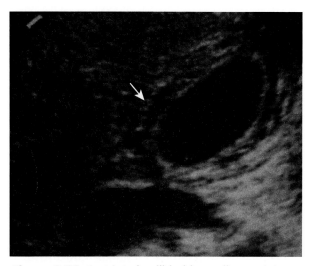

Figure 9.23 A striated gallbladder wall containing intramural edema (arrow) is one of the major signs of acute cholecystitis on ultrasound.

of cholelithiasis, maximum pain during compression over the gallbladder (the so-called sonographic Murphy's sign), and the presence of intramural edema in the gallbladder wall. Pericholecystic fluid may also be present, but is not individually a sensitive or specific sign. Intramural edema appears as a solitary band or multiple bands of lucency within the gallbladder wall (Figure 9.23). When multiple bands are present (also called a striated appearance) or edema is focal in location, it is most specific for the diagnosis of acute cholecystitis.

Gallbladder wall thickening also occurs in acute cholecystitis, but is more echogenic than intramural edema. Wall thickening (greater than 3 mm) may be due to a variety of etiologies including acute cholecystitis. The most common causes are a partially collapsed or physiologically contracted gallbladder, chronic cholecystitis, hepatitis, and metabolic disturbances such as hypoalbuminemia and ascites. Wall thickening without intramural edema should not be considered suggestive of acute cholecystitis. Be especially vigilant in patients with ascites; many will have a thickened gallbladder wall that is not due to acute cholecystitis. Gallbladder wall varices (acting as a portal venous collateral pathway) can mimic intramural edema on gray-scale images. They are typically more serpiginous than bands of edema and should reveal a typical venous flow pattern on color flow or power Doppler.

Power Doppler ultrasound may be of some value in detection of acute cholecystitis. Traditional color flow Doppler appears to be inadequately sensitive to the hyperemia and increased vascular flow seen in the acutely inflamed gallbladder. Power Doppler, however, may be useful for the diagnosis of acute cholecystitis if linear bands of hyperemia are seen. Criteria will undoubtedly be refined over the next several years.

Computed tomography is not generally used as a screening test for acute cholecystitis. It can be helpful in detecting the complications of acute cholecystitis and distinguishing these from gallbladder carcinoma. Cholecystitis may be seen to produce bands of low attenuation within the gallbladder wall due to edema, gallbladder wall thickening, pericholecystic inflammatory stranding, changes of perihepatitis, and numerous other findings.

Gallbladder carcinoma may look quite similar, but will usually show more focal mass effect or soft-tissue extension into the adjacent liver or pericholecystic fat.

Complications of acute cholecystitis

Complicated acute cholecystitis may be categorized as gangrenous cholecystitis, emphysematous cholecystitis, empyema of the gallbladder, perforation of the gallbladder, and Mirizzi syndrome. Choledocholithiasis may also occur in patients with acute cholecystitis and will be discussed further in the section on Biliary Tract Imaging in this chapter.

The term *gangrenous cholecystitis* is used to describe the presence of severe gallbladder inflammation with mural necrosis, but does not necessarily indicate clostridial infection. Because of the severe inflammation, patients with gangrenous cholecystitis are at increased risk of perforation. We have seen many patients in whom attempts have been made to remove gangrenous gallbladders laparoscopically. Frequently, the gallbladder is too friable to remove this way and conversion to open cholecystectomy is required. In patients with gangrenous cholecystitis, temporizing in the hopes of avoiding an emergency cholecystectomy is usually not advised.

Sonography is not very specific for the diagnosis of gangrenous cholecystitis unless desquamated mucosa appearing as intraluminal linear membranes is present. Pronounced intramural striations indicative of severe edema may also be present when there is gangrenous change, but is a far less specific sign. On cholescintigraphy, a band of increased tracer accumulation may be seen at the edge of the liver where it abuts the gangrenous gallbladder. This finding has been called the rim sign and most likely is due to perihepatitis (Figure 9.24).

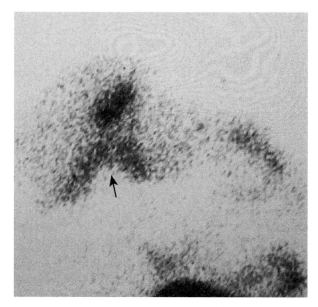

Figure 9.24 Cholescintigram using ^{99m}Tc-DISIDA shows the "rim sign" (arrow) indicating increased tracer accumulation where the gallbladder abuts the liver. This sign is very suggestive of gangrenous cholecystitis.

Emphysematous cholecystitis represents severe acute cholecystitis caused by a gas-forming organism. In about one third of patients, *Clostridia welchii* or *C. perfringens* are isolated from the infected bile. In the remaining patients other gas-forming organisms are the culprits. Emphysematous cholecystitis tends to occur in elderly patients, a significant number of whom are diabetic. Because of this association, small-vessel disease and gallbladder ischemia may play a contributory role. Like patients with gangrenous cholecystitis, patients with emphysematous cholecystitis are at substantially increased risk for perforation.

On sonography, emphysematous cholecystitis may be diagnosed as "dirty" (indistinct), shadowing arising from the gallbladder wall or lumen (Figure 9.25). Small foci of gas may produce "ring-down" or reverberation artifact. If there is marked accumulation of intramural gas, the gallbladder lumen may be entirely obscured by shadowing and reverberation artifact. It is important not to confuse reverberation from focal gas accumulation within the gallbladder wall with that of adenomyomatosis, one of the hyperplastic cholecystopathies. The latter will produce the typical ring-down artifact of reverberation, but will not demonstrate gas on CT scans or plain abdominal radiographs.

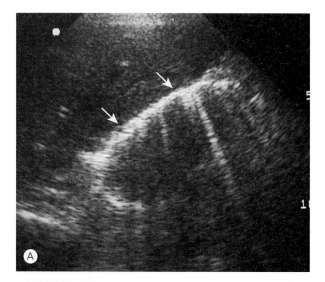

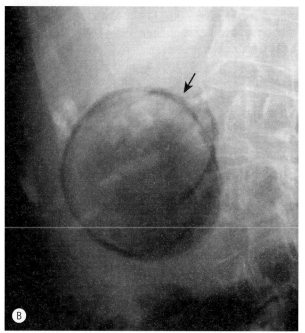

Figure 9.25 A) Ultrasound exhibits an echogenic gallbladder wall (arrows) with reverberation artifact. While not a specific appearance, the finding is suggestive of acute emphysematous cholecystitis. B) A plain abdominal radiograph confirms gas in the gallbladder wall (arrow).

Whenever sonographic findings are suggestive of emphysematous cholecystitis, the clinician should not hesitate to get a plain abdominal film, especially in diabetics. If positive, the film will show either circumferential, "bubbly" lucencies in the gallbladder wall, or a featureless extra-intestinal collection representing the gallbladder lumen (Figure 9.25). It is unusual for adjacent bowel loops or the gastric antrum to be mistaken for a gas-filled gallbladder, because the gallbladder does not exhibit peristalsis and has a characteristic location within the plane of the hepatic major fissure. If, however, there is confusion, CT can help. Gas in the gallbladder lumen may produce sufficient artifact and reverberation so as to render the gallbladder nearly invisible.

Gas formation may originate in the gallbladder wall, but it can rapidly spread into the gallbladder lumen, pericholecystic tissue, or hepatoduodenal ligament. The latter represents serious spread of infection, which is likely to require an extensive open cholecystectomy because pus usually coexists with the escaping gas. If the cystic duct is not completely occluded by an impacted stone or inflammation, or if accessory cholecystohepatic ducts are present, gas and bacteria may escape into the intrahepatic biliary ductal system. This may prompt the development of generalized cholangitis. Once the diagnosis of emphysematous cholecystitis is established, cholecystectomy should be performed as soon as possible. If the patient cannot tolerate surgery, percutaneous cholecystostomy may be considered as a temporizing maneuver, but cannot be used in lieu of surgery given the likelihood of underlying gallbladder ischemia.

Gallbladder empyema represents a distended gallbladder filled with viscous pus. Static bile is an excellent culture medium for organisms; an infected, inflamed gallbladder with an impacted cystic duct stone will quickly evolve into an empyema if cholecystectomy is not performed. Empyema identified on cross-sectional studies represents a relative contraindication to the laparoscopic cholecystectomy unless the gallbladder exhibits minimal wall edema and little distension.

Impressive gallbladder distension is common in empyema. The dilated gallbladder may extend inferiorly into the pelvis. Ultrasound usually shows a distended gallbladder full of non-shadowing echogenic debris, which may be sludge, pus, or mucosal exudate. It is typically very viscous and may not "settle out" as occurs with uninfected sludge. On CT, the suppurative gallbladder contents may have slightly greater attenuation than normal bile. Gallbladder distension, wall thickening, perihepatitis seen as reduced hepatic attenuation, and surrounding inflammatory stranding may be seen extending into the pericholecystic and mesenteric fat (Figure 9.26).

Gallbladder perforation usually occurs as an indolent process in the context of chronic cholecystitis. If the stone enters the duodenum, it

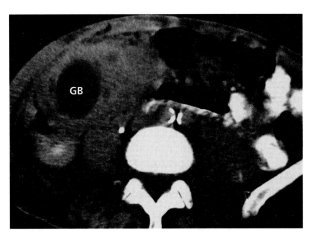

Figure 9.26 Computed tomography scan shows a dilated, thick-walled gallbladder (GB). Inflammatory mesenteric stranding is seen extending across the midline. At surgery gallbladder empyema was proven.

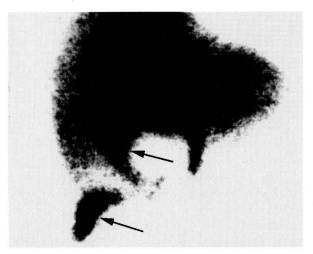

Figure 9.27 Cholescintigram using ^{99m}Tc-DISIDA shows extravasated tracer (arrows) tracking around a photopenic gallbladder. In the setting of acute cholecystitis this finding suggests gallbladder perforation.

may migrate distally and produce bowel obstruction, the so-called gallstone "ileus" (see p. 161). Gallbladder perforation can also occur in the setting of acute cholecystitis, although this is uncommon since symptomatic stones are so aggressively removed in the laparoscopic cholecystectomy era. Recognition that perforation has occurred is important because the presence of bile leakage is a relative surgical emergency. It is also a relative contraindication to laparoscopic cholecystectomy. The mortality of perforation can be quite high, especially if generalized sepsis ensues.

Ultrasonography or CT will often demonstrate a pericholecystic fluid collection with non-specific features in patients with perforation. Percutaneous aspiration may be needed to distinguish between a biloma and pericholecystic abscess that does not contain bile. In some cases stones will be seen outside the gallbladder on CT or plain films. The gallbladder lumen may become difficult to identify on ultrasound as bile leakage decompresses it into the peritoneal cavity. Ultrasound image quality may further be compromised by the presence of an adjacent small-bowel sentinel loop in the area of bile leakage. Nuclear cholescintigraphy offers the most specific appearance for perforation, demonstrating extravasation of tracer from the perforated gallbladder (Figure 9.27).

Mirizzi syndrome occurs when a stone impacts in the cystic duct and causes severe inflammation. The classical description included a fistula from the inflamed cystic duct into the common hepatic duct. A localized inflammatory mass may surround the fistula. When the surgeon sees a duct coming out of an inflammatory mass, the natural tendency is to believe the inflammatory mass is the gallbladder, and to ligate the duct in the mistaken belief that it is the cystic duct. In fact, in Mirizzi syndrome, the duct being ligated is the common hepatic duct.

Mirizzi syndrome should be considered whenever acute cholecystitis and biliary obstruction are simultaneously present. To specifically make the diagnosis, a stone should be seen straddling the junction of the cystic and common hepatic duct. We have had better luck seeing this on CT than on ultrasound. Inflammatory reaction in the hepatoduodenal ligament will be evident on both studies, and in fact can serve to obscure the ductal findings. Dilated intrahepatic bile ducts and intramural edema within the gallbladder wall will also be identified. Intraoperative cholangiography or preoperative ERCP should be used to confirm the diagnosis, or any time that the common hepatic duct anatomy is not clear. In addition, laparoscopic cholecystectomy may be ill advised as separating the cystic duct from the common hepatic duct may be difficult.

Other gallbladder diseases

Acute acalculous cholecystitis Acute gallbladder inflammation in the absence of stones is found in a small minority of patients undergoing cholecystectomy. Although many predisposing factors have been associated with acute acalculous cholecystitis, this disease is most commonly recognized in trauma and intensive care unit patients. Ischemia is a frequent element of this condition. Gallbladder distension resulting from hyperalimentation, hypotension, mesenteric ischemia, altered portal venous and bile flow associated with mechanical ventilation, and vasculitis may all produce gallbladder ischemia. Immunocompetent patients may get bacterially induced acute acalculous cholecystitis from spread of gastroenteritis via the portal circulation. In the immunocompromised patient, cytomegalovirus and cryptosporidiosis have also been suggested as a cause.

The role of imaging in acalculous cholecystitis is a subject of frequent debate. Cholescintigraphy, ultrasound, and CT have all been proposed as being the best technique to evaluate this disease, but the data are not entirely consistent; we do know that imaging in acute acalculous cholecystitis is not as sensitive or specific as in acute calculous cholecystitis. To make the diagnosis, it is important to maximize the detection of inflammatory changes in the gallbladder wall or occlusion of the cystic duct. On sonography, efforts should be made to elicit the sonographic Murphy's sign and scrutinize the gallbladder wall for edema. Unfortunately, eliciting Murphy's sign in intensive-care patients may be difficult. Pericholecystic fluid in the absence of generalized ascites is also helpful. Computed tomography with high levels of circulating contrast medium can demonstrate similar findings, such as low-attenuation intramural edema and perihepatitis in the adjacent liver parenchyma.

Chronic acalculous cholecystitis
Chronic acalculous cholecystitis is a poorly understood entity that may be associated with biliary pain and which often, but not always, resolves with cholecystectomy. Chronic acalculous disease probably represents an early stage of cholesterol gallstone formation when bile is lithogenic but macroscopic stones are not yet present. Gallbladder function and ejection fraction may be impaired. The gallbladder wall may show changes of chronic cholecystitis. Some surgeons accept the concept of chronic acalculous cholecystitis and are willing to perform cholecystectomy based on symptoms in the face of a reduced ejection fraction on cholescintigraphy, and others are not.

Adenomyomatosis
Adenomyomatosis is one of the hyperplastic cholecystopathies. It occurs in patients with chronic cholecystitis who get gall-

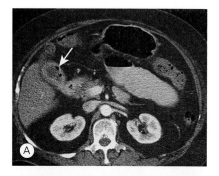

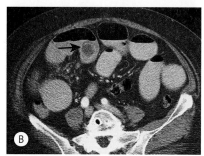

Figure 9.28 A) Air bubbles (arrow) are seen within the gallbladder. These are due to a fistulous tract from the gallbladder to the intestine. B) A faintly calcified gallstone (arrow) is seen within the mid-small bowel. The small bowel is dilated and fluid filled. The findings suggest gallstone ileus.

bladder-wall thickening and submucosal herniation of the epithelium to form Rokitansky–Aschoff sinuses. The sinuses may be seen on ultrasound as small cystic spaces or more commonly as echogenic foci containing small stones or lithogenic sludge. When the latter occurs ring-down due to reverberation artifact is common. The gallbladder may be constricted in these areas.

Gallstone ileus
Gallstone ileus occurs in the setting of chronic cholecystitis and refers to the erosion of a gallstone into the gastrointestinal tract with subsequent development of bowel obstruction (not ileus). These large stones may pass, producing minimal symptoms, or obstruct at narrow portions of the gastrointestinal tract such as the duodenum, ligament of Treitz, ileocecal valve, sigmoid colon, or any area of stricture (Figure 9.28). We have seen gallstones obstruct in areas of Crohn's disease, diverticulitis, and even above a carcinoid.

Radiographically, gallstone ileus is characterized by air in the biliary tree, intestinal obstruction, and the presence of a radiopaque gallstone surrounded by intestinal gas. The diagnosis on plain film is highly suggestive, but is especially compelling on

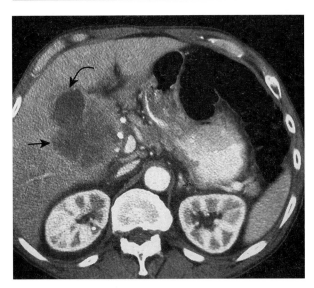

Figure 9.29 The thick-walled gallbladder (curved arrow) is engulfed by a soft-tissue mass (arrow). While this could be a hepatic tumor involving the gallbladder, it is far more likely that the findings represent gallbladder carcinoma spreading into the adjacent liver.

CT because the stone and the intestinal obstruction transition zone are so well seen.

Carcinoma of the gallbladder Carcinoma of the gallbladder usually arises in patients with long-standing chronic cholecystitis. Porcelain gallbladder (calcification in the gallbladder wall) is also a significant risk factor. Carcinoma may present as an intraluminal polypoid mass, focal or diffuse gallbladder wall thickening, or as a large bulky mass engulfing the gallbladder and spreading into adjacent structures. Masses are readily visualized on ultrasound, but wall thickening may be more subtle and mimic cholecystitis. On CT gallbladder carcinoma shows variable enhancement with intravenous contrast (Figure 9.29). Acute cholecystitis often will produce a homogenous, uniform band of low-attenuation edema in the gallbladder wall on CT. Tumor tends to be more nodular and irregular with a more well-defined soft-tissue component on CT and areas of enhancement mixed with low attenuation. Both diseases produce low attenuation perihepatitis and streaky "tentacles" in the fat of the hepatoduodenal ligament.

Although imaging may understage some gallbladder cancers, it seldom overstages them. It is important to look for nodular local invasion of the liver as well as for distant hepatic metastases. Computed tomography and MRI excel at this and also may visualize portal, celiac, and pancreatico-duodenal adenopathy. Evidence of common hepatic duct obstruction from adenopathy or direct invasion of the tumor into the porta hepatis is frequently present and may require percutaneous or endoscopic drainage.

Biliary tract imaging

Imaging approach to biliary obstruction

The patient with biliary obstruction is usually jaundiced, but occasionally presents with constitutional symptoms and only alkaline phosphatase elevation. Most patients who are jaundiced will have dilated ducts as jaundice occurs relatively late in the natural history of obstruction. The imaging plan for suspected biliary obstruction requires that the radiologist and clinician understand the questions that need to be answered to make a diagnosis and plan for subsequent therapy. In painless jaundice, the radiologist assumes that the clinician can assign a level of confidence to the liver-enzyme picture. If the bilirubin and liver enzymes are equivocal, sonography or MRCP is generally the screening test which is employed. If positive, it may suggest the need for CT or direct cholangiography. If negative, the enzymes and even imaging should be repeated in a few days to look for evolving changes which may better characterize the process. If, after this conservative approach, ultrasound and MRCP do not make the diagnosis, diagnostic ERCP may be necessary.

In elderly patients with painless jaundice and where the clinician is confident that a classic obstructive pattern is present, we generally go directly to CT for initial evaluation at our institution. This is especially true if there is any element of weight loss or back pain to suggest pancreatic cancer. Computed tomography, and to a lesser extent transabdominal ultrasound, provide a wealth of information on, for example, the extent of the tumor, the feasibility of surgical biliary bypass, the feasibility of biopsy and non-surgical drainage. The most important information regarding the feasibility of resection or surgical bypass is the location of the upper edge of the tumor. If the tumor extends up into the intrahepatic ducts, surgical bypass (except for the technically difficult intrahepatic cholangiojejunostomy) is not possible. If this information cannot be determined cross-sectionally, cholangiography is indicated. Certainly, evidence of advanced disease tempers our enthusiasm for doing anything except a biopsy to establish the diagnosis. If specific clinical indications such as cholangitis or severe pruritus are present, palliative drainage should be considered. If surgery is imminent, we do not "routinely" preoperatively drain the bile ducts.

It is not so easy to be dogmatic about the approach to biliary colic. If fever is present, acute cholecystitis versus choledocholithiasis with secondary cholangitis are the two main considerations. If that is the case, cholescintigraphy or ultrasound is an acceptable means of beginning the patient's evaluation. If characteristic findings of acute cholecystitis are not present, it is important to look for evidence of bile-duct obstruction. Scintigraphy is very sensitive for detecting altered biliary dynamics due to low grade obstruction. Unfortunately, in some centers the emergently performed "rule out acute cholecystitis" scintigram may not be sufficient to diagnose obstruction. The examination must be conducted so that ductal dynamics, especially wash out of activity on delayed images, can be visually scrutinized and, if possible, analyzed on the computer.

Sonography is the other choice for initial evaluation of patients with biliary colic. Only about two thirds of patients with common bile duct stones have those stones detected on sonography. Computed tomography is probably more sensitive than ultrasound in the detection of distal bile duct stones but has historically been under-utilized in the setting of suspected benign disease. The imprecise nature of ultrasound, and even CT, has led some gastroenterologists to believe that ERCP should be performed in every patient with a history of biliary colic or gallstone pancreatitis. With the advent of MRCP and increasing recognition that most 2- to 4-millimeter stones march down the bile duct into the duodenum, early diagnostic ERCP is becoming less common.

The approach to isolated alkaline phosphatase elevation will usually begin with ultrasound or CT. Elevation of alkaline phosphatase in the absence of jaundice either occurs due to low-grade (often early) obstruction of the central bile ducts or segmental (focal) biliary obstruction. Ultrasound in conjunction with cholecystokinin administration probably fares better than CT in detecting low-grade obstructive lesions of the bile duct. If alkaline phosphatase elevation is caused by segmental biliary obstruction, CT and ultrasound are both useful, with CT having the slight edge. Small pockets of minimally dilated intrahepatic ducts are often more obvious

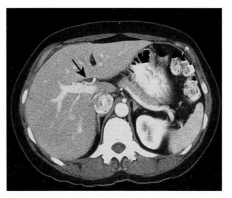

Figure 9.30 The normal common hepatic duct (arrow) is almost always well seen on high-quality sonograms and contrast-enhanced computed tomography scans.

on CT than ultrasound. The ability to use oblique or sagittal scan planes, however, helps ultrasound to localize the point of obstruction precisely. It is very common to see focally dilated ducts in patients with widespread liver metastases. Magnetic resonance cholangiopancreatography can also detect segmental obstruction, but is usually not necessary.

Unique aspects of biliary anatomy

On CT the hepatic arteries and the portal veins will normally be densely opacified with contrast material. Normal-size intrahepatic ducts will not be identifiable. Occasionally, the right or left hepatic duct may be seen as a low attenuation (near water density) structure anterior to its respective portal vein branch. It is important not to confuse small amounts of fat surrounding the hepatic vessels or lymphedema (in patients with ascites, abdominal trauma, or recent liver transplant) with dilated ducts. This type of edema usually surrounds the vessel circumferentially.

As the porta hepatis region is scanned, the common hepatic duct will be seen anterior to the hepatic artery and portal vein (Figure 9.30). In the axial plane, the hepatic artery may actually be seen coursing through the section. As with ultrasound, the common hepatic duct should not exceed 6 millimeters in diameter. The duct wall should be less than 1.0 to 1.5 millimeters in thickness. In patients who have sclerosing cholangitis, the duct wall may be symmetrically thickened. Cholangiocarcinoma typically thickens the duct assymetrically. As the common bile duct descends into the pancreas, it crosses over the duodenum and migrates progressively posteriorly on its way to the

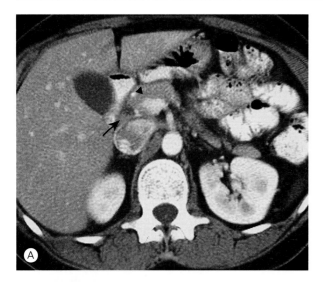

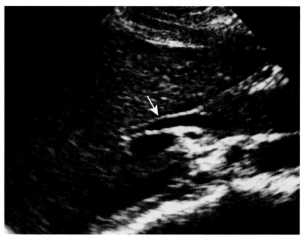

Figure 9.32 Sonography may view structures in parasagittal planes. This sonogram was obtained with the scan plane perpendicular to the right costal margin. This is the best view for visualizing the common hepatic duct (arrow). It is seen arching over the portal vein and extending inferiorly into the pancreatic parenchyma.

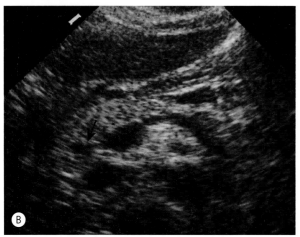

Figure 9.31 A) The normal distal common bile duct (arrow) is identified on computed tomography and (B) on sonography in the axial plane. It lies at the posterior margin of the pancreas. The enhanced gastroduodenal artery (arrowhead) is also seen on computed tomography.

ampulla. At the level of the ampulla of Vater, the duct may actually be seen crossing the pancreato-duodenal space to enter the duodenal wall. This space separates the pancreatic head from the duodenum and is normally filled with fat, the retroduodenal veins, and small peripancreatic lymph nodes. The gastroduodenal artery may be seen at the anterolateral edge of the pancreas. The common bile duct lies at the posterolateral margin of the pancreatic head (Figure 9.31).

When the bile duct is obstructed, its caliber will increase. It is important to scrutinize any transition zones that are present. When the duct is abruptly amputated with a very short transition zone, this often suggests the presence of neoplasm as the

underlying cause of obstruction. Stones within the duct will typically produce a bull's-eye appearance because of bile surrounding the stone just above its equator or meniscus.

Both the intra- and extrahepatic ducts may also be evaluated with ultrasound. The normal intrahepatic ducts are usually not evident, except as they contribute to the overall texture of the liver. When dilated, the ducts appear as sonolucent, tubular, branching structures in both longitudinal, coronal, and sagittal planes. The ducts may be followed as they converge centrally on the common hepatic duct. The common hepatic duct is best evaluated by placing the transducer perpendicular to the right costal margin. This view allows the duct to be seen as it crosses anterior to the right portal vein in virtually all patients (Figure 9.32). The hepatic artery will be seen as a round structure in cross-section, between the duct and portal vein. In approximately one fourth of patients who have a completely replaced accessory right hepatic artery, the artery will pass behind the portal vein. This is a common anatomic variant that can usually be delineated by following the artery back to the aorta or by using Doppler ultrasound.

The normal duct can be seen descending from the liver and passing over the duodenum as it migrates posteriorly into the pancreatic head. The normal common hepatic duct should not exceed 6 millimeters in diameter anterior to the right portal vein. This diameter is also used as the upper limit of normal size, even in patients who have undergone prior cholecystectomy. While several large population studies suggested that the bile duct dilates following removal of the gallbladder, this has subsequently been shown not to be true by analyzing examination of the same patient before and after cholecystectomy. After the age of 50 years, 1 millimeter can be added per decade of life to the maximum allowable diameter.

Diseases that commonly cause biliary obstruction

Pancreatic cancer Focal enlargement of the pancreas (mass effect) is the hallmark of pancreatic carcinoma on cross-sectional studies. Because the resolution of these studies has improved, it is increasingly common to identify small tumors. Over two thirds of pancreatic carcinomas arise in the pancreatic head. Almost all will obstruct the pancreatic duct, and the majority will involve the bile duct. On sonography, pancreatic carcinoma will be relatively sonolucent compared with the normal pancreatic parenchyma. Based on echo-texture alone, it is impossible to distinguish focal chronic pancreatitis (which may be lucent or echogenic) from carcinoma. On CT, carcinoma tends to produce focal low attenuation and will enhance with iodinated contrast material less than the normal pancreas. Chronic pancreatitis may produce similar changes, but usually results in more diffuse abnormality of the gland and frequently exhibits calcification. A small minority of tumors will show attenuation similar to that of the normal pancreas after contrast. An even smaller number will appear hyperdense. Since visualization of tumors depends on differential enhancement of tumor versus normal pancreas, achieving high levels of circulating contrast is extremely important on CT.

Computed tomography, ultrasound, and MRI may all be used to trace the dilated bile duct and pancreatic duct as they abruptly terminate in a mass. Concomitant involvement and obstruction of the bile duct and pancreatic duct has been called the double-duct sign (Figure 9.33). It is not specific for pancreatic or ampullary carcinoma; chronic pancreatitis may produce similar changes in a small minority of patients. There may be secondary changes of chronic pancreatitis, but usually there are not. If the patient appears to have local disease that may be amenable to resection, it is important to determine the length of bile duct that will be available for biliary bypass. This can be done on

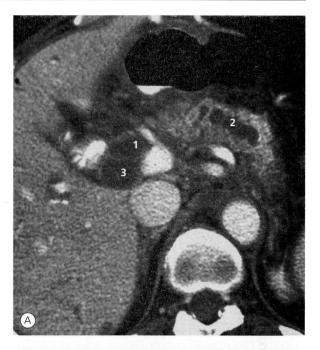

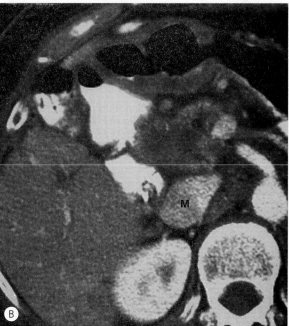

Figure 9.33 Computed tomography has the advantage of not only identifying the bile duct and pancreatic duct, but also the surrounding structures. A) The dilated common hepatic duct (1), pancreatic duct (2), and gallbladder neck (3) are seen. B) This section, 1 centimeter further caudad, shows a pancreatic mass (M) obstructing the ducts and gallbladder. This variation of the double-duct sign was caused by pancreatic carcinoma in this patient.

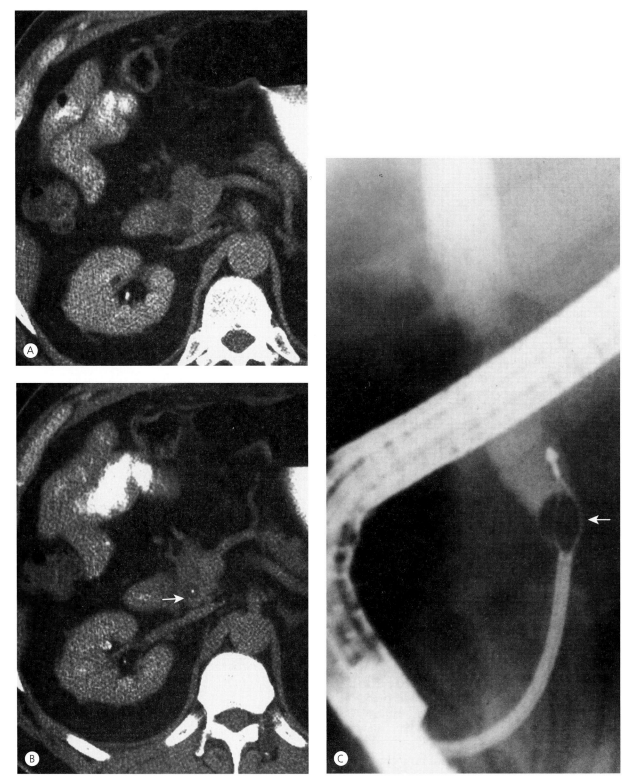

Figure 9.34 Multi-slice computed tomography has the advantage of allowing sections to be made thinner or repositioned even after the scan has been acquired. A) In this patient a mildly dilated common bile duct is identified within the pancreatic head. B) By repositioning the section just below the one shown in Figure 34A, a small, calcified nidus (arrow) is seen suggestive of a calculus. C) A stone (arrow) is confirmed on endoscopic retrograde pancreatography.

CT by reformatting the ducts in a sagittal or coronal orientation, or the patient may be sent for MRCP.

Choledocholithiasis Choledocholithiasis is the most common cause of biliary obstruction without a mass. Computed tomography will make the diagnosis in roughly 80% of cases. The most useful criteria are focal duct dilatation, visualization of intraductal, high-density material indicative of stone calcification, and the presence of a target or halo within the duct. The latter is due to visualization of a bile meniscus usually just above the equator of the stone. Thin sections and reconstruction of overlapping sections by using helical CT has further improved the accuracy of stone detection with CT (Figure 9.34). Ultrasound, in contradistinction, only results in detection of half to two thirds of stones. Failure to see discrete shadowing and obscuration of the distal duct by duodenal gas are common pitfalls. While CT has improved in its detection rate, MRCP and ERCP are still more accurate modalities for stone visualization.

Cholangiocarcinoma Cholangiocarcinoma in most patients will produce subtle mass effect. At presentation most tumors are only 1 to 1.5 centimeters in diameter and can be detected only on cross-sectional studies after careful scrutiny of the duct caliber and contour (Figure 9.35). Most tumors will result in a focal stenosis of the duct, but polypoid and scirrhous or infiltrative morphologies also occur. Roughly 50% of cholangiocarcinomas can be expected to occur at the bifurcation (Klatskin tumor) and extend superiorly to involve the right and left hepatic ducts. The association of cholangiocarcinoma with sclerosing cholangitis, choledochal cysts, pyogenic/Asian cholangiohepatitis, and any cause of biliary stasis is well known.

On sonography, cholangiocarcinoma is usually echolucent compared with liver parenchyma. Because of the flexible viewing positions afforded by ultrasound, the duct may be followed directly into the mass. On dynamically enhanced CT, cholangiocarcinoma is typically hypovascular. In a minority of patients it can be iso- or even hyper-attenuating compared with liver parenchyma. The latter is especially prone to occur in patients with intrahepatic cholangiocarcinoma. Computed tomography will often show focal ductal dilatation involving just the ducts of the right or left lobe if the mass is asymetrically straddling the duct bifurcation. If the tumor is narrowing the common

hepatic duct or is extending superiorly to involve the right and left hepatic ducts, generalized biliary dilatation will be present. Delayed images (10 to 15 minutes after the contrast injection) may demonstrate hyperdense vascular staining in these tumors because of slow vascular flow (Figure 9.36).

Cholangiography and cross-sectional studies all play a role in determining whether the ductal anatomy will allow surgical resection. If the tumor involves the bifurcation and has isolated the right and left ductal systems, it will not be resectable in most centers. Care should be taken in looking at CT scans for this finding or a MRCP should be performed, If the tumor involves the common hepatic duct but spares the right and left hepatic ducts, it may be amenable to choledocho-jejunostomy. Because it is the upper margin of the tumor that is important, contrast must be placed above the stricture should ERCP be performed. This, of course, will also necessitate establishing drainage if a high-grade stricture is present. Ultrasound, CT, or MRI may visualize the surrounding structures and determine if metastatic spread has occurred. Involvement of the portal vein, or spread to the adjacent liver are common causes of non-resectability.

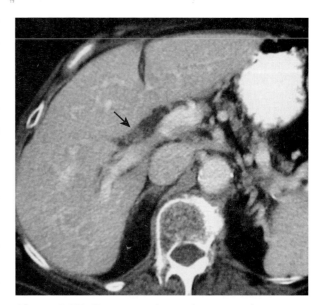

Figure 9.35 Contrast-enhanced computed tomography scan shows a small mass (arrow) involving the common hepatic duct. Other sections showed dilated intrahepatic bile ducts. The finding is very suggestive of a cholangiocarcinoma of the Klatskin type. These tumors are often small and subtle at presentation.

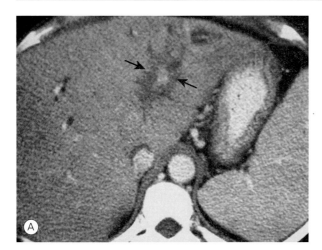

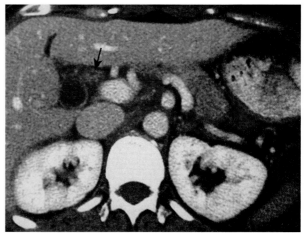

Figure 9.37 Normally the bile-duct wall is paper thin. If duct-wall thickening is present (arrow), considerations include primary sclerosing cholangitis or scarring from prior infection or surgery. This patient was found to have inflammatory bowel disease and primary sclerosing cholangitis.

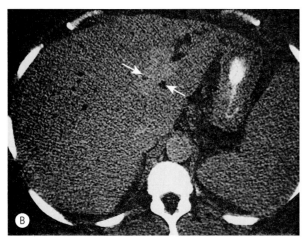

Figure 9.36 Delayed enhancement may be a helpful sign in detecting cholangiocarcinoma. A) A portal venous phase scan reveals low-attenuation tumor (arrows) surrounding the left portal vein. Note the peripheral dilated ducts "above" the tumor. B) A delayed scan 10 minutes later reveals delayed enhancement (arrows) in the area that was previously low attenuation. This pattern of enhancement is very suggestive of intrahepatic cholangiocarcinoma.

Primary sclerosing cholangitis Sclerosing cholangitis also seldom produces mass effect on cross-sectional studies with the possible exception of patients with multifocal fibrosclerosis in whom fibrotic masses occur in locations like the retroperitoneum and peripancreatic space. In most patients, CT and ultrasound will both reveal focal "pockets" of dilated intrahepatic ducts in patients with primary sclerosing cholangitis. Significant symmetrical thickening of the extrahepatic duct wall (2 to 4 mm) may also be seen on ultrasound

and CT (Figure 9.37). Ductal pseudodiverticula, although common, are below the resolution of CT or ultrasound. Lobar atrophy and the changes of secondary biliary cirrhosis may be present in long-standing disease. Small stones, which may be calcified, may develop from stasis above strictures. Adenopathy in the porta hepatis is often associated with primary sclerosing cholangitis. If any asymmetric duct-wall thickening or a focal mass is present, a secondary cholangiocarcinoma may be present. This usually requires endoscopic, percutaneous, or even open biopsy to definitively prove. When it comes to mapping the extent of primary sclerosing cholangitis and looking for subtle evidence of progression there is still no substitute for direct cholangiography.

Asian cholangiohepatitis Asian cholangiohepatitis due to *Clonorchis sinensis* or *Fasciola hepatica* is common in southeast Asia and occasionally seen in immigrants to the US from that part of the world. In some cases, parasites are not present, but persistent secondary bacterial infections and strictures develop resulting in a similar clinical picture to primary sclerosing cholangitis.

Computed tomography and ultrasound images of Asian cholangiohepatitis may also be similar to primary sclerosing cholangitis. Focal pockets of dilatation above strictures, duct-wall thickening, and stones or debris within the ductal system occur. The presence of multiple calcified stones and high-density debris within the ducts favors Asian cholangiohepatitis over primary sclerosing cholangitis; in the latter intrahepatic stones are less common and they often lack dense calcification.

Choledochal cysts Choledochal cysts are relatively rare in the US. They are far more common in Japan and the Far East. On CT and ultrasound, the various types of choledochal cysts have a predictable appearance based on their morphology.

- Type 1 cysts, which are by far the most common, are seen as an area of cystic or fusiform dilatation of the common bile duct. There is usually relatively little dilatation above or below the cyst.
- Type 2 cysts exhibit a diverticulum that lies adjacent to and in communication with the duct. Both Type 1 and 2 cysts are easily diagnosed on both CT and ultrasound. The bile-duct wall is usually paper thin; an area of focal thickening may suggest the development of a secondary cholangiocarcinoma.
- Type 3 cyst (choledochocele) is somewhat more difficult to diagnose on CT and ultrasound. Because Type 3 cysts represent dilatation of the intraduodenal segment of the duct (with partial prolapse into the duodenum), its visualization is variable depending upon the degree of distension and contrast opacification of the duodenal contents.
- Caroli's disease, Type 4, and Type 5 cysts are rare, but may give rise to confusing appearances. Multiple intrahepatic cysts may overlap in appearance, with the appearance of primary sclerosing cholangitis, multiple cholangitic abscesses, and other cystic lesions of the liver including multiple biliary hamartomas and autosomal polycystic kidney disease. When superimposed infection, cirrhosis, and secondary cholangiocarcinoma occur, the CT and ultrasound appearance may be even more confusing. Seeing multiple intrahepatic cystic spaces with areas of bile duct dilatation is suggestive of cystic dilatation of the intrahepatic ducts, but cholangiography and often biopsy of the liver is needed to sort out the diagnostic considerations. Patients with Caroli's disease may also have renal tubular ectasia (medullary sponge kidney) with stones and cystic changes in the kidney.

Pancreatic imaging

Computed tomography is the dominant modality for screening evaluation of the pancreas for neoplasms and complications of pancreatitis. It allows visualization of the entire gland far more frequently than conventional transabdominal ultrasound. Magnetic resonance imaging is increasingly being used to evaluate the pancreas, but its role is generally limited to studying patients with contrast allergies, renal failure, or in whom the diagnosis is unclear using cross-sectional modalities or ERCP.

As described earlier in this chapter, helical CT clearly has advantages over conventional scanning for evaluation of the pancreas. Both oral and intravenous contrast agents are needed to produce an optimum examination of the pancreas. The gastrointestinal tract may be opacified with either dilute barium, water-soluble iodinated contrast, or a negative opacification agent such as water. In patients in whom neoplasm is the primary concern, negative opacification of the duodenum may be helpful in recognizing invasion of the duodenal wall. In the setting of pancreatitis, we generally administer dilute barium so as not to confuse unopacified loops of bowel for peripancreatic fluid collections. Pre-contrast, non-helical sections are obtained first to localize the pancreas prior to the helical scan. Contrast is then injected at a rate of at least 3 mL/sec for a total dose of 130 to 150 mL. Images are obtained in the pancreatic phase at approximately 40 seconds and again at 65 seconds in the portal venous phase. The pancreatic phase optimizes contrast differences between the normal pancreas and possible neoplasm. The entire liver will be included on the portal venous phase helical scan.

Pancreatic neoplasms

Pancreatic carcinoma Pancreatic carcinoma is one of the most lethal neoplasms afflicting mankind; nearly 25 000 cases are reported each year in the US with less than 5% long-term survival. Even at presentation, the lack of a true capsule surrounding the tumor results in diffuse retroperitoneal infiltration and encasement of the splanchnic vessels in most patients. Computed tomography plays two important roles in the evaluation of pancreatic carcinoma: it detects the presence of neoplasm and accurately stages it in most patients.

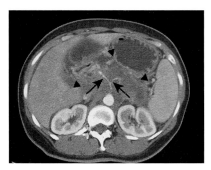

Figure 9.38 Unresectable pancreatic carcinoma. Contrast-enhanced axial computed tomography image through the pancreas reveals a hypodense, non-enhancing solid mass (arrowheads) replacing most of the pancreas and encasing vessels of the celiac axis (arrows). There is also retroperitoneal lymphadenopathy surrounding the aorta.

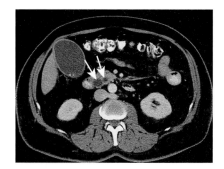

Figure 9.39 Carcinoma of the ampulla of Vater, resulting in the double-duct sign. A contrast-enhanced axial computed tomography scan through the abdomen, shows prominent biliary and pancreatic ducts. A mass in the region of the ampulla of Vater (not shown) was present distally, resulting in this appearance of the double-duct sign (arrow).

The hallmark of pancreatic carcinoma is focal enlargement with an asymmetric glandular contour. At times the tumor may infiltrate the entire gland and produce diffuse enlargement. Secondary acute or chronic pancreatitis can also develop from pancreatic duct obstruction by the neoplasm. In these cases the gland may enlarge even further and the presence of edema may cause the radiologist to overestimate the volume of the tumor. Most pancreatic cancers are of lower attenuation than normal-enhancing pancreatic parenchyma (Figure 9.38). Since helical scans are performed while the circulating contrast level is high, we are increasingly identifying small tumors that do not enlarge the contour of the gland, but which represent an area of reduced attenuation in the absence of clinical pancreatitis.

Carcinoma will often produce the so-called double-duct sign (Figure 9.39). This refers to concomitant obstruction of the bile duct and pancreatic duct. The diagnosis of malignant obstruction on CT is suggested when a focal tumor mass is present in association with abrupt amputation of the bile duct and pancreatic duct. As on cholangiography, an abrupt transition zone at the level of a biliary or pancreatic-duct stricture suggests malignancy.

Resection of pancreatic carcinoma will be precluded in patients with hepatic metastases, nodal involvement beyond the field of resection, or vascular encasement. Encasement of the major vessels greater than 180 degrees of circumference implies that the tumor is not resectable. The presence of overt caliber change of the superior mesenteric artery, celiac artery, portal vein, or superior mesenteric vein even more strongly

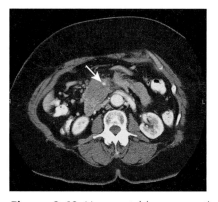

Figure 9.40 Unresectable pancreatic head carcinoma. Contrast-enhanced axial computed tomography scan through the pancreatic head shows an irregular hypodense mass in the head of the pancreas, encasing the superior mesenteric artery (arrow). The mass was also encasing the superior mesenteric vein (not shown).

suggests vascular encasement (Figure 9.40). Benign or well-encapsulated tumors may compress a vessel without encasing it; in our experience however, with pancreatic cancer the tumor is almost always adherent to the vessel when a caliber change is identified. When indistinct fat planes around a vessel are present, the tumor may be non-resectable, but this is not a definitive sign. Three-dimensional rendering of helical CT data may help clarify involvement of major vessels by tumor when uncertainty exists on the axially displayed sections. The three-dimensional model also serves as a preoperative vascular road map to the surgeons in lieu of a conventional arteriogram. If portal-vein encasement is limited to 1 to 2 centimeters in length, grafting the vessel may be considered if no other disease is identified. Endoscopic ultrasound provides similar information to CT, but cannot assess distant disease. Nevertheless, we do not hesitate to recommend EUS in equivocal cases where CT cannot definitively assess the status of the portal or superior mesenteric vein.

Regardless of the imaging technique that is used, we have adopted an approach that has worked well in our attempt to distinguish surgical candidates from those with more advanced disease. If the patient has distant disease sites (hepatic metastases or regional nodes outside the field of possible resection), these, along with the primary tumor, will be percutaneously biopsied. If distant disease is not present, our major focus in determining resectability will be the splanchnic vessels. We deliberately err on the side of "undercalling" vascular involvement, in borderline cases, so as not to exclude patients from their one chance for cure. In this setting EUS or MRI may be of value.

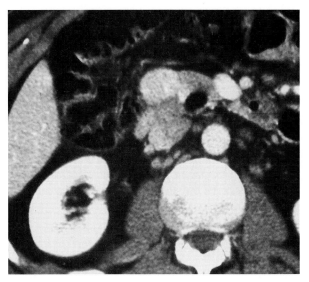

Figure 9.41 Islet cell tumor. Contrast-enhanced computed tomography scan through the head of the pancreas shows a well-defined hyperdense solid mass (arrow).

Islet-cell tumors The islet cells of the pancreas may give rise to a wide variety of functional and non-functional endocrine tumors. The functional tumors are generally small, may be multiple, and become symptomatic owing to their hormonal activity. The islet-cell tumors include insulinomas, gastrinomas, glucagonomas, VIPomas, and somatostatinomas. The non-functional tumors typically are larger in size, producing symptoms only when they have compromised adjacent structures such as the gastrointestinal tract, bile duct, or pancreatic duct.

The hallmark of islet-cell tumors is their hypervascularity. Helical scanning results in high levels of circulating contrast, and hypervascular tumors are much more easily seen to be of higher attenuation than the surrounding gland (Figure 9.41). This is especially pronounced during the arterial phase of contrast rather than the pancreatic phase. Hepatic metastases from islet-cell tumors are also typically hypervascular.

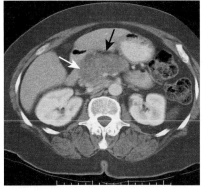

Figure 9.42 A 70-year-old woman with microcystic adenoma in the region of the head of the pancreas. Contrast-enhanced axial computed tomography scan through the pancreatic head, showing a large non-enhancing mass replacing the head of the pancreas (arrows). The mass contains multiple small cysts which do not enhance.

Cystic neoplasms There are two distinctly different types of cystic neoplasms of epithelial origin occurring in the pancreas: the microcystic adenoma and the mucinous cystic neoplasm.

Microcystic adenomas are benign and tend to occur in elderly women. Tumors are equally distributed throughout the gland. The lesions tend to be large at the time of presentation. Multiple small cysts with a prominent radial distribution are

identified. A central fibrotic scar with calcification may also be seen. When helical scans are performed, the cyst septations often show enhancement. The cysts do not enhance and stand out as negative defects against the overall background of enhancing normal pancreatic parenchyma (Figure 9.42). The mass may displace or compress the major splanchnic vessels, but frank encasement or thrombosis is unusual.

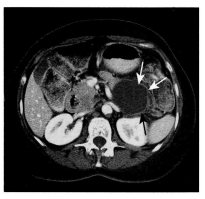

Figure 9.43 Mucinous cystic adenoma. Contrast-enhanced computed tomography scan through the mid-abdomen, showing a large non-enhancing cystic mass in the tail of the pancreas (arrows). No metastases were present at the time of diagnosis.

Mucinous cystic neoplasms tend to occur in a slightly younger age group. This lesion is far more common in women than men. Most lesions are large at presentation, and have a propensity for involvement of the pancreatic tail. Whenever a mucinous neoplasm is identified, it must be presumed malignant and excised unless distant metastases are present. The CT diagnosis can be difficult, but several key differences exist in the appearance of this lesion as compared to microcystic adenoma. The mucinous cystic neoplasm will usually have one or more dominant cysts, which is up to several centimeters in diameter (Figure 9.43). Mural nodules, a prominent soft-tissue component, or a "shaggy" cyst wall may be present. The soft-tissue components may show dramatic enhancement associated with tumor vascularity. While calcification is less common than in microcystic adenoma, we have seen several mucinous malignant lesions with scattered calcifications.

Despite recent advances, it is unlikely that CT can uniformly distinguish benign from malignant cystic neoplasms. While the appearance of some lesions clearly suggests microcystic adenoma, there is considerable overlap in the appearances of cystic lesions. We have seen patients with clusters of pancreatic pseudocysts that have closely mimicked the appearance of cystic neoplasms. The converse, a cystic neoplasm mimicking a pancreatic pseudocyst, is also all too common. Whenever a possible cystic neoplasm is identified, and there is no evidence of advanced disease on CT, an aggressive surgical approach is recommended. In patients who are elderly or refuse surgery, careful follow-up with CT is recommended.

Acute and chronic pancreatitis

Acute pancreatitis Acute pancreatitis results from leakage of pancreatic enzymes and secretions, causing autodigestion and diffuse inflammation of the pancreatic gland. Spreading of the inflammatory process to the surrounding structures and fat is facilitated by lack of a pancreatic capsule. The two most common causes of acute pancreatitis in the US are cholelithiasis and ethanol abuse. Other etiologies include trauma (the most common cause in children), infection, ERCP, drugs, pancreas divisum, and ductal obstruction secondary to tumors. Roughly 10% of cases remain idiopathic. Although the diagnosis of acute pancreatitis is mostly made using clinical and laboratory parameters, an increasing number of patients coming through the emergency room are worked-up radiographically, typically to establish the prognosis and evaluate for complications.

Ranson criteria, which combine five parameters at admission and six parameters 48 hours following admission, are used to assess the systemic effects of pancreatitis and hence the severity of the disease process. The higher the number of positive risk factors, the higher the morbidity and mortality. Patients who have less than three positive signs usually have mild pancreatitis and no associated mortality. Patients with six or more positive signs will most likely have severe necrotizing pancreatitis and have an associated mortality rate of over 50%. For patients having scores between three and five however, staging the severity of pancreatitis is frequently indeterminate. The more recent APACHE II (Acute Physiology and Chronic Health Evaluation) scoring system, which uses 12 physiologic measurements to assess the severity of the disease, appears to be more accurate in staging acute pancreatitis. Similar to Ranson's criteria, mortality and morbidity increase with higher scores. In addition to predicting the severity of the disease, the APACHE II system allows better monitoring of the patient during hospitalization.

Contrast-enhanced CT scan using protocols tailored to the pancreas is a safe and accurate method to evaluate the severity and extent of pancreatitis. Imaging of acute pancreatitis using contrast-enhanced CT scan is usually performed using thin cuts through the pancreas prior to and following the administration of intravenous contrast agents. Preferably patients are also given positive oral contrast such as barium to opacify adjacent loops of small bowel. In many cases, patients will be on bowel rest and no oral contrast is administered. Computed tomography can differentiate the milder edematous form of pancreatitis from the more severe necrotizing form of the disease. The greater the necrosis and areas devoid of parenchymal enhancement, the poorer the outcome. Patients who have less than 30% necrosis of their gland have no associated mortality, whereas involvement of 50% or more of the pancreas have a mortality rate of roughly 25%. Together with APACHE scoring, an accurate imaging and physiologic picture may be obtained.

Approximately one third of patients with mild pancreatitis will have a normal CT scan. The remaining patients will have an edematous, enlarged but homogeneously enhancing gland. This could be focal or diffuse, involving the entire gland. The contour may be irregular with surrounding inflammatory stranding and thickening of the fascial planes. The inflammation is greatest in the anterior pararenal space and transverse mesocolon. As inflammation extends laterally it will thicken Gerota's fascia (Figure 9.44). Ultrasound evaluation will show diffuse or focal enlargement of the gland, assuming there is no significant associated small-bowel ileus, which considerably limits the examination. The gland appears typically isoechoic or hypoechoic relative to liver (Figure 9.45). In addition, sonographic evaluation may show cholelithiasis as the etiology to the pancreatitis.

In more severe acute pancreatitis, there are considerably more surrounding inflammatory changes with fluid collection formation within and surrounding the gland. These fluid collections can dissect along fascial planes from the retroperitoneum (anterior pararenal and perirenal spaces) to involve the mesentery and the rest of the abdominal organs. Both CT and ultrasound can demonstrate extrapancreatic fluid collections (Figure 9.46). Computed tomography is particularly good at diagnosing necrotizing pancreatitis and shows lack of enhancement of the necrotic pancreas, a finding which cannot be appreciated with sonography. In the absence of infection or other complications, necrosis is the most significant indicator of morbidity and mortality.

Infected necrosis and pancreatic abscess formation are two severe complications of acute pancreatitis.

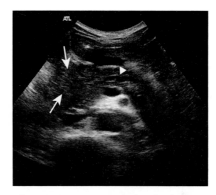

Figure 9.45 Transabdominal ultrasound in a young man with acute epigastric pain. The pancreatic head is enlarged with indistinct margins (arrows). Incidental note is made of the prominence of the pancreatic duct (arrowhead).

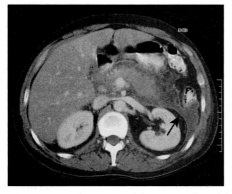

Figure 9.44 38 year-old man with mild acute pancreatitis. Contrast-enhanced, axial computed tomography scan of the abdomen shows an enlarged edematous pancreas with surrounding inflammatory changes and free fluid. The fluid extends into the anterior pararenal space on the left, resulting in thickening of Gerota's fascia (arrow).

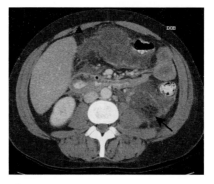

Figure 9.46 Severe acute pancreatitis. Contrast-enhanced axial computed tomography scan through the mid-abdomen showing extensive inflammatory changes in the left retroperitoneal space (arrow). Some of the fluid and inflammatory changes have dissected along fascial planes out of the retroperitoneum into the mesentery (arrowhead).

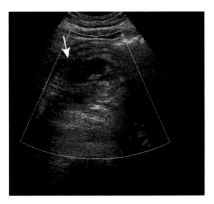

Figure 9.47 Pancreatic abscess. Transabdominal ultrasound shows a complex cystic mass in the region of the head of the pancreas (arrow). This mass was aspirated under ultrasound guidance. Purulent material was obtained and the patient was taken to the operating room for surgical debridement.

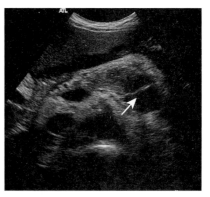

Figure 9.49 Pancreatic pseudocyst. Transabdominal ultrasound shows a well-defined, round, complex fluid collection in the region of the tail of the pancreas (arrow).

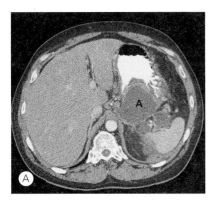

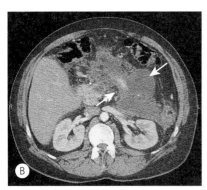

Figure 9.48 Pancreatic abscess. Contrast-enhanced computed tomography scan of the abdomen showing A) thick-walled cystic fluid collection in the lesser sac (A) with surrounding inflammatory changes. B) more irregular-appearing abscesses are noted in the retroperitoneum in the region of the body and tail of the pancreas (arrows).

Both require surgical debridement. Mortality rates approaching 100% have been reported for untreated pancreatic abscess. Sonographically, one will see a thick-walled heterogeneous complex cystic mass with internal debris. Echogenic foci will be seen when there is associated intraluminal gas (Figure 9.47). On CT the presence or new development of gas within a pre-existing, thick-walled, well-defined fluid collection suggests the diagnosis (Figure 9.48), but may also be seen if a spontaneous fistula to the gastrointestinal tract has developed. Rarely, sterile necrosis may show the presence of gas. Ultrasound or CT-guided aspiration prior to surgery may be performed in uncertain cases.

Other complications of acute pancreatitis include pseudocysts, pseudoaneurysms involving the splenic or gastroduodenal artery, and thrombosis of the splenic vein or superior mesenteric vein. Pseudocysts usually occur 4 to 6 weeks following acute pancreatitis. They are the result of maturation of the acute intra- or peripancreatic fluid collections, which develop in the acute phase of the disease. Neither CT nor ultrasound can determine the age of a pseudocyst. On CT and ultrasound they are characterized by a thick fibrous wall in contra-distinction to the much thinner wall of the acute fluid collections (Figures 9.49, 9.50). The contents are typically simple resulting in a homogeneous appearance, unless there is superimposed hemorrhage or infection. Just as the fluid collections in the acute phase, these pseudocysts can dissect along fascial planes to extend out of the retroperitoneum to invade the intraperitoneal cavity (Figure 9.51) and its contents or even the mediastinum. Cysts

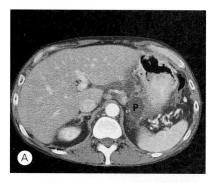

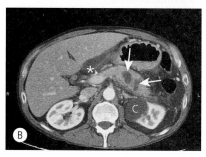

Figure 9.50 Computed tomography scan of pancreatic pseudocysts (same patient as shown in Figure 9.49). Contrast-enhanced axial computed tomography scan of the abdomen reveals A) thin-walled cystic extra-pancreatic pseudocyst (P), and B) two small pseudocysts within the body and tail of the pancreas (arrows) and a third one posterior to the lateral segment of the left of the liver (*). Incidental note is made of a left renal cyst (C).

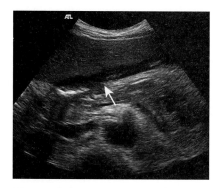

Figure 9.51 Intraperitoneal pseudocyst. Abdominal ultrasound through the head of the pancreas reveals an oblong cystic fluid collection (arrow) corresponding to a pancreatic pseudocyst, which has dissected out of the retroperitoneum.

that are less than 6 centimeters in size tend to resolve spontaneously, whereas the larger ones require percutaneous drainage or surgical debridement if superinfected.

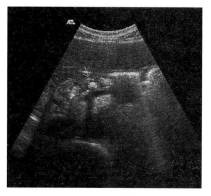

Figure 9.52 Chronic pancreatitis. Abdominal sonogram showing multiple pancreatic calcifications (white arrow) in a patient with chronic pancreatitis.

Chronic pancreatitis Acute and chronic pancreatitis are two separate disease entities, with the latter infrequently being associated or resulting from repeated bouts of acute pancreatitis. Rather, it is secondary to prolonged exposure to inflammation resulting in fibrosis and gradual destruction of the gland. Etiologies include ethanol abuse, hyperlipidemia, cystic fibrosis, hyperparathyroidism, lupus, and cholelithiasis. Early age of onset of the disease is associated with the hereditary form, which is autosomal dominant and is complicated later by development of adenocarcinoma.

On sonography, the pancreas will appear heterogeneous with areas of increased and decreased echogenicity, corresponding to areas of calcification and fibrosis and areas of inflammation respectively (Figure 9.52). The pancreas is usually atrophic, but may be enlarged if extensive fibrosis is present. The main pancreatic duct will be irregularly dilated and contain innumerable small calcifications resulting from calcium carbonate deposition. These findings are similarly depicted on non-contrast enhanced CT scans (Figure 9.53). Intraductal calcifications are present in roughly 50% of cases. Other findings will include fluid collections, focal masses and biliary ductal dilatation in 30% of cases. The diagnosis can be difficult when chronic pancreatitis presents as a focal mass, which can sometimes be indistinguishable from a carcinoma. Further evaluation of these challenging cases is usually needed with MRI, ERCP, or even percutaneous biopsy. Complications of chronic pancreatitis are similar to the ones mentioned for the acute form of the disease, namely pseudocyst formation and splenic and portal venous obstruction.

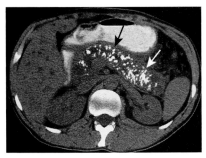

Figure 9.53 Computed tomography scan of chronic pancreatitis. Unenhanced computed tomography scan through the pancreas shows a dilated pancreatic duct with multiple intraductal calcifications of varying sizes (arrows).

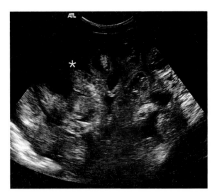

Figure 9.54 Ascites. Ultrasound of the right lower quadrant of the abdomen shows free-flowing ascites (*) between loops of small bowel in a patient with portal hypertension.

Pancreas divisum

Pancreas divisum is the most common anatomic variant of the pancreas. While its relationship is controversial, it is seen in association with idiopathic pancreatitis in roughly 25% of cases. It is characterized by the presence of two separate, non-fused ducts, the dorsal and ventral ducts, draining an incompletely fused gland. The embryonic dorsal duct drains the largest portion of the pancreas, which consists of the tail, body and superior-anterior part of the head directly into the duodenum through the small accessory minor papilla. The shorter, embryonic ventral duct drains the uncinate process and the posterior-inferior portion of the head of the pancreas. It joins the common bile duct to drain through the major papilla into the duodenum. It is postulated that the accessory papilla is too small to appropriately drain the large amounts of exocrine secretions from the larger dorsal pancreas into the duodenum. This would result in repeated bouts of pancreatitis, which appears to involve the neck, body, and tail of the pancreas with relative sparing of the uncinate process. Computed tomography may show a fat plane between the two moieties or less commonly, the two separate draining ducts. Magnetic resonance pancreatography also can show the ductal anatomy, especially if dilatation of the dorsal duct is present.

Mesenteric and peritoneal-space imaging

The peritoneal cavity and mesentery are best evaluated using contrast-enhanced CT scans of the abdomen and pelvis. Ultrasound evaluation is usually limited by the presence of bowel gas and peristalsis. Ultrasound can also be very difficult in patients with a large body habitus. Magnetic resonance imaging is generally not necessary, but offers high sensitivity in the detection of peritoneal tumor implants.

The various potential spaces that form the peritoneal cavity are best visualized on CT when fluid, air, or soft-tissue processes distend and delineate those spaces. All of the potential spaces of the peritoneal cavity communicate with each other. The right subphrenic space communicates with the anterior and posterior (Morison's pouch) subhepatic spaces. The left subphrenic space communicates with the left subhepatic space. On the right, the subphrenic and subhepatic spaces communicate with the pelvic peritoneal cavity through the right paracolic gutter. On the left, the left phrenicocolic ligament prevents free communication between the subphrenic and subhepatic spaces and the left paracolic gutter. It is this ligament that partially prevents pancreatic enzymes from tracking into the left paracolic gutter in acute pancreatitis.

Ascites

Ascites may be associated with a variety of conditions such as portal hypertension, congestive heart failure, hypoproteinemia, inflammatory processes, and neoplasms. Bile, chyle, and blood can also accumulate within the peritoneal cavity. Sonographic evaluation of patients with ascites is performed with the patient in the supine position using a 3.5 or 5 MHz sector probe. Since ascites distributes mainly because of gravity, the most dependent portions of the abdomen, such as the pouch of Douglas, the ileocecal region, and the paracolic gutters, must be carefully examined for

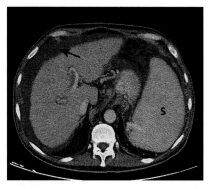

–Figure 9.55 Patient with portal hypertension and ascites. Contrast-enhanced computed tomography scan through the upper abdomen reveals ascites surrounding a cirrhotic liver (arrow). There is also splenomegaly (S).

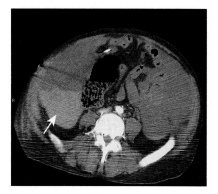

Figure 9.56 Hemoperitoneum in a trauma patient. Computed tomography scan through the lower abdomen reveals free fluid within both lower quadrants. The denser fluid in the dependent portion (arrow) corresponds to acute blood.

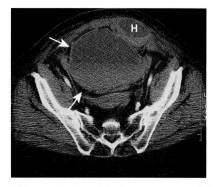

Figure 9.57 Pelvic hematoma with hematocrit level. Computed tomography scan through the pelvis showing a large pelvic hematoma (arrows) with a fluid-fluid level with more acute blood in the inferior aspect. Also present is a left rectus sheath hematoma (H).

small amounts of fluid. Scanning patients in the decubitus position may help determine whether the ascites is loculated or free flowing. A massive amount of ascites will displace loops of small bowel, spleen, and liver centrally within the abdomen.

Simple ascites will appear sonographically as homogeneous anechoic fluid (Figure 9.54). The presence of septations, internal echoes, or debris indicates superimposed infection or blood. Ultrasound can also be used to guide paracentesis in cases of small amounts of free-flowing ascites or if the fluid is loculated. On CT, simple free-flowing ascites is homogeneously low in attenuation density (Figure 9.55). In addition to evaluating the size and extent of the ascites, CT can help make the diagnosis by demonstrating the etiology of the ascites such as a cardiomegaly and prominent hepatic veins in congestive heart failure, enlarged inflamed pancreas in pancreatitis, or a cirrhotic liver in portal hypertension.

Hemoperitoneum

Hemoperitoneum refers to the presence of blood within the intraperitoneal cavity. Most common causes include trauma and postoperative complications. Other etiologies include over anticoagulation, rupture of a hemorrhagic ovarian cyst or ectopic pregnancy, perforated duodenal ulcer, bleeding from tumors such as hepatic adenoma, and mesenteric ischemia.

On ultrasound, hemoperitoneum will have a slightly more echogenic appearance than simple ascites. Blood will tend to accumulate around injured organs such as around the liver and spleen. A small amount of echogenic free fluid in the pelvis may

indicate bowel injury. Early after bleeding into the peritoneal cavity CT of the abdomen and pelvis will show blood which has the same appearance as simple ascites. Within hours, as clot formation takes place and the hemoglobin becomes more concentrated, the attenuation of the fluid increases to reach levels between 30 and 90 HU (Figure 9.56). A hematocrit level may be demonstrated within a loculated peritoneal fluid collection or cyst when fresh blood accumulates within a more subacute or chronic hematoma (Figure 9.57). Active bleeding may show actual extravasation of intravenous contrast.

Pneumoperitoneum

Pneumoperitoneum, or intraperitoneal free air, most commonly results from perforation of a

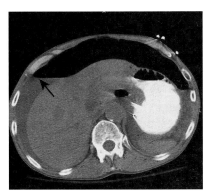

Figure 9.58 Postoperative pneumoperitoneum. Unenhanced computed tomography of the upper abdomen shows a large air–fluid level anterior to the liver and stomach (arrow). The hydro-pneumoperitoneum was postoperative in nature.

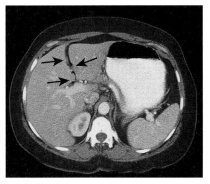

Figure 9.59 Intraperitoneal free air, small amount. Contrast-enhanced computed tomography scan of the abdomen in a trauma patient shows tiny foci of free air in the porta hepatis and in the fissure for the ligamentum teres (arrows).

hollow viscous as seen with a perforated duodenal ulcer, diverticulitis, or ischemic/infarcted bowel. Other etiologies include iatrogenic causes such as surgery or endoscopy following paracentesis and biopsy, and penetrating trauma. Patients who are found to have free air on CT examination usually will present through the emergency department with a painful, diffusely distended and rigid abdomen. Computed tomography, by far, is the favored imaging modality to detect the presence of free air (Figure 9.58) and also to determine the site of perforation and hence etiology.

A retrospective review of 40 cases of surgically proven spontaneous gastrointestinal-tract perforations was recently performed in our department. This study concluded that CT was far more accurate than plain film and was accurate in 90% of cases in estimating the site of perforation based on a number of findings, including extravasation of contrast material, bowel-wall thickening, abscess formation, fat stranding, and distribution of air. The findings can, however, be extremely subtle and one might miss tiny foci of extraluminal air, which will tend to collect in the porta hepatis and along the falciform ligament (Figure 9.59). Larger amounts of air will collect anterior to the liver and may form an air–fluid level if there is associated ascites or hemoperitoneum. Perforation of the second portion of the duodenum, ascending and descending colon, and sigmoid are more likely to produce retroperitoneal air than free air. Pneumoperitoneum secondary to surgery can be present for up to 7 days, but should gradually decrease and resolve by postoperative day 10 in most cases.

Abscess and peritonitis

Etiologies of abdominal abscess or peritonitis include contamination during surgery, complication of trauma, bowel perforation associated with diverticulitis or appendicitis, Crohn's disease, pancreatitis, and pelvic inflammatory disease with tubo-ovarian abscess. Evaluation with ultrasound is usually a good screening tool for diagnosing subphrenic and perihepatic abscesses. Overlying bowel gas and large body habitus are limiting factors. Postoperative pneumoperitoneum or free air secondary to bowel perforation cause reflection of the sound waves obscuring the underlying organs. When an abscess is identified, it has the appearance of a round or oval complex cystic mass, which may have a thick irregular wall, internal thick septations, as well as internal echogenic debris. When possible, ultrasound-guided percutaneous aspiration or drainage is performed for diagnosis.

Computed tomography with contrast is superior to ultrasound in the postoperative patient as well as for localization of small interloop abscesses. Computed tomography is accurate in detecting intra-abdominal abscesses in roughly 95% of cases. The typical CT appearance of an abscess is that of a homogeneous or complex fluid collection with a thick or thin enhancing wall. The presence of gas or air–fluid levels within the collection confirms the diagnosis. Surrounding inflammatory fat stranding, thickening of fascial planes or ascites help in making the diagnosis. Small interloop abscesses can mimic fluid-filled, small-bowel loops. Percutaneous drainage or aspiration can be performed under CT guidance. This is a safe and

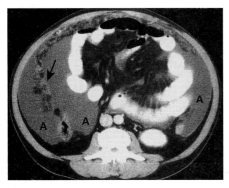

Figure 9.60 Tuberculous peritonitis. Contrast-enhanced computed tomography scan of the mid-abdomen shows ascites (A) and nodular thickening of the peritoneum (arrow). There is enhancement of the peritoneum.

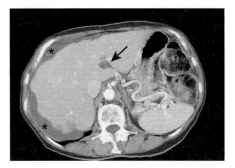

Figure 9.62 Pseudomyxoma peritonei in a patient with mucinous adenocarcinoma of the appendix. Contrast-enhanced computed tomography scan through the liver shows perihepatic lowdensity material (*) causing scalloping of the margins of the liver. There are also implants extending in the fissure for the ligamentum venosum (arrow).

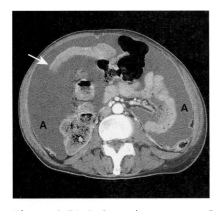

Figure 9.61 Peritoneal metastases. Contrast-enhanced computed tomography scan of the abdomen reveals ascites (A), enhancement of the peritoneum, and enhancing nodular peritoneal implants (arrow) in a patient with metastatic lung cancer.

Solid peritoneal and mesenteric masses

Peritoneal metastases Metastases are the most common solid masses involving the peritoneum. Peritoneal carcinomatosis and omental caking refer to diffuse seeding of the peritoneum and omentum respectively. While ultrasound may shows these lesions when they are surrounded by ascites, CT generally fares better in visualizing small lesions or lesions immediately adjacent to bowel. Most common peritoneal implants result from primary neoplastic carcinomas involving the gastrointestinal tract such as the stomach, colon, or pancreas or from pelvic malignancies such as ovarian carcinoma. The implants appear as mildly enhancing areas of nodularity or peritoneal thickening (Figure 9.61). There may be associated pseudomyxoma peritonei (Figure 9.62). Metastases will implant first in the most dependent portions of the abdomen, namely the pelvic cul-de-sac as well as to mesenteric attachments such as the sigmoid mesentery and root of the small bowel mesentery at the ileocecal region (Figure 9.63). Another frequent site for metastatic peritoneal implants is the perihepatic space resulting in scalloping of the margins of the liver.

Omental caking refers to diffuse infiltration and thickening of the omentum most commonly seen with metastatic ovarian carcinoma and non-Hodgkin's lymphoma. A stellate pattern may be seen when there is diffuse tumor infiltration of the mesentery resulting in thickening and tethering of the perivascular bundles due to extensive fibrosis. This is often seen with small-bowel carcinoid tumors, and the stellate mesenteric implant is usually calcified.

relatively easy procedure depending on the location of the abscess within the abdomen. Interposition of bowel or vascular structures precludes percutaneous drainage.

Bacterial peritonitis usually results from perforated acute appendicitis, diverticulitis, perforated ulcer or carcinoma, and acute cholecystitis. On CT, there is focal or diffuse thickening and enhancement of the peritoneum. Ascites, which may be high in attenuation density, is an associated finding. Tuberculous peritonitis in AIDS (Figure 9.60) produces nodular thickening and enhancement of the peritoneum, as well as multiple lymph nodes containing low-density centers secondary to caseation necrosis.

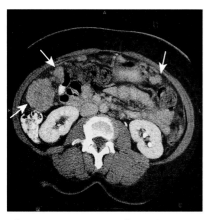

Figure 9.63 Omental ovarian metastases. Contrast-enhanced computed tomography scan through the mid-abdomen in a patient with ovarian cancer. The computed tomography reveals soft-tissue omental peritoneal masses (arrows) in the right lower quadrant surrounded by fluid.

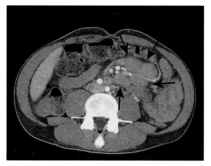

Figure 9.64 Non-Hodgkin's lymphoma with mesenteric lymphadenopathy. Contrast-enhanced computed tomography scan through the mid-abdomen shows multiple, large, round, soft-tissue masses in the small bowel mesentery (arrows) displacing loops of bowel and sandwiching mesenteric vessels.

Hematogenous spread of metastases within the peritoneal cavity occurs along the mesenteric arteries to reach the antimesenteric border of the bowel. Computed tomography findings include thickening of the mesentery, serosal implants along thickened bowel wall, and small ulcerations. The most common tumors to cause this appearance are melanoma and carcinoma of the lung and breast. Do not mistake mesenteric varices for serosal implants.

Lymphadenopathy Adenopathy may appear as a mesenteric mass. Nodal enlargement suggestive of neoplastic involvement is diagnosed when individual nodes exceed 1 centimeter in the long axis. Peritoneal lymphomatosis refers to extensive confluent extranodal involvement of the mesentery and omentum by non-Hodgkin's lymphoma. Roughly half of patients with non-Hodgkin's lymphoma have mesenteric lymph node involvement at presentation compared to only 5% of patients with Hodgkin's lymphoma. The CT appearance varies from that of many enlarged mesenteric lymph nodes to numerous, large, soft-tissue masses abutting and displacing adjacent bowel (Figure 9.64).

The presence of multiple small mesenteric lymph nodes is a non-specific finding which can be seen with a constellation of other processes such as inflammatory, infectious, and infiltrative diseases. These include Whipple disease, MAI (Figure 9.65), Crohn's disease, AIDS, and mastocytosis. Children and young adults may have multiple, borderline-size lymph nodes in mesenteric adenitis.

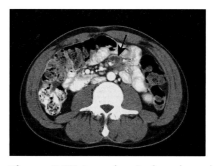

Figure 9.65 Low-density lymph nodes in a patient with MAI. Contrast-enhanced computed tomography scan of the abdomen shows low-density lymph nodes (arrow) in a HIV-positive patient with MAI.

Primary peritoneal tumors Primary tumors of the peritoneum are rare. Desmoid tumors, which are associated with Gardner's syndrome, are a form of mesenteric fibromatosis. Desmoids are locally invasive, soft-tissue enhancing masses that have spiculated margins on CT (Figure 9.66). Sonographically, they have the appearance of solid, hypoechoic masses with acoustic shadowing resulting from fibrous collagenous strands. Associated findings include adenomatous polyps of the stomach and colon, osteomas, and pancreatic periampullary carcinomas.

Benign and malignant lipomatous tumors are usually recognizable by the typical CT appearance of a fat-density mass. Pleomorphic liposarcoma may, however, appear of low but not fat attenuation. Most liposarcomas have enhancing soft-tissue components. Other primary peritoneal neoplasms

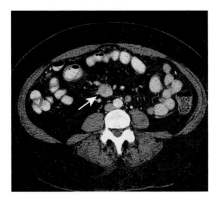

Figure 9.66 Desmoid tumor. Contrast-enhanced computed tomography scan of the lower abdomen reveals a soft-tissue density mass with spiculated margins (arrow) representing a desmoid tumor.

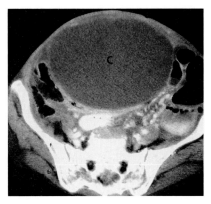

Figure 9.67 Mesenteric cyst. Contrast-enhanced computed tomography scan of the pelvis shows a large, well-defined cystic mass in the pelvis displacing surrounding loops of bowel (C).

are rare and include malignant fibrous histiocytoma and desmoplastic small round cell tumor. Both have a non-specific CT appearance, consisting of soft-tissue density masses, which may contain central areas of necrosis and hemorrhage. Papillary serous carcinoma is a rare primary peritoneal tumor affecting older women. On CT, the appearance mimics that of metastatic serous ovarian papillary carcinoma except that the ovaries are normal. Computed tomography shows multiple, calcified, large, soft-tissue masses invading the peritoneum and omentum.

Cystic peritoneal masses

Benign cysts Mesenteric and omental cysts are benign cystic lesions of uncertain etiology. Most do not produce symptoms unless they are large and compress adjacent structures. Mesenteric cysts usually arise from the small-bowel mesentery while omental cysts are found adjacent to the bowel. These cysts differ from enteric duplication cysts histologically because they lack a mucosal layer. Duplication cysts can arise anywhere along the gastrointestinal tract and usually do not communicate with the bowel lumen. Sonographically, these cysts are unilocular simple-appearing cysts. They may contain thin septations. On CT findings include a small or large well-defined round, fluid density mass (Figure 9.67). Peritoneal pseudocysts are secondary to chronic pancreatitis and are most commonly located in the lesser sac, but they can dissect anywhere within the peritoneal cavity. The pseudocyst may contain thick walls and septations, and findings of chronic pancreatitis may be present on CT and ultrasound.

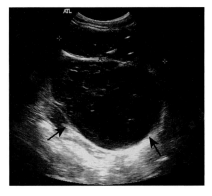

Figure 9.68 Lymphocele. Ultrasound of the pelvis shows a complex, cystic mass (arrows) with thick internal septations. This lymphocele was post-surgical in nature and decreased in size on subsequent imaging following sclerotherapy.

Lymphoceles, which are usually retroperitoneal in location, can occasionally be found within the intraperitoneal cavity. They are lymph-containing collections which can be small or large, resulting from disruption of lymphatics secondary to trauma or surgery. Their sonographic and CT appearance is that of a simple or complex cystic structure (Figure 9.68). Unless infected, there is no enhancement of the wall or septations. They can resolve spontaneously over time or respond to sclerotherapy, which consists of tetracycline instillation.

Cystic neoplasms Cystic neoplasms include mesenteric teratomas and cystic mesotheliomas. Mesenteric or omental teratomas are extremely rare. Cystic mesotheliomas can be benign or malignant. The benign mesotheliomas are not associated with asbestos exposure. While not malignant, they tend to recur following surgical resection. On CT and ultrasound, multiple cystic masses are usually identified. Malignant peritoneal mesotheliomas are associated with asbestos exposure and are rare neoplasms. They may be associated with pleural involvement or may occur alone. The CT appearance may mimic tuberculous peritonitis or peritoneal carcinomatosis when there is irregular and nodular thickening and enhancement of the peritoneum. A multilocular cystic mass with enhancing mural components is more typical.

Gastrointestinal-tract imaging

Contrast-enhanced CT examinations using intravenous as well as oral contrast agents can visualize the gastrointestinal lumen, wall, and adjacent organs. While endoscopic ultrasound shares these attributes, its depth of penetration is limited to only a few centimeters beyond the gastrointestinal wall. Common indications for CT examination of the alimentary tract include staging of neoplastic processes and evaluating their response to treatment; evaluating the extent and etiology of bowel obstruction; evaluating complications of Crohn's disease; establishing the presence of postoperative leaks status – post bowel anastomoses; and characterizing a palpable mass. Computed tomography is also a useful tool in evaluating for the presence of intra-abdominal free air secondary to spontaneous gastrointestinal-tract perforation or trauma.

Esophagus

Imaging of the esophagus using CT scans usually entails performing a contrast-enhanced CT scan of the chest preferably with intravenous contrast, although not required, and positive oral contrast agents such as barium coupled with gas-producing granules to distend the esophageal lumen. The normal esophageal wall measurement varies from 3 to 5 millimeters in thickness. The esophagus is mainly air filled, hence the presence of too much fluid, air–fluid level, or a diameter of greater than 1 centimeter usually indicates the presence of a distal obstruction or motility disorder such as presbyesophagus or achalasia.

Esophageal tumors Leiomyoma is the most common of the benign esophageal tumors. Other benign tumors include lipomas, neurofibromas, schwannomas, and fibrovascular polyps. With the

exception of esophageal lipoma, which has the characteristic CT density of fat, the other benign tumors appear as focal, intraluminal, or intramural masses of soft-tissue density, resulting in eccentric wall thickening. Benign tumors usually do not cause any disruption of the surrounding mediastinal fat planes. The definitive diagnosis is confirmed endoscopically, at which time directed biopsies could be performed.

Squamous cell carcinoma and adenocarcinoma of the esophagus appear identical on CT except for the distal predilection for adenocarcinoma arising from Barrett's esophagus. Computed tomography is often performed in esophageal cancer patients to get the "lay of the land" and detect remote disease, while EUS is more accurate in determining transmural spread. Computed tomography excels at evaluating extension to mediastinal structures such as the tracheobronchial tree, aorta, pericardium, and pleura. It also can accurately detect pulmonary metastases. Celiac adenopathy adjacent to the celiac axis is common in distal esophageal cancer and can be reliably detected with CT. Endoscopic ultrasound may also evaluate the celiac nodes in patients with favorable anatomy. The findings on CT suggestive of malignant esophageal tumors consist of irregular wall thickening, an eccentric esophageal lumen due to the presence of an obstructing mass, dilatation and fluid above the level of obstruction, invasion of adjacent mediastinal structures, and regional and distant liver and lung metastases (Figure 9.69).

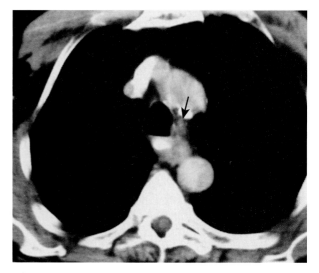

Figure 9.69 Contrast-enhanced computed tomography scan shows eccentric thickening of the esophagus due to esophageal carcinoma. Irregular stranding (arrow) of the mediastinal fat was due to tumor spread. Adenopathy was seen at other levels.

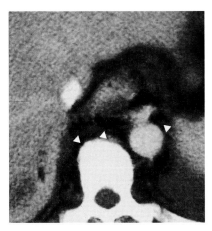

Figure 9.70 Gas in the mediastinum (arrowheads) and a small amount of contrast are present just behind the normal esophagogastric junction. The patient proved to have Boerhave's syndrome.

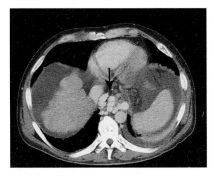

Figure 9.71 Gastroesophageal varices in a patient with portal hypertension. Contrast-enhanced computed tomography through the lower chest shows multiple, enhancing, tubular structures at the gastroesophageal junction, (arrow) compatible with varices. There is associated ascites and a cirrhotic nodular liver.

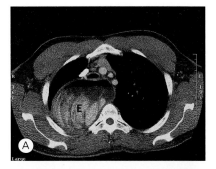

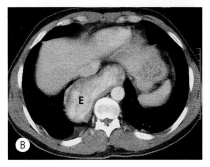

Figure 9.72 Achalasia. Contrast-enhanced computed tomography scan through A) the chest and B) upper abdomen. Both images show severe dilatation of the esophagus, which occupies a large portion of the posterior mediastinum (E). An air–fluid level is noted in A, while in B the esophagus is mostly contrast filled (E).

Other malignant tumors such as esophageal lymphoma are rare, being more commonly diagnosed in patients with AIDS. Their CT appearance is characterized by diffuse wall thickening with or without ulcerations and the presence of bulky mediastinal lymphadenopathy. Leiomyosarcomas can have the same appearance on CT as leiomyomas, except for the fact that they are usually larger and more exophytic.

Miscellaneous disorders Boerhave's syndrome (Figure 9.70) is increasingly being imaged with CT. Pneumomediastinum, extravasation of oral contrast material, and loculated mediastinal fluid collections may readily be appreciated. Esophageal varices are seen in patients with portal hypertension and have a characteristic CT appearance, consisting of multiple, tubular enhancing structures in the esophagogastric region (Figure 9.71). Associated signs of portal hypertension will usually be obvious including other portosystemic collaterals. Esophageal diverticulum and duplication cysts can readily be identified on CT. They both have a well-defined cystic appearance. The one feature that helps distinguish between the entities is that esophageal diverticula communicate with the lumen and may contain air whereas duplication cysts typically do not. Computed tomography may show an extremely enlarged esophagus which will occupy most of the posterior mediastinum. The differential diagnosis usually includes achalasia (Figure 9.72), Chagas' disease, scleroderma, or a gastroesophageal-junction tumor causing distal obstruction.

Stomach

When the stomach is being evaluated using CT, it is important that the lumen be well distended and free of debris. Patients are instructed to refrain from taking any solid foods after midnight the night before the examination. Oral contrast or

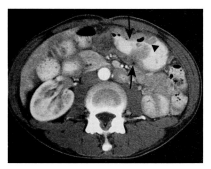

Figure 9.73 Adenocarcinoma of the stomach. Contrast-enhanced computed tomography scan of the upper abdomen shows severe thickening of the wall of the body of the stomach (arrows) with narrowing of the lumen (arrowhead).

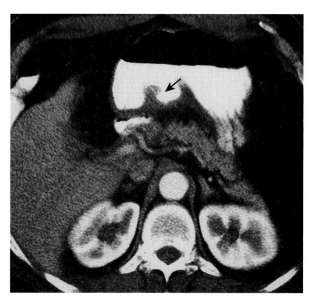

Figure 9.74 Ulceration within a gastric mass (arrow) is present. This is the computed tomography equivalent of the Carmen meniscus sign described in upper gastrointestinal series many years ago.

water is given to obtain adequate distension of the stomach cavity with or without gas-producing granules. Intravenous contrast material is essential for evaluation of the gastric wall and characterization of suspected masses. The normal thickness of the gastric wall should not exceed 5 millimeters. A food-filled or under-distended stomach is all too common and can simulate a mass or inflammatory process. Scanning patients in the prone or decubitus position can help resolve problematic cases.

Inflammatory conditions Computed tomography is not routinely used to assess or evaluate gastritis or peptic ulcer disease. Computed tomography findings are non-specific and may consist of diffuse wall and rugal fold thickening. A layered or "halo" appearance has been described, characterized by a low-density submucosa from edema and an enhancing mucosa secondary to hyperemia. *Helicobacter pylori* infection and non-steroidal anti-inflammatory drug use are the two most common etiologies for this appearance. Massive thickening of the gastric rugae may be seen in association with the Zollinger–Ellison syndrome, eosinophilic gastritis, and Menetrier's disease. In Zollinger–Ellison syndrome, an associated pancreatic islet-cell tumor may also be present as a subtle hypervascular mass. Giant gastric ulcers may be seen on CT, but most peptic ulcers are too small to be identified.

Neoplasms The most common malignant neoplasms involving the stomach are adeno-carcinoma, lymphoma, and stromal tumors. Computed tomography is recognized as the most accurate diagnostic tool for overall staging of the disease, but as for esophageal carcinoma, EUS is

better at assessing the degree of transmural spread. Adenocarcinomas can appear on CT as segmental wall thickening (Figure 9.73), an exophytic or ulcerating mass, or a diffuse infiltrating process due to linitis plastica or scirrhous gastric carcinoma. When a deep ulcer is present, it is usually retracted into the lumen and has a tumor shelf present at its base (Figure 9.74). This is the so-called Carmen meniscus sign. Computed tomography frequently shows spread of the disease via ligamentous attachments. Extension to the liver and porta hepatis is through the gastrohepatic ligament; to the transverse colon is through the gastrocolic ligament or transverse mesocolon; and to the spleen is through the gastrosplenic ligament. Distant metastases to the liver, lungs, and peritoneal cavity are also well visualized. Although the stomach is a common site for non-Hodgkin's lymphoma in AIDS patients, its overall incidence is low. Lymphoma tends to produce more significant wall thickening than gastric adenocarcinoma, is less prone to ulcerate, and will usually have associated lymphadenopathy. Lymphoma may ulcerate and even perforate after chemotherapy.

Small bowel

To evaluate the small bowel properly, opacification with oral contrast agent is needed to achieve adequate distension of the lumen. The administration of intravenous contrast is also preferred to better visualize and evaluate the bowel lumen and its vascular supply. This is especially true when excluding bowel ischemia or infarction. In addition, unopacified or collapsed loops of small bowel can mimic any type of soft-tissue density mass. In the setting of suspected small-bowel obstruction or possible perforation, water-soluble contrast may be given by mouth or via the patient's nasogastric tube. Some radiologists now prefer no oral contrast in the setting of obstruction, and take advantage of the copious fluid in the small bowel as a negative contrast.

Small-bowel tumors Small-bowel tumors are uncommon, the incidence ranges from 3% to 6% of all malignancies of the gastrointestinal tract. Computed tomography can detect small-bowel tumors in most cases and usually can stage the disease. Enteroclysis may be more accurate in detecting small lesions, but cannot assess the surrounding structures. The most common benign tumor is leiomyoma which is usually seen protruding into the lumen and which may ulcerate. Some leiomyomas are exophytic, extending well beyond the bowel wall. Lipomas also occur and are of fat density on CT.

Malignant tumors include adenocarcinomas, lymphoma, and carcinoid tumors. Adenocarcinoma tends to occur in the proximal small bowel, lymphoma in the distal small bowel, and carcinoid in the ileocecal region. On CT adenocarcinoma will be seen as a focal mass with an irregular contour and possibly frank ulceration on the mucosal surface (Figure 9.75). Lymphoma, as elsewhere in the gastrointestinal tract, produces nodular wall thickening, nodules of varying size, and at times aneurysmal dilatation of the small bowel from tumor necrosis. Carcinoid tumors tend to be small

and difficult to detect, but the associated desmoplastic reaction within the mesentery can readily be identified. This is characterized by a stellate, often calcified retractile mass in the small-bowel mesentery sometimes resulting in tethering of adjacent loops of bowel.

Small-bowel obstruction Computed tomography has largely replaced plain films and the small-bowel follow-through in the setting of obstruction. The CT diagnosis of small-bowel obstruction relies on identifying a transition zone, above which the loops are dilated. Beyond the transition point the bowel is decompressed (Figure 9.76). The differential diagnosis for small-bowel obstruction is lengthy, including adhesions, hernias, and obstructing tumors. Inguinal hernias may be responsible for obstruction and are readily visualized on CT (Figure 9.77). Other etiologies are intussusception, volvulus, foreign bodies, and stricture. Bowel obstruction secondary to adhesions usually occurs in the clinical context of prior surgery; an abrupt transition from dilated to

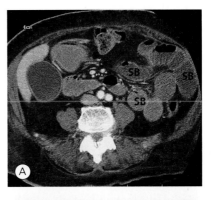

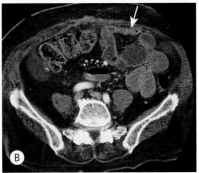

Figure 9.76 Small-bowel obstruction due to adhesions. A) Contrast-enhanced computed tomography scan of the pelvis shows multiple, dilated, fluid-filled loops of small bowel (SB). B) The transition zone is identified (arrow), beyond this point the small bowel is decompressed.

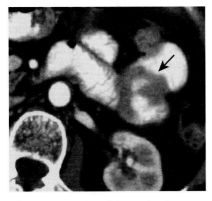

Figure 9.75 Small-bowel adenocarcinoma (arrow) seen as a soft-tissue mass stricturing the jejunum.

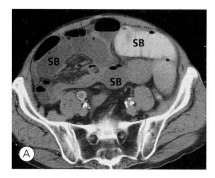

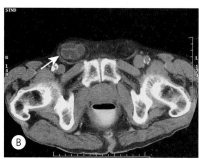

Figure 9.77 Incarcerated inguinal hernia causing small-bowel obstruction. A) Contrast-enhanced computed tomography scan through the pelvis shows multiple, contrast- and fluid-filled dilated loops of small bowel (SB). B) a right inguinal hernia is identified (arrow), responsible for the small-bowel obstruction. Beyond the hernia the bowel was decompressed.

decompressed bowel and failure to identify an obstructing mass or ischemic loop is suggestive. When closed-loop obstruction has occurred, ischemia may be present. The CT findings of ischemia include ileus, wall thickening, poor enhancement on contrast-enhanced studies, and pneumatosis intestinalis. Edematous and hemorrhagic changes are noted within the mesentery and ascites may or may not be present (see colon ischemia).

Crohn's disease Crohn's disease is a granulomatous colitis, which may involve the entire gastrointestinal tract from the mouth to the anus. However, it involves most commonly the terminal ileum (Figure 9.78), the ascending colon (Figure 9.79), and the rectum. It is characterized by the presence of erosions, ulcers, non-caseating granulomas, and inflammation of the entire thickness of the bowel wall. Presenting symptoms usually consist of abdominal pain, diarrhea and weight loss, and fever. Upper gastrointestinal series with small-bowel follow through and enteroclysis are the two main imaging modalities which can assess the degree and extent of mucosal involvement.

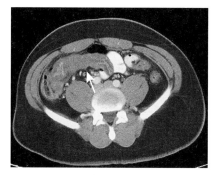

Figure 9.78 Crohn's disease involving the terminal ileum. Contrast-enhanced computed tomography scan of the lower abdomen shows severe thickening of the wall of the terminal ileum (arrow) in this patient with known Crohn's disease.

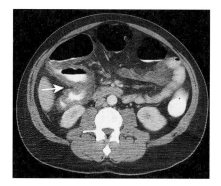

Figure 9.79 Crohn's disease involving the ascending colon. Contrast-enhanced computed tomography scan through the lower abdomen reveals circumferential thickening of the wall of the ascending colon (arrow). No abscesses or fistulae were identified.

The main role of CT in the evaluation of Crohn's disease is to assess the extramural manifestations and complications such as abscess formation and fistulae. Computed tomography findings include circumferential wall thickening, stranding and focal accumulation of the mesenteric fat referred to as "creeping fat", and skip lesions with intervening normal bowel segments. Bowel perforation is usually confined resulting in phlegmonous changes and small interloop abscess formation. Sinus tracts and fistulae can also be identified as contrast- or air-filled irregular linear bands between loops of bowel or bowel and other viscera (Figure 9.80). Infectious conditions that affect the distal small bowel and proximal colon (such as tuberculosis, *Yersinia enterolitica*, and cytomegalovirus) may radiologically mimic Crohn's disease.

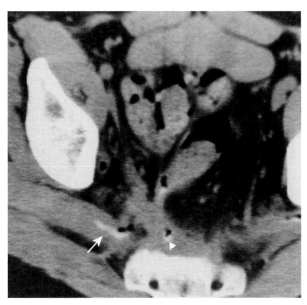

Figure 9.80 Multiple fistulae are seen extending to the pre-sacral space. A small air bubble and contrast are present (arrowhead). Contrast is also seen tracking into the gluteus muscle (arrow).

Appendix

Computed tomography and ultrasound are increasingly being used to image the patient with suspected acute appendicitis. In the surgical literature a 20% misdiagnosis rate is considered acceptable for patients undergoing laparotomy for symptoms of appendicitis. Imaging may help reduce this misdiagnosis rate. Considerable debate exists on how to most effectively evaluate the appendix. Computed tomography is the pre-eminent technique with ultrasound a close second. Most experts would recommend using sonography to initially evaluate young children, pregnant women, and women of childbearing age under approximately 150 pounds in weight. In women over 150 pounds, the ability to identify and compress the appendix may be limited, but still may be possible depending on the body habitus. Regardless of whether ultrasound or CT is used, a clearly negative or positive study is of great value in the patient with equivocal signs and symptoms. At some centers, routine use of CT or ultrasound in suspected appendicitis is being advocated.

When ultrasound is used to evaluate the appendix, a 5 or 7.5 MHz probe should be used. Modest compression of the tissues on the right lower quadrant is essential to displace adjacent bowel loops and gas which could obscure the appendix. The lower abdomen is imaged in both

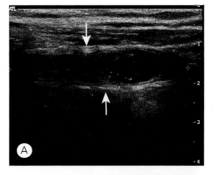

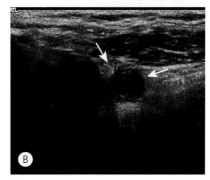

Figure 9.81 Acute appendicitis. A) Longitudinal and B) transverse ultrasound of the appendix. The appendix is thick-walled, dilated, and non-compressible (arrows) in this patient with proven acute appendicitis.

transverse and longitudinal planes. If normal, the appendix is not visualized in 90% of patients. If it is seen, the lumen should be no more than 6 millimeters in diameter. Its wall should be paper thin. There are times when adjacent bowel loops make it difficult to evaluate the appendix or differentiate appendiceal abnormalities from those of the adnexa. Fluid-filled loops are especially challenging and can mimic appendiceal abscess or sequelae of pelvic inflammatory disease.

Computed tomography is more likely to result in a diagnostic study in male and larger patients. Considerable debate has occurred regarding the optimal CT technique for assessing the appendix. The group at Massachusetts General Hospital has popularized the focused examination for appendicitis. Focused means sections that are limited to the right lower quadrant and that are performed without oral, rectal, or intravenous contrast. While not using any contrast may make the examination more efficient in the emergency setting, we remain advocates of full contrast studies for appendicitis. Our confidence level is always higher imaging the appendix with contrast, and too many patients with lower abdominal pain due to diseases other than appendicitis may go undiagnosed by a focused or limited examination. It is very important that

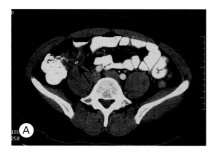

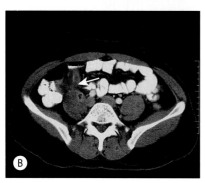

Figure 9.82 Acute appendicitis with appendicolith. A) Contrast-enhanced computed tomography scan through the pelvis shows an appendicolith in the proximal appendix (arrow). B) The appendix is dilated, fluid-filled distally and thick-walled (arrow). There is surrounding inflammatory stranding.

the distal small bowel and colon are opacified with dilute barium and that intravenous contrast is injected at least at 2 mL/sec.

What are the sonographic findings of appendicitis? The presence of a non-compressible, blind-ending, tubular structure in the right lower quadrant is highly suggestive of acute appendicitis. Its transverse diameter should not exceed 6 milllimeters (Figure 9.81). If inflammation is severe, multiple alternating hypo- and hyperechoic layers will be seen within the appendiceal wall. An echogenic appendicolith may been seen within the lumen. Some individuals have used power Doppler ultrasound to show hyperemia. This may be of value if the appendix is severely inflamed, but may not be helpful in cases where the appendix has become ischemic. Most recent series have shown sensitivity approaching 90%, with slightly higher specificity.

There are many CT findings in acute appendicitis that may be identified. Seeing a dilated appendix with a thickened wall and surrounding inflammatory stranding is almost pathognomonic of appendicitis. As on ultrasound, a diameter greater than 6 millimeters is suggestive of dilatation (Figure 9.82). On CT the diameter is measured from the outer edge of the lumen. Appendiceal wall

thickening is diagnosed whenever the wall exceeds 2 millimeters in thickness. The most valuable secondary sign of appendicitis is stranding of the peri-appendiceal mesenteric fat. Stranding may appear as individual tentacles within the fat or as a diffuse hazy appearance. In reviewing CT scans, it is important to compare the peri-appendiceal fat to fat elsewhere in order to detect subtle stranding and density differences.

Another sign of appendicitis is the "arrowhead" sign. This refers to contrast media funneling between each side of a thickened cecum and coming to a point at the edematous orifice of the appendix. When dilute barium is given, it may be difficult to distinguish barium from an appendicolith. If a wider window setting is used, it may be possible to detect a calcified nidus of different attenuation than the barium in the lumen of adjacent loops (Figure 9.82). The presence or absence of air or contrast material within the lumen is of questionable value. In some patients, failure to see contrast at the tip of the appendix in the face of a well-opacified base may be indicative of distal appendicitis.

If the appendiceal wall has a "bubbly" appearance, this may be evidence of appendicitis with pneumatosis indicative of ischemia.

Some of the secondary signs seen in appendicitis such as thickening of adjacent small bowel, lymphadenopathy, and right hydroureter are also seen in Crohn's disease. Since Crohn's can also involve the appendix, a good clinical history is essential. It is important to remember that only the combination of appendiceal dilatation and wall thickening allows the imaging diagnosis of appendicitis to be suggested with high specificity. Another frequent fooler is appendagitis, which results from torsion of an epiploic appendage. The latter represents a small, fatty appendage on the serosal surface of the colon. When inflamed it may give rise to a whorl-like mesenteric stranding in the area of inflammation.

Complicated appendicitis implies the presence of an abscess (Figure 9.83), extraluminal gas bubbles, or severe phlegmonous change. It is distinctly unusual to see significant, free, extraluminal air in patients with appendicitis, but this can occur. In some patients the appendiceal tip is retroperitoneal and therefore a small amount of air or pus may accumulate in the retroperitoneum. If extensive intra- or retroperitoneal abscess is seen, it may need to be drained percutaneously prior to surgery. If an inflammatory mass is seen, the patient may benefit from preoperative antibiotics.

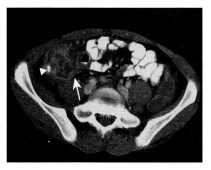

Figure 9.83 A mixed-attenuation appendiceal abscess (arrow) is seen occupying much of the right lower quadrant. A high-density appendicolith (arrowhead) is engulfed by the abscess.

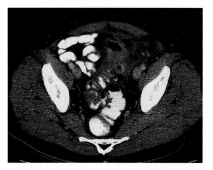

Figure 9.84 Contrast-enhanced computed tomography scan reveals moderate inflammatory stranding due to acute sigmoid diverticulitis.

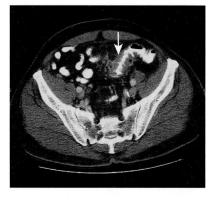

Figure 9.85 Acute sigmoid colon diverticulitis. Contrast-enhanced computed tomography scan through the pelvis shows a thick-walled sigmoid colon (arrow) with luminal narrowing and inflammatory stranding in the sigmoid mesentery.

Colon

The colon is well visualized on CT and is distinguished from the small bowel based on many different anatomical characteristics such as its more peripheral location, the presence of tenia coli, appendices epiploicae and haustra, and its caliber. In addition, the ascending and descending colon are retroperitoneal in location while the transverse colon remains intraperitoneal. The diameter of the colon varies, with the cecum being the largest segment having a diameter of roughly 9 centimeters. When the colon is adequately distended either by air, water, or positive contrast material its wall is barely perceptible and should be no greater than 3 millimeters.

Diverticulitis In many respects, CT has become the primary method for identifying the presence of diverticulitis. Diverticulitis results from perforation and/or inflammation of a diverticulum. Approximately 5% to 10% of affected patients are over 45 years of age and 80% are over the age of 85 years. The vast majority of symptomatic patients will exhibit inflammatory stranding in the pericolonic fat and bowel-wall thickening with associated diverticula. These patients get treated conservatively with antibiotics and get better. There appears to be good correlation between the degree of inflammation seen on CT and the patient's symptoms.

In mild cases there may be only a vague or hazy increase in density of the surrounding fat (Figure 9.84). As for mild appendicitis, comparing the fat in the suspected region of diverticulitis with the fat elsewhere within the abdomen allows subtle changes to be detected. It is not unusual to see areas of inflammation delimited by portions of the sigmoid mesocolon or by other compartmental boundaries, such as the lateral conal fascia. Some cases of diverticulitis may present with gas surrounding the kidney. In these patients, the gas enters the perirenal space via the open end of Gerota's fascia. Although diverticulitis occurs most commonly in the descending and sigmoid colon, it can involve the right colon and mimic acute appendicitis. Identifying diverticula may help in making the diagnosis, although if it is occluded by inflammation it may not be seen. With increasing inflammation, diffuse wall thickening and stranding occur (Figure 9.85).

The presence of an extraluminal fluid collection adjacent to the site of inflammation indicates the presence of a peridiverticular abscess which is seen in 30% of the cases (Figure 9.86). Percutaneous or surgical drainage of the abscess reduces morbidity. Other complications such as colovesical fistulae and perforation are well identified on CT. When air

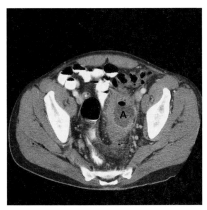

Figure 9.86 Peridiverticular abscess. Contrast-enhanced computed tomography scan of the pelvis reveals a thick-walled cystic collection containing air (A) with surrounding inflammation. There was associated sigmoid colon diverticulitis (not shown).

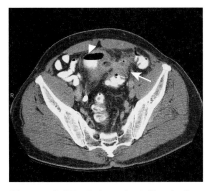

Figure 9.87 Colovesical fistula from sigmoid diverticulitis. Contrast-enhanced computed tomography scan through the pelvis. There is a colovesical fistula, as evidenced by the presence of air in the urinary bladder (arrowhead) and the adjacent sigmoid colon diverticulitis (arrow). This patient did not have an indwelling Foley catheter to account for the intraluminal air in the bladder.

is noted within the bladder (in the absence of an indwelling Foley catheter) and there is thickening and inflammatory changes noted in close proximity to the diseased bowel segment, a colovesical fistula is almost always present (Figure 9.87). These enterovesical fistulae tend to involve the left posterior aspect of the bladder. This is in contradistinction to the fistulae associated with Crohn's disease, which are located on the right anterior-lateral aspect of the bladder since the terminal ileum is most commonly involved with the disease process.

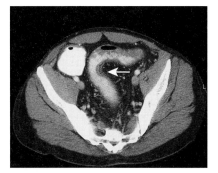

Figure 9.88 Ulcerative colitis. Contrast-enhanced computed tomography scan of the pelvis shows mild thickening of the wall of the sigmoid colon (arrow), which is symmetrical and more diffuse than the thickening seen in patients with Crohn's disease.

Inflammatory colitis The appearance of a wide range of inflammatory conditions of the colon have been described in the literature. These include ulcerative colitis, typhlitis and radiation colitis; infectious etiologies such as bacterial or viral causes including pseudomembranous colitis; and ischemic disease. Based on the amount of wall thickening, the distribution of the disease throughout the colon with or without involvement of small bowel, and the presence of extraluminal complications such as fistulae or abscesses, most radiologists can make a confident diagnosis in the appropriate clinical context. The colonic changes seen in Crohn's disease are similar to those described for the small bowel.

As on endoscopy, the CT distribution of disease provides useful information. Ulcerative colitis consistently involves the rectum, and may be diffuse throughout the colon or confined to the left side. It is extremely rare to only involve the right colon, a finding that is more characteristic of Crohn's disease. The wall thickening seen with ulcerative colitis is usually less than in Crohn's disease and is typically more diffuse and symmetrical (Figure 9.88). A target-like appearance to the bowel wall (the "halo sign") is more commonly seen in patients with ulcerative colitis. This appearance results from fat deposition within the submucosal layer of the bowel wall. This will manifest on CT as a thickened and low-density submucosa surrounded by a higher density serosa (Figure 9.89). Other colitides with severe mucosal inflammation can also display this finding. In addition, patients with ulcerative colitis usually have a shortened and ahaustral colon. Abscess formation and fistulous tracts are more common in Crohn's disease (Figure 9.90) and rare in ulcerative colitis.

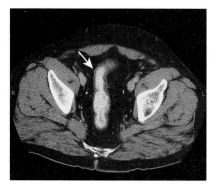

Figure 9.89 "Halo sign" in ulcerative colitis. Contrast-enhanced computed tomography scan of the pelvis shows a thickened, hypodense submucosa surrounded by a hyperdense serosa (arrow) resulting in the "halo sign" or target-like appearance seen in this patient with known ulcerative colitis.

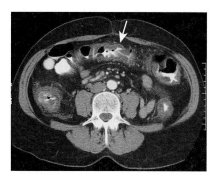

Figure 9.91 Pseudomembranous colitis. Contrast-enhanced computed tomography scan through the lower abdomen shows extensive, diffuse thickening of the wall and haustra of the transverse colon. Contrast is seen trapped between the thickened haustra resulting in the "accordion sign" (arrow).

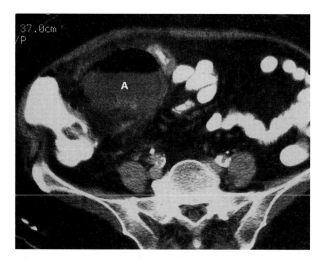

Figure 9.90 A large abscess (A) due to Crohn's disease is present. Note the adjacent, thickened, abnormal, distal ileal loop.

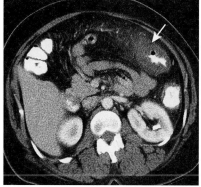

Figure 9.92 The distal transverse colon ("watershed area") is markedly thickened (arrow) and there is mild mesenteric stranding. Other areas of the colon were normal. While these findings are not specific, they are suggestive of ischemia.

Pseudomembranous colitis is an important diagnosis to make because of its high morbidity and mortality if left untreated. The presence of the *Clostridium difficile* toxin within the patient's stool is the key to making the diagnosis. Unfortunately, the presenting symptoms are non-specific and in many cases the radiologist is the first one to suggest the diagnosis. Computed tomography demonstrates a dilated colon with extensive wall thickening, which may be circumferential or eccentric. In severe cases, the "accordion sign" might be present. This results from contrast material being trapped between considerably thickened haustra that take on a pleated appearance (Figure 9.91). The entire colon is typically involved. However, in roughly 30% to 40% of cases the disease might be confined to the ascending colon.

Ischemic colitis, which can be secondary to vascular occlusions or hypovolemic states, has a predilection for the descending colon. Extension to the watershed portions of the colon, namely the sigmoid colon or splenic flexure, may occur (Figure 9.92). This pattern of colonic involvement is more common in the elderly population, while in younger patients the right side of the colon is the most affected. The CT findings are non-specific, including wall and fold thickening. The wall may be hypodense due to edema, or hyperdense if mural

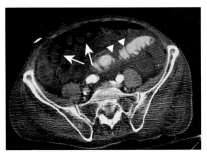

Figure 9.93 Pneumatosis is seen involving the distal small bowel and right colon (arrows). Thickening of the sigmoid is also present (arrowheads). The patient had extensive ischemia at surgery.

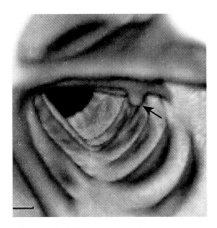

Figure 9.94 Virtual colonoscopy showing a small sessile polyp (arrow).

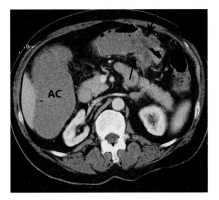

Figure 9.95 Colon cancer. Contrast-enhanced computed tomography scan through the mid-abdomen shows irregular and asymmetrical thickening of the wall of the left transverse colon with a soft-tissue mass extending into the lumen (arrows). This mass was causing obstruction of the colon proximally as evidenced by the dilated ascending colon (AC).

hemorrhage is present. When contrast is administered enhancing loops may be seen next to unenhancing ischemic or edematous loops (Figure 9.93). Computed tomography also shows thrombi in the involved vessels in cases of occlusive ischemia. Acute and chronic complications can also be identified on CT, consisting of pneumatosis intestinalis and strictures (Figure 9.93).

Colon carcinoma As elsewhere in the gastrointestinal tract, CT plays a major role in detecting distant spread of colon cancer. It is not yet fully established as a screening technique for colon cancer, but has been shown to be useful in high-risk populations. The typical virtual colonoscopy or CT colonography examination requires bowel preparation that is less vigorous than that for barium enema. The colon is insufflated with air or carbon dioxide and thin-section CT images are obtained in the prone and supine positions. The images are reviewed in axial, sagittal, and coronal planes for evidence of polyps or mass lesions. Some centers

will reconstruct a fly-through "virtual" view to aid in diagnosis (Figure 9.94). In the future computer-assisted diagnosis programs may also be of value. Some centers administer glucagon to reduce peristalsis or give intravenous contrast as a problem solver to distinguish a polyp from stool.

Computed tomography plays an important role in evaluating local spread and liver metastases in patients with colon cancer. When staging colorectal cancers prior to surgery, CT has been shown to have accuracy rates varying from 48% to 77%. The greatest limitations of CT reside in its inability to discriminate metastatic from hyperplastic lymph nodes based on size criteria and difficulty in assessing the degree of tumor spread through the bowel wall. Colorectal carcinoma on CT appears as an irregular, soft-tissue density mass arising from the wall and extending into the lumen (Figure 9.95). When the mass is large, central low density may be visible corresponding to central necrosis. The mass may present as focal asymmetrical wall thickening or as a true "apple-core" lesion; the latter can result in luminal narrowing and partial or complete bowel obstruction (Figure 9.96). Caution must be taken not to confuse this finding with diverticulitis. Computed tomography can also demonstrate complications of colorectal cancer, which include obstruction, fistula formation, and perforation.

Local spread of the disease is characterized by extension of the tumor into the pericolonic fat and loss of the fat plane between the colon and the invaded structure. In the pelvis, CT allows for potential invasion of the bladder, vagina, prostate

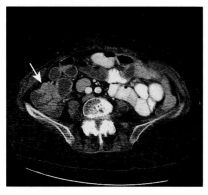

Figure 9.96 Cecal carcinoma. Contrast-enhanced computed tomography scan of the pelvis shows an irregular enhancing soft tissue mass in the cecum (arrow). This was incidentally discovered after scanning this patient for what appeared to be a small-bowel obstruction on plain radiographs of the abdomen. The patient had multiple pulmonary metastases (not shown).

and seminal vesicles, and pelvic sidewall and muscles. Unfortunately, the true meaning of pelvic sidewall invasion is not clear nor is it based on anatomic abnormality of specific structures. Nevertheless, for staging rectal carcinoma, CT detection of adjacent organ or pelvic muscle invasion is comparable to that achieved with MRI when thin sections are obtained and water is used as a negative rectal contrast agent. Endoscopic ultrasound is still best at assessing the spread through the layers of the rectal wall. Distant metastases from colorectal cancer include involvement of the liver, the lungs, and less likely adrenal glands and

bones. Liver metastases are more common in tumors arising from the colon and upper rectum because they both drain via the portal vein. Liver metastases are typically hypovascular lesions, best visualized in the portal venous phase of enhancement.

Conclusion

Computed tomography and ultrasound are both extremely important gastrointestinal imaging techniques. A close working relationship between gastroenterology and radiology promotes the best patient care.

Further reading

Fishman EK, Jeffrey BR (eds). *Spiral CT: Principles, Techniques, and Applications*, 2nd edn. Baltimore MD, Lippincott Williams & Wilkins, 1998.

Gore RM, Levine MS (eds). *Textbook of Gastrointestinal Radiology*, 2nd edn. Philadelphia PA, WB Saunders, 2000.

Sanders RC, Miner MS (eds). *Clinical Sonography: A Practical Guide*, 3rd edn. Baltimore MD, Lippincott Williams & Wilkins, 1997.

Zeman RK, Brink J, Costello P, Davros WJ, Richmond B, Silverman PM. *Helical/Spiral CT: A Practical Approach*. New York, McGraw Hill, 1994.

Zeman RK, Burrell MI. Gallbladder and Bile Duct Imaging: A Clinical Radiologic Approach. New York, Churchill-Livingstone, 1987.

Index